THE CARE OF OLDER P.
ENGLAND AND JAP/
A COMPARATIVE STU

STUDIES FOR THE SOCIETY FOR THE SOCIAL HISTORY OF MEDICINE

Series Editors: *David Cantor*
Keir Waddington

TITLES IN THIS SERIES

THE CARE OF OLDER PEOPLE:
ENGLAND AND JAPAN,
A COMPARATIVE STUDY

BY

Mayumi Hayashi

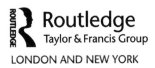

Routledge
Taylor & Francis Group

LONDON AND NEW YORK

First published 2013 by Pickering & Chatto (Publishers) Limited

Published 2016 by Routledge
2 Park Square, Milton Park, Abingdon, Oxfordshire OX14 4RN
711 Third Avenue, New York, NY 10017, USA

First issued in paperback 2015

Routledge is an imprint of the Taylor & Francis Group, an informa business

BRITISH LIBRARY CATALOGUING IN PUBLICATION DATA

Hayashi, Mayumi, author.
The care of older people: England and Japan, a comparative study. – (Studies for
the Society for the Social History of Medicine)
1. Older people – Institutional care – Great Britain. 2. Older people –
Institutional care – Japan. 3. Older people – Institutional care – Government
policy – Great Britain. 4. Older people – Institutional care – Government
policy – Japan.
I. Title II. Series
362.6'1'0941-dc23

ISBN-13: 978-1-138-66478-4 (pbk)
ISBN-13: 978-1-8489-3417-7 (hbk)
Typeset by Pickering & Chatto (Publishers) Limited

CONTENTS

ACKNOWLEDGEMENTS

This book began life as a PhD thesis, awarded by the University of East Anglia in 2010. I am immensely indebted to a number of people who have encouraged and advised me during the course of my research. First and foremost, I would like to express my heartfelt thanks to Steven Cherry, a supervisor as helpful and insightful as one could wish for. His unstinting support, unwavering encouragement and immense store of knowledge, as well as constructive criticism, unquestionably contributed to refining the dissertation on which this book is based. I am most grateful to him. My examiners, Pat Thane and Jill Robinson, both offered encouragement, as well as advice and criticisms, which helped me to take the research further. I would like to thank Pat Thane in particular for her continuing support and her belief in this project.

I wish to acknowledge and thank all those who participated in my fieldwork research in Norfolk, United Kingdom and Ogaki City, Japan. They willingly offered their time and hospitality and contributed positively and enthusiastically to my research. I regret that it has been possible to use only a fraction of the material they provided. I am also grateful to many archivists and librarians for their help with identifying and accessing the documents, particularly in Norfolk Record Office, Norfolk Heritage Centre, Gifu Record Office and Gifu Public Library. Special thanks are due to Adult Social Services (now Community Services) of Norfolk County Council for granting me accelerated access to materials, which are subject to a fifty-year restriction or still held at the County Hall archives; and to the staff at Yorokaen and Kusunokien homes in Ogaki, for allowing me to access documents kept privately on the premises.

My thanks are also due to the Leverhulme Trust, who provided a postdoctoral fellowship which enabled me to undertake the revisions that were needed to prepare the dissertation for publication. I would also like to record my very sincere thanks to the Institute of Gerontology, King's College London for appointing me to a fellowship, and for providing so stimulating and supportive an environment in which to work. I am deeply grateful to Ruth Willats for her meticulous help in preparing the manuscript of this book for publication.

I would like to express my genuine thanks to all those friends who have helped in a variety of ways to facilitate my work. A special debt of gratitude is owed to Claire and Martin Daunton, who have taken a generous interest in my study and provided me with encouragement, valuable advice and research material. Above all, my thanks must go to my parents and sisters for their constant support and encouragement and unfailing interest in my study throughout. I hope that this book goes some way towards repaying them. Finally, the book originated in my experiences of caring, along with my family, for my grandfather, Toneo Hayashi, during the last years of his life until he passed away in 2005, aged 84 years. I dedicate the book to him.

NOTES ON THE TEXT

Language Conventions and Style
- All Japanese words are romanized according to the modified Hepburn system used in *Kenkyusha's New Japanese–English Dictionary*.
- Where Japanese terms are incorporated into the main body of the text, they appear in italics, followed by the author's English translation in round parenthesis, for example *obasuteyama* (granny-dump mountain) and *tatami* (straw mats).
- Unless otherwise stated, all translations from Japanese are by the author.
- People's names are given in the English order, with the surname following the given name.

Note Entries
- Titles of Japanese publications are translated by the author into English. The original Japanese titles can be found in the Works Cited.
- The statement 'Japanese translation available' refers the reader to the Japanese Translations section of the Works Cited.
- All interviewees are anonymized. Their oral testimonies are identified using one random letter per interviewee, followed by his/her title and position and the date of the interview.

Other Conventions
- Please be aware that in this volume one 'billion' refers to one million million, and not to one thousand million as in normal US practice.

LIST OF FIGURES AND TABLES

INTRODUCTION

Diversity and Challenges

Societies throughout the world are ageing. In 1900 around 5 per cent of the population of the United Kingdom and Japan were aged 65 years or over. By 2010 this had risen to 17 per cent and 23 per cent respectively.[1] This trend is set to continue; by 2050 the proportion of over-65s is forecast to be 24 per cent in the UK and 36 per cent in Japan.[2] Japan currently has one of the longest-lived populations in the world, but its total population is expected to shrink from 128 million to 87 million by 2060, the lowest since 1953.[3] However, demographic projections are fallible: in the 1930s Enid Charles and Eva Hubback noted that the birth rate in Britain was below replacement levels. This suggested a long-term population decline, but the trend reversed after the Second World War.[4] Japan's projections may also prove to be wrong, but the implication is that the demographic 'double-squeeze' will reduce the ratio of producers to dependants from 2.8:1.0 to 1.2:1.0 by 2060.[5] This will have repercussions for all strata of society.

The British and Japanese governments face pressing challenges in providing long-term care for older people. In July 2012 the British government published a white paper in response to the 2011 Dilnot Commission's Report on Funding of Care and Support, which recommended that affordable and sustainable funding was needed to replace what it described as a 'confusing, unfair and unsustainable' system.[6] In the white paper the government acknowledged the need for reform but did not settle the funding arrangements.[7] Japan's Long-Term Care Insurance (LTCI) scheme of 2000 has commodified care and extended it beyond traditional family practice.[8] Yet skyrocketing expenditure and public funding constraints have already necessitated rationing, tighter eligibility criteria and higher user fees. This has added to the inequality between the well off and poorer older people – something that is also seen in Britain.[9]

The two governments are monitoring each other's developments and initiatives. In 2008 the UK had some 460,000 long-term places (4.7 per cent of the

65-plus), including nearly 350,000 private sector places and 16,000 long-stay hospital beds.[10] In addition, thousands of 'housing with care', sheltered housing or assisted housing accommodation projects give older people the opportunity to live independently, but with the assurance of 24-hour care and support on site if required. This has proved popular as it offers a more homely substitute for the traditional home. In 2010 Japan had 1.3 million residential places (4.5 per cent of the 65-plus population) under its LTCI scheme, with an additional 200,000 private residential places for the well off and 60,000 in means-tested accommodation for disadvantaged older people.[11] Over half a million hospital beds were mainly occupied by long-stay older patients. (Japan has the world's highest hospital beds to general population ratio and the greatest average length of stay in hospital.[12]) In total, 7 per cent of older people in Japan were in institutional accommodation, refuting the popular assumption that Japan retains a strong family care ethos.

In spite of this, in both Britain and Japan many older people requiring care and support remain wholly or substantially dependent on their family. For some this is their preferred option, but others have no choice. Most people consider residential care a last resort, a sentiment deeply rooted in the legacy of the English Poor Law and of Japanese cultural traditions. Residential care bears a stigma, associated with the workhouse in England and in Japan with the Confucian legend of *obasuteyama* (literally, granny-dump mountain) whereby unwanted parents were abandoned and left to die by their cold-hearted sons.[13] This has deterred older people and their families from seeking residential care, while those already in residential care and their families frequently experience a sense of failure or guilt.

Overall, residential care for older people in both countries is varied in its form, delivery and how it is perceived, and suggests the robustness of its historical legacy. This in turn has informed public and policy discourse.

Gaps in Knowledge and Understanding

Considerable work has been published in Britain and Japan. Many texts focus on current or recent national policies and trends, and accept policy or ideological frameworks as representative of residential care models, administration and practice theories. Longer-term historical studies, based on archival and empirical research, or regional or local data or testimony, are few. The dearth of Japanese sources in English translation is reflected in the lack of comparative literature.

Together, these have contributed to a consensus which suggests that overall residential care for older people in both countries has improved, or when placed in a comparative context, that Britain's residential care is more 'advanced' than Japan's 'lagging' equivalent. This reflects the policy and ideological goals of each country, realized in improvements in general welfare standards and also in Western-derived theoretical frameworks which are commonly used in comparative welfare or social policy research.[14]

The result is often overgeneralized or even misleading accounts of residential care, which focus on an ideal model and overlook the many homes failing to meet the 'ideal'. The latter include very basic homes, where mostly female older residents continue to suffer stigma associated with the English workhouse and the Japanese *obasuteyama*. The same is true of bleak, crowded hospital wards, where privacy and autonomy are denied, and older patients are institutionalized for long periods. The focus on ideal models may also risk ignoring poor practice in care homes classified as excellent, but in which older people fall victim to overworked or callous carers or are exploited by profit-driven home owners. In short, there are significant gaps in our knowledge of residential care for older people in both countries.

Aims, Rationale and Contributions

This book addresses these gaps and deficiencies. It offers a survey of residential care, tracing its origins in each country and recognizing the cumulative impact of traditions and cultural norms, past decisions and commitments in helping to arrive at the present situation. It argues that future planning should acknowledge historical precedents. The book establishes and considers the distinctive features of the English and Japanese residential care systems in the context of perceived needs.

As such, the book challenges beliefs, including the role of the family, which, it is argued, is less supportive in Japan than is generally supposed.[15] The aim is to consider how residential care is actually delivered. Instead of using models and ideological compartmentalization, it acknowledges developments in their own right, given the cultural and policy contexts. It therefore adopts a multilayered approach, to provide studies at the macro (national), meso (regional) and micro (case) levels. Beginning with an overview of national policy in the two countries, it then takes a regional example for each country since the 1920s, stressing the interaction of national and local priorities, influences and practices, examining the life experiences and practice in actual institutions.

The overarching themes of the book are three-fold. First, it investigates how far residential care has improved at three organizational levels: central government, local authorities and specific institutions. Second, it identifies and analyses the factors that promoted these goals or prevented them from being implemented. Finally, it considers the responses to and consequences of these obstacles. While acknowledging the risks of overgeneralization and simplification, as well as the diversity and complexity within and between the two countries, the book offers a comparative and cross-national dimension. This is reflected in the structure of the book, which features three paired English and Japanese chapters. This approach highlights distinctiveness and commonalities, continuities and changes. Britain and Japan developed comparable post-war welfare states, and both experienced an ageing population albeit at different rates and scales, something that is reflected in their policy developments and cultures and traditions. These are considered in the Conclusion, which focuses on the research findings and their implications for current problems, policy debates and discourse, again recognizing the cultural and policy contexts in each country.

Although data for the UK are sometimes referred to when discussing general trends and national performance, most of the interpretative analysis and empirical case studies concern England. The countries that make up the UK have, to varying degrees, separate legal traditions and policies as well as varied cultural and socio-economic backgrounds. The UK is also increasingly a multicultural society, which makes it difficult to generalize, so the oral histories (Chapter 5) focus on the residential life and observations of a white English population. Finally, there is a growing awareness that the category 'older people', 'the elderly' or 'the aged' ignores the complexity of a broad age group. However, the terms are used in this book to refer to all people aged 65 or over to facilitate comparisons between the two countries over time and in each period, unless otherwise specified.

Research on the Care of Older People in Britain and Japan

Growing interest in old age has resulted in considerable published work in Britain and Japan as well as around the world. Until recently, this has tended to concentrate on old age as a social problem or burden of dependency, involving 'a predictable cause of need, with a more or less predictable chronological starting point, requiring remedy from the communal purse'.[16] Reflecting this, studies of the residential care of dependent older people requiring high levels of care and support have attracted interest, yet the focus has been mainly on 'flagship' statutory provision. This fails to acknowledge the diversity within the mixed economy of care, including voluntary or informal care.[17] Similarly, although the importance of integrated care, linking health and social care needs, has been recognized in both countries, residential care has received less attention than community care. Residential or long-term care in health care settings is largely overlooked or examined separately. The result is that the health/social care divide is maintained.[18] What is more, although residential care is sometimes thought of as a form of extended community care within social care, book titles such as *Residential Versus Community Care* imply otherwise.[19]

With governmental policies since the 1960s favouring de-institutionalization, community care has become the preferred option, with residential care depicted in terms of 'rejection' and 'segregation', or subject to approaches focusing on 'what is wrong with institutions'.[20] In the United States, Erving Goffman's

Asylums raised the problem of mentally ill older people in nursing homes.[21] In Britain, Russell Barton's *Institutional Neurosis* suggested that mental hospitals themselves created this illness.[22] Barbara Robb's *Sans Everything* painted a bleak picture of conditions for older, chronically ill patients in psychiatric hospitals, as did Michael Meacher's *Taken for a Ride*.[23]

At the same time an anti-psychiatry movement contributed to de-institutionalization, its British advocates including the psychiatrists David Cooper and Ronald Laing, under the influence of the French philosopher Michel Foucault.[24] Peter Townsend's *The Last Refuge* similarly presented evidence that residential homes failed to offer 'the advantages of living in a "normal community"', features of which (notably family association) were studied by Peter Willmott and Michael Young.[25] In Japan, institutions for older people have also tended to be viewed negatively.[26] Yet there were fewer works on the subject in Japan before 1990, reflecting a lesser interest among Japanese scholars. For example, a translation of Goffman's *Asylums* (1961) into Japanese did not appear until 1984.[27]

Meanwhile, some British scholars were arguing that more residential care places were necessary, given the expected growth in the numbers of very old people. Emily Grundy and Tom Arie regarded this as vital for those who required round-the-clock support and lived alone.[28] Others suggested that there would always be a minority who could most appropriately be cared for in an institution.[29] Isobel Allen and her colleagues further argued that as significant numbers of older people made an 'active "positive choice"' to enter (private) residential homes, this should not be regarded as a 'last resort'.[30] For the most part, though, discussion centred on contemporary issues in relation to policies and principles. Historical surveys were used only to contextualize influential viewpoints in care development, rather than to trace the actual form and delivery of residential care.

To some extent these approaches reflected research funding trends, particularly in Britain, with

> the distribution of research interests in gerontology ... governed by utilitarian values and a pragmatism born of dependence upon government and voluntary agencies for funding. It is unfortunate that the current situation does not permit the growth of understanding which is not tied to immediate action.[31]

Yet more than two decades ago, Anne Digby emphasized the importance of a historical perspective:

> on a broader front, certain policy issues, dilemmas, problems and choices do recur in social welfare. To forget the past record of these events is to force each generation to relearn what should already be known, and thus make future developments less satisfactory than they might be. Equally undesirable, however, has been the tendency in some quarters to manufacture a fictitious past; to create a past golden age of mythical virtues which present policy can seek to emulate. Through each of these ahistorical tendencies, current debate on social welfare is made less informed and cogent.[32]

Among important contributions from other British historians has been Pat Thane's groundbreaking *Old Age in English History*, which, drawing on material from the pre-modern era onwards, challenged current assumptions about the declining status and economic 'burden' created by older people, and revealed the important role that they have always played.[33] David Thomson presented detailed statistical work on residential care trends for older people in England since the 1840s, and Robin Means and Randall Smith published a history of welfare services for older people, including residential care, from 1939 to 1971 (subsequently updated to the 1990s).[34] In Japan, Yoshimasa Ikeda and Kyuichi Yoshida have provided histories of Japanese welfare and philanthropy since the Middle Ages, and Yuji Ogasawara contributed a history of residential care for older people since 1880 (*Fifty-Year History of National Council of Elderly Homes*), which remains the definitive historical synopsis.[35]

Although the emphasis on historical and longer-term perspectives is welcome, its top-down approach may have led to the oversimplification of local variations and practice, whereas practice 'sometimes develops in a policy vacuum, in that policy does not meet real needs. There is an evident gulf between intention and implementation.'[36] It is all too easy to assume that local delivery of care reflects national policy and ideology or that care has improved across the whole country.

One option is to shift the emphasis from centre to locality. Keith Wrightson, for example, argued that 'the thick context of local study ... can do much to make concrete and accessible the abstractions and generalizations of historical interpretation.'[37] While there are still very few regional studies in Japan, British scholars have been more active. Amelia Harris looked at social services provision for older people in thirteen local authorities across Britain.[38] Muriel Brown adopted a historical perspective in four English local councils from 1948 to 1965, tracing developments and changes and exploring the relationship between central legislative intention and local administrative measures.[39] However, these regional studies mainly reflected the viewpoints of local authorities, treating the latter as the minimum unit and rarely touching on grassroots provision and services, or the views of residents and staff.

Others have gone further. English-language studies of Japanese residential homes for older people include one by the Chinese anthropologist Yongmei Wu of a long-term care complex for older people in a Tokyo suburb, taking a participant observation approach.[40] Using a similar methodology, Diana Lynn Bethel has depicted the lives of residents in an old people's home in rural northern Japan, and Leng Leng Thang has examined a pioneering age-integrated facility, which accommodated both nursery children and older people.[41] Earlier, Jeanie Kayser-Jones provided a comparative and international perspective by examining a long-term care institution in Scotland and one in the United States.[42] Although providing insights into institutional life through the eyes of the residents and staff, these studies typically reflect the current situation and problems and lack a historical perspective. Above all, there is little comparative work examining Britain and Japan.

Yasuko Ichibangase has emphasized the value of institutional histories, arguing that 'an institution is not merely an organization or building. It is the very daily living place of the residents'.[43] Accordingly, she provided a detailed history of Japan's first public mixed almshouse for the destitute and sick in Tokyo from 1872 to 1972.[44] Many British historians in recent decades have moved beyond 'bricks and mortar' depictions of workhouses, hospitals and asylums.[45] Yet most deal with the nineteenth century, and there are comparatively few twentieth-century studies. Work written by managers or founders of residential homes is limited when compared, for example, to mental hospital histories by psychiatrists or superintendents.[46] In particular there are very few studies of Japanese old people's almshouses, 'mainly because of the lack of such almshouses in quantitative terms and the consequent dearth of relevant source material'.[47] Drawing on privately held records, Keiso Imura produced histories of five charitable old people's almshouses in southern Japan during 1930–45 (later published as *History of Old People's Almshouses in Japan*). His introduction emphasized that 'the belated research into the history of old people's almshouse in Japan can be enriched by accumulating the histories of individual almshouses'.[48]

Finally, research trends can be examined in an international and comparative perspective. G. Esping-Andersen's *The Three Worlds of Welfare Capitalism*, for example, stimulated academic debate on comparative welfare systems more than two decades ago.[49] This review does not focus on welfare typologies but considers briefly the two countries examined, since Esping-Andersen classified Britain and Japan in different regime models. He positioned Britain as a 'liberal' regime, characterized by means-tested assistance, limited universal transfers and social insurance schemes. Japan was closer to the 'conservative-corporatist' regime model, where social rights are based on employment record and contributions, and the responsibility for welfare is vested in the family rather than the state.

The regime typology approach has contributed to the clustering of various welfare states, yet the typologies can be problematic, since they usually refer only to one point in time and do not take changes into account. A welfare state might be reshaped according to the changing roles of different sectors involved in welfare provision.[50] Britain is one example of 'regime-shifting': social democratic in 1945, contemporary Britain is now described as a 'rather uneasy mix of universalism and the market'.[51] Another shortcoming comes from the positioning of non-Western countries, with Japan usually placed within a variety of existing welfare regime models, conceptualized from a Western framework rather examined on its own terms. Since it rarely sits comfortably within such typologies, the Japanese welfare system is consequently depicted as 'unique' or 'exceptional'.[52] Esping-Andersen's own revision suggested that Japan was a 'hybrid' of liberal-residual and conservative-corporatist types, while Catherine Jones and others have offered a typology of welfare states extended to include a 'Confucian welfare state' or 'East Asian welfare model'.[53]

While the typology debate is unresolved, one consequence is the more prominent inclusion of Japan, along with Britain, in such comparative analysis, with cross-national studies of social policy and welfare published in both countries in recent decades.[54] Yet comparative work on residential care for older people, using a longer-term, historical perspective and including regional or grassroots case studies, is needed. Most comparative texts merely touch on the subject or present it in subsections within welfare, health care and social policy themes.[55] Here American scholars have been more active. A prominent example is Susan Orpett Long's well-received edited collection *Caring for the Elderly in Japan and the US*, but even this gives comparatively little attention to residential care as such, and the focus is mainly on current affairs and problems as well as national trends.[56] Again, residential care is only addressed within broader provision for older people, and the focus is mainly on current affairs and problems as well as national trends. In short, the lack of data in comparative studies arises because the work has been produced by native scholars and is restricted to specific countries and languages.

These somewhat isolationist tendencies may have contributed to the dearth of relevant Japanese literature in English translation. Conversely, it is all too easy to accept the contextualization of a nation's residential care within Western-derived theoretical frameworks, based on ideology or regime typology in comparative welfare and social policy research. Such approaches may not sufficiently acknowledge national or regional influences or be sensitive to socio-economic features, experiences and traditions. Similarly, details and trends in elderly residential care may be subsumed within discourse on the ageing of the population or concerning more general welfare provision and policy directives, resulting in overgeneralized or even misleading interpretations.[57] Thus, notions of Japan's residential care having lagged behind the English equivalent have been common, with Japan's performance assessed unfavourably against the more 'advanced' English model. Or, taking a particular feature, the investigation of less 'homely' environments and lack of personal privacy or space for living and possessions within multi-bedded accommodation is viewed as a problem in English care arrangements and therefore an even greater one in Japan.

From this literature review, it can be surmised that while there is no shortage of scholarly material, much of it lacks historical focus, with very few empirical historical studies at regional or grassroots levels. Above all, these works have largely been produced by native scholars and are restricted to specific countries and languages. A principal aim of this book is thus to address these deficiencies by adopting a different approach and methodology.

Methods and Approach

This volume takes an empirically grounded historical approach, informed by a cross-national dimension. It thereby offers the beginnings of a more rounded understanding of residential care for older people in England and Japan. It follows a multilayered methodology, stepping down from national surveys in each country, to regional case studies, to examples of institutions in one region of each country. The regions cannot be regarded as representative of the respective countries, and when placed in a transnational context may be of limited applicability. Rather, those selected partly reflect their relative ease of access and their rich research materials and facilities.[58] The coverage of urban and rural districts within each region also highlights different or contrasting interpretations and consequently actual developments. The regions – the county of Norfolk and Gifu Prefecture – have much in common. Both are rural and large; they have sparse, largely homogeneous populations, with above-average proportions of people aged 65-plus, many of whom are conservative in outlook and adhere to traditions and cultural values. Their main towns accounted for 15–20 per cent of their total populations during the study period. Neither region is considered exceptional, but is reasonably indicative of rural regions within their respective countries and hence can be thought of as reasonably comparable.

The regional case studies examine how national policies and objectives were implemented by their authorities. Sensitive to specific regional contexts, this approach reveals interpretations and practice, and the complex processes of implementation and variations, which are not necessarily clear from a state-led single narrative. The case examples also acknowledge cultural traditions and experiences; moreover, the local examples offer insights into the residential life and practice from older residents' and staffs' perspectives. These narratives are often understated or marginalized, but they are vital because they reveal attitudes and practices that do not necessarily reflect official policy goals or accord with popular discourses. This methodology is acknowledged by historians and social scientists alike. To quote Steven Cherry, the approach 'acknowledges that various national perspectives may lead to overgeneralization and ignore significant diversity, but that local or micro studies may be simply too narrow to generalize from and are more vulnerable to the distortions of specific or even chance circumstances'.[59]

Most texts on residential care for older people do not adopt this approach, so a particular strength of this book is the use of oral testimony, drawing on interviews with staff, relatives and older residents themselves. This adds a personalized dimension to the study, bringing out the experiences and authentic voices of older residents, who are otherwise 'hidden from history'.[60] Paul Thompson has eloquently described the value of this approach:

> Reality is complex and many-sided; and it is a primary merit of oral history that ... it allows the original multiplicity of standpoints to be recreated ... witnesses can now also be called from the under-classes, the unprivileged, and the defeated. It provides a more realistic and fair reconstruction of the past ... The scope of historical writing itself is enlarged and enriched ... History becomes, to put it simply, more democratic.[61]

Critics have castigated memory as 'an unrealistic historical source' or claimed that oral testimony is inevitably subjective or selective.[62] Nonetheless, oral history can paint a broader picture since the interviews often confirm each other or offer an alternative view, while visits to the local care homes and observation of everyday life there have helped to contextualize interviewees' own accounts.

The Structure of the Book

The book is presented in three parts, featuring paired chapters of broadly comparable studies at the national, regional and local institutional levels for England (Chapters 1, 3 and 5) and Japan (Chapters 2, 4 and 6). Chapters 1 and 2 set the scene by providing a historical overview of the development of residential care for older people from the Elizabethan Poor Law of 1601 in England and from the Meiji Restoration of 1868 in Japan. Based on official reports and statistics, and supplemented by key studies, each chapter examines government policy and objectives, legislation and regulations, and implementation and national performance both quantitatively and qualitatively. Each focuses on statutory, residential care provision as laid down by legislation and post-war welfare arrangements, and considers alternatives, including informal (family) care, long-stay hospitals, private and voluntary homes, and community care. The latter are of considerable significance, given the increasingly diversified and complex form and delivery of residential care in both countries, as are recent trends, including privatization, renewed attention to the social/health care divide, and the relative role of the state and family. Also explored is the importance of legacy and stigma, associated with the English workhouse and Japan's *obasuteyama*.

Chapters 3 and 4 turn to regional perspectives, with Norfolk and Gifu Prefecture taken as examples. The two regions both represent rural and conservative-minded areas, which facilitate a comparative analysis. Drawing mainly on archival and local materials, the regional studies examine how national policies have been assimilated by the responsible bodies since the 1920s, acknowledging their individual contexts rather than shoe-horning them into national trends. Whether their experiences have any significance at the national level and have any particularly influential features are also considered.

Before the 1974 local government reform in England and Wales, 146 county or county borough councils were responsible for residential care for older people. Norfolk comprised three councils: Norfolk itself and the more urban Norwich and Great Yarmouth county boroughs. Norfolk and Norwich are considered separately here, prior to the 1974 reform and creation of the enlarged unitary Norfolk county. In contrast, Japan had a two-tier administrative structure, with forty-seven upper prefectural (regional) authorities responsible for overall provision and some 800 local authorities or councils (cities, towns and villages) dealing with everyday administration, determined by the provisions of the 1951 Social Services Reform Act. This remained essentially unchanged during the period examined. Since the local authorities were too small and varied in size to be representative and have few official records available to the public, this study deals with the upper Gifu Prefecture, examining its twenty-six local authorities collectively and taking a number of 'snapshots' in selected local authorities.

Chapter 3 suggests that Norfolk's county and county borough councils oversaw contrasting transitions from the workhouse to the 'small' home, which could be seen in their wartime experiences and subsequent policy interpretations, although both authorities initially developed residential care provision in line with national averages. Perversely, their early successes were effectively penalized by ministerial policy in the 1960s and early 1970s, which directed loans for capital projects to local authorities that had not created sufficient residential places. This put counties and councils with enough places at a disadvantage, even when those places were in former workhouses (as in Norfolk) or in older, converted small homes (as in Norwich). This set back Norfolk's closure programme of its former workhouses and Norwich's modernization programme.

Chapter 4 examines similar themes in Gifu, extending the period reviewed to the 1990s to cover its later expansion of statutory residential care provision, which lagged behind the rest of Japan. This arose from its specific regional features, notably the prefecture's restrictionist policy, which regarded family care as a cost-free asset that ought to take priority over public welfare. This limited residential care to needy older people without family support. A discernible expansion in prefecture nursing homes from the 1980s did not indicate the end of official restrictionism, but reflected central government targets and the prefecture's acceptance of the initiatives of local leaders and wealthy philanthropists, underpinned by central government subsidies. Taken together, the regional studies shed light on the problems and complexities of implementing central legislation, national policy and aspirations, in the light of available resources, local traditions, socio-demographic trends and perceptions of need.

Chapters 5 and 6 present detailed institutional studies, examining how national policy objectives impacted on grassroots practice and residents' lives. They focus on the delivery of quality care. Each chapter has two sections. The first covers the period 1945–73, examining a former workhouse or almshouse and its replacement in each region. The methodology is similar to that of the regional studies, recovering the history of the selected institutions and drawing on archival and local records to examine whether a 'homely' home and improvements in residential life and practice have been achieved. These are considered in relation to the physical environment, amenities and services, and the quality of care provided by care workers, which simultaneously reveal the extent to which the Poor Law legacy, stigma and pre-war measures and mentalities have survived. The second section provides a more dynamic history of local residential care based largely on in-depth interviews. In both the English and Japanese sections, the voices reveal not only positive aspects of residents' life experiences in outdated psychiatric hospitals or 'bottom-of-the-pile' basic homes, but also the negative features in improved or 'ideal' homes. The implication that residential care 'models' devised by policymakers may not suit everyone is relevant to current debates and future planning, something taken up in the Conclusion. Overall, the institutional studies reveal the great diversity and complexity of residential life and practice, casting doubt on whether a truly 'representative' or 'model' practice or home exists.

Finally, key findings and their implications for each country are reviewed in a cross-national and comparative context and at each national, regional and grassroots institutional level. The analysis highlights commonalities and differences, continuities and changes, achievements and failings in the two systems, avoiding simplistic judgements and considering also the cultural and policy context of each country. These are linked to current policy trends and debates, again in a cross-national context. The study ends with a plea for future planning for the ageing populations of England and Japan to be based on the evidence of real experience at home and elsewhere, since the major issues, dilemmas and problems recur and transcend national boundaries.

1 THE ENGLISH CONTEXT

This chapter and Chapter 2 give an overview of the development of residential care for older people in England and Japan respectively, tracing it to its origins in each country. Each focuses on statutory residential care provision under the country's Poor Laws and post-war welfare arrangements. This chapter discusses the English workhouse, the legacy and stigma associated with it, post-war statutory residential care provision under the 1948 National Assistance Act, and finally alternatives.

Origins: The Poor Law Workhouse from 1601

Forms of institutional care for the needy in England, including the destitute, sick or disabled elderly, can be traced back to the Middle Ages, when monastic communities ran infirmary almshouses for the sick and houses of pity for the destitute. This ended with the dissolution of the monasteries under Henry VIII between 1536 and 1539, but was revived in different form with the establishment first of poor houses or houses of correction and later with the 1834 Poor Law.[1] By that date voluntary hospitals were providing medical care for the acute sick poor, but not longer-term institutional care for the chronic sick or infirm, including the elderly.[2] The latter, along with paupers of all ages, sometimes received alms or were granted allowances or indoor relief, increasingly in the 'mixed' workhouses established by the 1834 Poor Law. It was not until the early twentieth century that the special needs of older people were acknowledged, with more places provided and separate legislation.

Workhouses were viewed with fear and loathing and described ominously as 'the Bastille' or 'old Basty'.[3] If these perceptions were fuelled by Dickens's novels, excesses such as the Andover scandal of 1846, where inmates' meagre rations were stolen by the workhouse master and they were reduced to eating bones they were supposed to crush for fertilizer or starve, were real enough.[4] Although the 1948 National Assistance Act repealed the Poor Law, many workhouse buildings served as homes or 'hostels' for older people, and even among their modern replacements, it is arguable whether the stigma of the Poor Law workhouse was fully eliminated.

The Elizabethan or 'Old' Poor Law of 1601, which was based on a series of statutes enacted between 1597 and 1601, represented the first national framework for welfare policy. This was a means of dealing with the vulnerable in society, who were considered vagrants, beggars or criminals and associated with public disorder, though their conditions were in reality brought about by economic and social change.[5] While efforts were made to discipline able-bodied paupers, the needs of the sick, elderly, widowed, deserted and orphans were recognized. The legislation made every parish responsible for its own poor, funded by a property-based poor rate. Unpaid overseers of the poor were appointed annually by the local justices of the peace, and distributed 'competent sums of money for and towards the necessary relief of the lame, impotent, old, blind and such other among them being poor and not able to work'.[6]

How rigorously the legislation was enforced is unknown, but it was probably slow to be implemented. Moreover, practice varied widely and the workhouses reflected this, varying significantly in size, type, administration and conditions. The first official returns of 1776 listed around 2,000 workhouses, with a capacity to house up to 90,000 inmates. The smallest accommodated just two and the largest in excess of 500, but most housed between twenty and thirty.[7]

Inside the workhouses,

> diet and comfort, though always Spartan, probably exceeded what the pauper might obtain outside, and while large numbers of poor houses [workhouses] were ramshackle, insanitary and undisciplined, some others were well endowed, with infirmaries and a high degree of regulation ... husband and wife were parted ... [but] ... This was by no means universal practice, and Liverpool workhouse even housed married couples apart from the main building.[8]

Some parishes, such as Harrington, in Cumberland, sent claimants to the workhouse rather than give them outdoor relief on the grounds that 'the poor have such a dislike to this mode of provision that it is expected that this new system will lower the rates very considerably'.[9] This method would later be formulated as the 'less eligibility' and 'workhouse test' measures under the 1834 Poor Law. Variations were found between parishes in the form of their outdoor relief even following the introduction of the 1795 Speenhamland system, which supplemented wages based on the number of children in a family and the price of bread, as well as providing essential maintenance and other material benefits.[10] The same was true with variations in the balance between indoor and outdoor relief recipients, although generally there were few indoor relief recipients, with just 8 per cent (83,000) of all paupers on indoor relief in 1802–3.[11] However, this small group absorbed approximately one quarter of all relief expenditure, suggesting that 'workhouse inmates were probably the hard core of the pauper population', whereas roughly a third of all paupers were relieved only occasionally.[12]

How did the elderly fare? It is difficult to identify them, since 'old age was not a *de facto* reason to give relief. Rather, the claims of the elderly had to be substantiated with supplementary causes of poverty and destitution such as sickness, disability or underemployment.[13] Nonetheless, the 1802–3 official returns indicated that 166,400 (16 per cent of all paupers) were aged 60 or over and sick, 1.8 per cent of the total population at a time when 8 per cent of the total population in England and Wales were aged 60 or above.[14] Some historians have suggested that 'up to a third of the elderly ... received parish relief', absorbing up to a half of all local Poor Law resources.[15]

Given such great local variations, the Old Poor Law has been the subject of widely differing interpretations. What Sidney and Beatrice Webb saw as an imposition – 'Relief of the Poor within a Framework of Repression' or 'Charity in the Grip of Serfdom' – may also have offered welcome allowances and a modicum of 'humanity and flexibility' in adapting to local conditions.[16] Thus Geoffrey Oxley saw 'an effective, comprehensive and flexible system for the relief of the deserving poor – the aged, the sick, one-parent families and so on'.[17] However limited in its scope, the Old Poor Law affirmed national responsibility for providing the destitute and vulnerable with basic subsistence – 'a welfare state in miniature'.[18] Focusing on the old, David Thomson concluded that the Poor Law was more generous than the contemporary English welfare state, although Pat Thane noted that it 'remained overwhelmingly residual in character': 'only a small minority [of the aged] received anything approaching full subsistence'.[19]

The 1834 'New' Poor Law introduced a far stricter approach to the able-bodied poor through the principle of 'less eligibility' by reference to the 'workhouse test', which meant 'that his [the pauper's] situation on the whole shall not be made really or apparently so eligible as the situation of the independent labourer of the lowest class'.[20] This was to be achieved in 'well regulated workhouses', with outdoor relief to the able-bodied eventually prohibited.[21] Consequently, it was envisaged that

> into such a house none will enter voluntarily; work, confinement, and discipline, will deter the indolent and vicious; and nothing but extreme necessity will induce any to accept the comfort which must be obtained by the surrender of their free agency, and the sacrifice of their accustomed habits and gratifications.[22]

Accordingly, oppressive conditions, humiliating regulations, segregation by age and sex, and uniformity characterized the system. Anne Crowther draws attention to the 'unrelieved tedium of the institutional life, which probably afflicted the inmates most'.[23] Relief thus came at the cost of the loss of human, civil and political rights.

Under a revised administrative framework, the autonomous parishes were amalgamated into 643 unions, and elected boards of guardians replaced overseers of the poor. Ostensibly, these new authorities had no discretionary powers within a framework of national regulations, enforced and controlled by a new central body.[24] The guardians were to establish a union workhouse. This was sometimes an existing facility but usually a new one was built, and by 1854 all but eighteen unions had their own workhouse.[25] Altogether, 725 workhouses offered 210,000 places, but the total workhouse population that year averaged just 112,000, and over 750,000 paupers continued to receive outdoor relief, suggesting its longevity but also partly reflecting official recognition of outdoor relief in 1852.[26]

The treatment of aged paupers was not given priority in the Royal Commission's Report. Indeed, the Commission recommended no change in the balance between indoor and outdoor relief for the non-able-bodied poor, which meant that the workhouses might house old and sick persons alongside able-bodied paupers. However, it did suggest 'the principle of separate and appropriate management', with inmates divided into at least four classes: the aged and impotent; children; able-bodied females; and able-bodied males.[27] Through such classification, 'each class might thus receive an appropriate treatment; the old might enjoy their indulgences without torment from the boisterous'.[28] Yet this proposal failed to materialize fully, since even in the early 1900s, 'of the 140,000 persons over sixty in Poor Law institutions, only a thousand or two ... are in the separate establishments'.[29] Nor was the 'appropriate' treatment of the aged fully implemented, since conditions in some mixed workhouses were 'defective in every particular':

> The inmates, over 900 in number, were congregated in large rooms, without any attempt to employ their time or cheer their lives. There was a marked absence of any human interest ... It could not be better described than as a 'human warehouse'. The dormitories ... were so full of beds as to make it impossible to provide chairs, or to walk, except sideways, between them ... it is impossible to conceive a more dismal and hopeless asylum for age.[30]

Attitudes and beliefs in Victorian England extolled self-help and independence, and destitution was seen as a personal failing or family irresponsibility. The unfortunate might be assisted, but had no entitlement beyond the poor law minima, tightened further from the 1870s: 'by 1890 the proportion of elderly persons who received some form of public assistance was less than half of what it had been in 1870 or earlier ... [and] the value [of outdoor relief] ... was only about half in 1890 of what it had been in the 1860s'.[31] Of the 2,100,000 persons aged 65 or more in the United Kingdom by 1900, 1,750,000 were living in poverty, with 613,000 in receipt of poor relief in the course of a year; another 600,000 perhaps were deterred from recourse to the guardians; and the remaining third endured a ceaseless struggle with poverty for at least three successive years.[32]

However, attitudes gradually began to change. Chronic and widespread poverty, the harsh treatment of paupers under the Poor Law, its association with industrial depression and political and social unrest, and the publication of official and social surveys all played a part. In 1895 the Royal Commission on the Aged Poor stated that many were undeniably poor but reluctant to ask for assistance because of the stigma attached to it.[33] Similarly, the social researcher Charles Booth stressed that 'old age stands out plainly as the prevailing cause of pauperism after 65', with nearly a third of the 65-plus age group in receipt of poor relief in 1892.[34] In evidence to the 1905–9 Royal Commission on the Poor Laws, Booth claimed that half the recipients of outdoor relief were aged 60 or over, of whom three-quarters were women.[35] He concluded, 'when we consider how many of the poor are old, we cannot escape the conclusion that poverty is essentially a trouble of old age'.[36] Wider investigations by Booth and the social reformer Seebohm Rowntree revealed that roughly 30 per cent of the population of London and York were living in poverty.[37] They concluded that rather than profligacy or idleness, poverty was caused by low pay, irregular employment, large families, illness, widowhood and old age. In short, evidence that destitution increased in old age cast doubt on the deterrent character of the Poor Law: if less eligibility and the workhouse test deterred the able-bodied poor, for the aged poor its logic was harsh and irrelevant, though quirkily successful. Charitable initiatives and work developed rapidly to remedy the situation, providing services to the aged frail and poor. To promote coordination between charities and further expansion, the Charity Organisation Society was established in 1869.

Towards the Break-Up of the Poor Law, 1900–45

The early twentieth century marked the beginning of the break-up of the Poor Law.[38] This involved a raft of legislation which introduced alternatives to the indiscriminate approach to pauperism, although the Poor Law was retained for the residuum. The legislation aimed to reduce reliance on the Poor Law and also to offer higher standards and more specialist services targeting the needs of different groups of people. Thus the 1908 Old Age Pensions Act provided a non-contributory weekly pension to persons aged 70 or over, subject to stringent means and character tests. The 1911 National Insurance Act sought to limit poverty caused by interruption of earnings due to sickness or unemployment, with the insurance principle extended under the 1925 Old Age and Widows and Orphans Contributory Pensions Act to cover other contingencies. Attempts to extend the 1911 Act culminated in the 1934 Unemployment Act. Home help provision started with the 1918 Maternity and Child Welfare Act and extended it to sick and frail older persons under the Ministry's 1944 Circular 179/44.[39] The development of children's homes, infirmaries, isolation hospitals and mental hospitals made it possible to separate more of the poor from the general mixed workhouse. In particular, the 1929 Local Government Act encouraged county and county borough councils (which replaced the guardians) to take over work-houses as general or specialized hospitals, with a third of workhouse infirmaries appropriated by 1938.[40]

E. P. Hennock has argued that welfare reform was prompted by revulsion against the harshness of the Poor Law and a determination to provide something more humane.[41] Nevertheless, the Poor Law remained a pervasive influence. Tellingly, 'the new developments tended to by-pass rather than replace or reform the basic poor law provision', which survived mounting criticism, the conflict-ing reports of the 1905–9 Royal Commission and post-war plans for social reform.[42] Although the 1929 Local Government Act dismantled its administra-tive structure and renamed workhouses as Public Assistance Institutions (PAIs) and Poor Law relief as Public Assistance, according to one critic, the 1929 Act 'did not "break up" the Poor Law ... Poor Law relief remained Poor Law relief and pauperism remained pauperism'.[43]

Consequently, the needs of frail older paupers were largely neglected between 1910 and 1946, something Townsend described as 'a conspiracy of silence on the subject'.[44] Whereas the total workhouse population more than halved from 275,000 to 127,000 between 1911 and 1946, the decline in the 65-plus popu-lation was more moderate, falling from 82,700 to 59,000 in this period; as a result, the proportion of the 65-plus workhouse population increased from less than a third (30 per cent) to almost half.[45] Some improvements were introduced. Included were better quality care provided by trained and qualified nursing staff, access to basic health care, restoration of electoral rights, and 'comforts', such as the right to wear their own clothes, to make and receive visits, to smoke and to eat other than the prescribed diet.[46] Starting in 1882, the charitable Brabazon Employment Scheme tried to 'cheer the lives of the old people in the work-house' by introducing handicrafts, with the products sold to purchase further comforts.[47] Even so, these changes barely altered the fearsome image of the work-house: as Booth remarked, 'almost any amount of suffering and privation will be endured by the people rather than go into it'.[48]

The Second World War brought considerable hardship and disruption; air raids killed many bedridden older residents and destroyed or severely damaged many workhouses, leaving the survivors severely disadvantaged.[49] Residents of undamaged workhouses and public hospitals were discharged to create 300,000 beds for the war wounded under the Emergency Medical Service (EMS) scheme.[50] Prominent among the displaced were the frail and chronic sick elderly. While those without permanent accommodation gravitated to public air raid shelters and rest centres not intended for permanent use, others, referred to alternative EMS hospitals, 'were ... shifted from one place to another'.[51] The EMS scheme also resulted in some middle-class older people being sent to workhouses, which accelerated the search for better or alternative institutional care. For example, voluntary organizations working for wartime older evacuees established at least 230 hostels for some 9,000 people by 1944.[52] Similarly, the Government Evacuation Scheme provided hostel accommodation for over 1,500 older homeless Londoners in 1941, with 150 hostels added for bedridden or frail people in reception or neutral areas in 1942.[53] Yet almost 60,000 older people remained in workhouses in 1944 in conditions summarized by Emily D. Samson, Secretary of the Old People's Welfare Committee (later Age Concern and now Age UK), as:

> large grim buildings erected in the early Victorian era as general mixed workhouses ... defy all efforts to produce anything akin to a homelike atmosphere ... 'inmates' – are generally accommodated in very large wards, and the homogeneity of the equipment, the precision of its arrangement and the scrupulous tidiness ... inevitably conduce to an institutional atmosphere.[54]

A letter to the *Manchester Guardian*, headed 'A Workhouse Visit', stated:

> On each chair sat an old woman in workhouse dress, upright, unoccupied. No library books or wireless. Central heating, but no open fire. No easy chairs. No pictures on the wall ... None was allowed to lie on her bed at any time throughout the day, although breakfast is at 7 a.m.; but ... three ... had crashed forward, face downwards, on to their immaculate bedspreads and were asleep ... I have learnt ... that old people in workhouses cannot be expected to demand their own rights ...[55]

Early in 1946 the Ministry of Health, in cooperation with the Nuffield Foundation, issued a survey of conditions in workhouses which confirmed that 'in large urban areas such institutions may accommodate as many as 1,500 residents of various types, including more than a thousand aged persons ... In some institutions rules are harsh or harshly administered'.[56]

The 1948 National Assistance Act: A New Departure?

In 1946 a small, interdepartmental group, the Break-up of the Poor Law Committee, was formed under Sir Arthur Rucker, Deputy Secretary to the Minister of Health. Its proposals contributed to the National Assistance Bill of 31 October 1947.[57] In introducing the bill, Aneurin Bevan, Minister of Health and Housing, celebrated 'a great departure in the treatment of old people. The workhouse is to go. Although many people have tried to humanize it, it is in many respects a very evil institution'.[58] J. Edwards, Parliamentary Secretary to the Minister, emphasized the 'profound significance, even if nothing else happens, that the Poor Law is dead', while in the House of Lords, Lord Henderson declared that many would 'hail the demise of the Poor Law'.[59] Whether, like Bessie Braddock MP, they thought 'of what we are repealing more than of what we are proposing' was less clear.[60]

The National Assistance Act came into force on 5 July 1948, when 'the existing poor law shall cease to have effect'.[61] It required county and county borough councils to provide 'residential accommodation for persons who by reason of age, infirmity or any other circumstances are in need of care and attention which is not otherwise available to them'.[62] The model Bevan envisaged was of homes for twenty to thirty persons, analogous to private residential hotels: older residents would be given 'the maximum of privacy and independence'; and to avoid stigma they would pay an economic rent 'so that any old persons who wish ... may go there in exactly the same way as many well-to-do people have been accustomed to go into residential hotels'.[63] Although claimants were still means-tested, financial criteria no longer determined eligibility to residential care, as 'persons for whom accommodation is provided under this Part of this Act shall pay for the accommodation'.[64] Most pensioners could pay for their accommodation and maintenance of twenty-one shillings a week from their twenty-six shillings basic old age pension, keeping five shillings to buy personal items.

Optimists claimed that the legislation 'marks the end of a whole period of the social history of Great Britain'.[65] They also detected a qualitative change in residential care 'from merely a provision of shelter to the provision of ... bodily care, health care, care for disabled, etc. ... real substantive reform'.[66] Newspaper headlines reflected this view: 'End of Poor Law, Hostels for Aged' and 'Private Rooms and All Necessary Services for 21s. a Week'.[67] But critics have argued that preoccupation with abolishing the Poor Law meant that the 1948 Act was not 'a forward-looking measure ... because the new provisions were based on past conceptions rather than on new thinking which was beginning to take shape'.[68] In other words, the Act focused on accommodation for the minority in need of 'care and attention'. Beyond the provision of an old age pension, alternative arrangements, such as community-based services for the majority who needed some assistance in their own homes, were left to voluntary organizations or private means. Local authorities were given no powers to develop community-based services; they were merely enabled to make grants to voluntary agencies.[69] Statutory provision for older people living at home was limited to home help and home nursing, again to be arranged through voluntary organizations, in association with local health authorities under the 1946 National Health Service (NHS) Act.[70]

This was understandable given the severe post-war restrictions. Yet compared with other client groups, older people appeared to be a low priority. As Julia Parker noted, 'the concern to maintain and foster family life evident in the Children Act was completely lacking in the National Assistance Act'.[71] This possibly reflected the belief that frail older persons could not manage in their own homes unless they were living with family members, or that existing community-based services could not offer sufficient support to enable older people to live independently.[72] Community-based provision was a second-best alternative, to be supplemented by families and voluntary agencies.[73] However, the earlier restriction of residential care to a minority who perceived it as undesirable encouraged older people to struggle at home on low incomes and with few community-based services, a policy which cost little and reinforced the core values of society.[74]

The Act had other shortcomings. First, with public expenditure restrictions, and other social or health services consuming scarce resources, continuing policy ambitions beyond 1948 was uncertain. Second, the Act failed to define the group to whom local authorities might offer residential accommodation; they were simply people 'in need of care and attention'. This excluded anyone with a physical impairment or personality disorder, as residential homes were not intended for people in need of medical treatment or nursing care.[75] The problem of policy interpretation increased as the number of hospital beds was reduced, aggravating disputes over the blurred boundary between free NHS health care and local authority means-tested social care. Finally, 'there was no clear guidance about the development of welfare schemes; little thought had been given to the sort of staff that would be needed for the developing services; and no attention was paid to the local administrative arrangements'.[76]

In short, the 1948 Act promised to provide something as close as possible to a 'normal' home for those in need of care and attention. However, the targeted group represented a small minority of less frail older people and excluded the frail or chronic sick along with many others able to live independently with some assistance. Above all, the retention of means-testing suggested the resilience of the legacy and stigma of the Poor Law and workhouse.

Delayed Responses, 1948–60

Residential arrangements on 5 July 1948 were complex. Of the 400 or so former workhouses in England and Wales, fewer than 100 were designated as hospitals under the 1946 NHS Act, and just over 100 became local authority (Part III) residential homes.[77] The rest were used as NHS hospital beds and as local authority residential places. As a result, 122,000 mainly aged and chronic sick residents of the old workhouses now became 82,000 NHS hospital patients while 40,000 were classified as Part III residents. With a further 8,000 Part III residents in local authority-supported voluntary premises or pre-existing local authority 'small' homes or hostels, the number of institutionalized older people of some kind was 130,000, or 3 per cent of England's 65-plus population. Of these, 94 per cent remained in former workhouses, and these temporary arrangements continued for much longer than is generally realized.

The first annual report of the Ministry of Health stated that 'local authorities are busy planning and opening small, comfortable homes, where old people, many of them lonely, can live pleasantly and with dignity'.[78] Yet continuing shortages of building materials and restrictions on capital investment hampered all new projects, and resource allocation prioritized industrial estates, new towns and family housing: 'it will be some years before local authorities cease to be handicapped by large and outmoded premises ... it will obviously be necessary to continue to use existing buildings for some years to come'.[79] One year later, purpose-built small homes 'had to be ruled out almost entirely'.[80] The first five-year plan (1949–54), based on local authorities' plans submitted to the Ministry, envisaged 52,000 new residential places, but just 21,000 had materialized by 1954, and former workhouses were still being used.[81] At the same time, waiting lists for residential places were growing and less than 20 per cent of applicants were successful.[82]

The Ministry of Health took a *laissez-faire* attitude towards local authorities.[83] There were no clear guidelines for committee arrangements for their services and for implementation of the five-year local plans for residential home provision. Almost three-quarters (72 per cent) of local authorities had welfare committees, but others had sub-committees of health committees or made no distinction for welfare within health committee provision.[84] Their proposals were 'unimpressive', reflecting the availability of former workhouses and other residential premises and local interpretations of perceived needs, informed by political culture or tradition, socio-economic and demographic trends, and current and potential resources.[85]

By the 1950s state officials, politicians and professionals agreed that it was better for older people to be assisted at home as 'a genuine economy measure, and also [as] a humanitarian measure'.[86] Similarly, Ministry of Health reports emphasized the 'importance of enabling old people to go on living in their own homes, where they most wish to be, and of delaying admission to residential care for as long as possible'.[87] Despite official endorsement of more voluntary input and coordination of statutory and voluntary agencies, progress was limited: in 1962 Peter Townsend and Dorothy Wedderburn estimated that 600,000 of the 5.8 million older people living at home had no access to the home help services they needed, while requests for 344,000 meal services were unmet.[88] Lack of labour, money, legislative power and coordination between the various sectors were problems, as were ambiguities concerning entitlement and charges for services.[89] There was also disquiet that state or voluntary assistance would undermine family responsibilities for the care of older relatives, although no evidence was presented to substantiate this.[90] Beliefs such as these often resulted in clients without family support being prioritized.[91] In short, faith in community care as the best option might be manipulated as a cost-effective way of delivering services and deflecting criticism of residential arrangements.

Problems were aggravated as demand for institutional care increased. Attempts to distinguish the 'sick' from those 'in need of care and attention' struck Iain Macleod, Minister of Health, as 'perhaps the most baffling problem in the whole of the National Health Service'.[92] More frail and dependent old people received care in residential homes simply because 'hospital beds for the chronic sick were also acutely scarce'.[93] This accentuated deficiencies in converted residential homes, notably the lack of ground-floor accommodation and lifts. Substantial modifications were required. Suitable premises were scarce. Consequently, in heavily populated areas where demand was high or sites were difficult to acquire, 'small' homes (for up to sixty residents) were permitted, offering more ground-floor beds, smaller day rooms and most beds in 4–6-bedded rooms.[94] Yet even these changes were delayed by restrictions on capital investment.

With shortages in both local authority residential places and NHS hospital beds, the two sectors looked to each other for care of the frail elderly. *The Times* noted that 'between "health" and "welfare" there is an administrative no-man's-land. Its inhabitants are mostly old people'.[95] Barnett Janner MP pointed out that 'the provisions of the two Acts [the NHS and the National Assistance Acts] do not overlap, and this creates a kind of "no man's land" between them'.[96] Suggested solutions included intermediate ('halfway') houses offering rehabilitation so that older people could return to their own home or go to a conventional residential home after rehabilitation, and for the more dependent elderly, 'special long-stay annexes' at hospitals, which could provide nursing care under medical supervision.[97] Yet the Ministry was reluctant to pursue initiatives like these.

One London survey suggested that 45 per cent of older hospital patients could manage in a residential home but remained in hospital due to a lack of alternative accommodation.[98] Similarly, the 1957 Boucher Report estimated that perhaps 4,500 mainly aged chronic sick patients in hospital would benefit from a residential home place. It considered that 'the number of beds for the chronic sick ... is sufficient in total if they are properly used and better distributed'.[99] 'Bed blocking' was also common in mental hospitals, where about 43,000 (29 per cent) patients were aged 65 or over.[100] Many of them were certified simply to secure accommodation for them. Norman Dodds MP estimated that 'altogether 95 per cent should not be certified'.[101] The Boucher Report suggested that 30 per cent of elderly mental hospital patients might be cared for in residential homes 'if the facilities had been available'.[102] The 1954–7 Royal Commission on the Law Relating to Mental Illness and Mental Deficiency concurred, and the 1959 Mental Health Act made criteria for compulsory admission to psychiatric hospitals more stringent and encouraged local authority residential home provision for the elderly mentally ill.[103] Yet without clear Ministry directives and guidance, local authority residential accommodation for the elderly mentally ill varied greatly: some integrated this group within conventional homes, whereas others provided designated homes or separate units (see Chapter 3).

One effect of the 1950s inquiries was to shift the definition of people 'in need of care and attention' under the 1948 Act from relatively active able-bodied persons to those with some physical or mental illness. The resulting reduction of hospital beds for older patients put more pressure on residential home provision, something that reflected anxieties over the relatively high cost of hospital care, which averaged £500 per annum per capita in 1953, compared to £180 in a residential home.[104] Moreover, it was generally agreed that 'it is more humane to nurse illnesses known to be terminal in the home where the patient has resided wherever possible'.[105] Attempts to redefine the frail and demarcate the roles of the hospital and residential home were also made by the Ministry of Health.[106] But the results were unsatisfactory, even though both sides increasingly made concessions and arranged swaps.[107] Forms of rationing also featured as 'residential homes should only be provided for the really frail and infirm elderly'.[108]

Overall, assumptions that community-based services, hospitals or halfway houses might compensate for the lack of residential homes or possibly replace them were gradually discarded. Nevertheless, aspirations for community care undermined faith in residential care, and 'so far as residential services for the aged and handicapped were concerned, Britain appeared to have been going through one long tunnel of an economic crisis between 1948 and 1958'.[109]

In 1960 former workhouses still 'accounted for just over half the accommodation used by county and county borough councils, for just under half the residents and for probably over three-fifths of the old people actually admitted in the course of a year'.[110] They housed 35,000 mostly aged and frail residents, a mere 4,000 fewer than in 1948.[111] According to Townsend's 1958 survey, based on thirty-nine former workhouses and their 9,000 or so residents, eleven were 'large' (250 residents or more), seventeen were 'medium' (100–249 residents) and eleven were 'small' (fewer than 100 residents).[112] Inadequate facilities were found in a third and another third were little better. Just 2 per cent of residents had single rooms, while 57 per cent slept in rooms with at least ten beds, and 16 per cent were in dormitories with twenty or more beds. Basic amenities were not only 'insufficient but they were often difficult to reach, badly distributed and of poor quality'.[113] In the worst examples,

> a few stained straw mattresses were being used ... fire-escapes were blocked by beds and one man slept in a bed on a landing. There were broken and dangerous floor boards, passageways surfaced with broken flagstones, and dormitories without any form of lighting ... cockroaches swarmed over the floors and earwigs over the bread ... washrooms, dining-rooms and W.C.s could only be reached across open yards ... A few dormitories – one with 74 beds – had been temporarily or permanently adapted from large, cold halls and chapels.[114]

The Ministry acknowledged that some former workhouse premises 'have shown little change since 1948' and that 'the vast majority ... however adapted ... can never provide a proper home for the elderly'.[115] Nonetheless, the large stock of former workhouse premises secured at least some care and security for a significant older population who otherwise had nowhere to go.

With the lack of a clear central policy, a number of authorities, including Norfolk (see Chapter 3), adopted a two-tier system for residential care arrangements. This involved new or adopted 'small' homes for less frail and well-behaved older people, and 'second-class' former workhouses for 'the chronic sick who need nursing and the anti-socials who have never lived in normal households ... [and] the hard core of low-grade people, the mentally defective and dirty people',[116] 'many [of whom] are satisfied with any cover for their head and are happier there. Even these places are better than some of them deserve'.[117] The use of former workhouses did not seem like an emergency measure, as reported in 1958:

> a few of the chief welfare officers ... planned to close a particular workhouse during the next three or four years ... but the majority said that ... [such] accommodation would be retained for 'at least ten years', 'at least twenty or thirty years' or for 'the foreseeable future'.[118]

Some authorities attempted to replace all existing workhouses as soon as possible and achieved this by the mid-1950s, among them Norwich (see Chapter 3), but they were the exception.

The problems of structural deficits in former workhouses and obsolete premises might be offset by the care offered, which ostensibly kept pace with rising statutory (minimum) guidelines. Significantly, any transition from a Poor Law workhouse to welfare service 'homely' residential homes meant that staff attitudes had to change. Although the Ministry emphasized the value of training courses, this was disappointingly slow to be introduced, and 70 per cent of matrons, wardens and superintendents still had no recognized qualification in 1956.[119] Although the 1959 Younghusband Report made important recommendations for social workers' training and deployment in fieldwork, references to the residential sector were brief and vague.[120] At the same time difficulties in recruiting and retaining residential staff because of poor working conditions were acknowledged.[121] Townsend's 1958 survey found that the ratio of residents to staff in former workhouses sometimes reached 17 to 1 during the day and 34 to 1 at night. Many staff were not 'imbued with the more progressive standards of personal care encouraged by the Ministry of Health', with some 'unsuitable, by any standards, for the tasks they performed ... with authoritarian attitudes ... who provoked resentment or even terror among infirm people'.[122] Overall, the workhouse mentality prevailed in the 1950s, reflected in the physical environment, the home ethos and the care provided by staff.

Expansion and Retrenchment, 1960–79

Spending caps on health and welfare projects were finally relaxed from 1959–60, and loan sanctions for residential homes then rose from £5.5 million in 1960–1 to £9 million in 1961–2, compared with a 1954–9 annual average of £4.2 million for health and welfare projects combined.[123] The 1962 Hospital Plan for England and Wales was presented as 'complementary to the expected development of the services for prevention and for care in the community'.[124] Local authorities were to review their services and prepare ten-year plans, including residential care provision for older people, with proposals from all local authorities summarized in 1963 as Health and Welfare: the Development of Community Care, which stated that 'their aim is to provide care in the community – at home, at centres, or, where necessary, in residential accommodation – for all who do not require the types of treatment and care which can be given only in hospitals'.[125] Here, residential care was defined as an alternative to long-stay geriatric hospitals or large, isolated institutions and a necessary last resort *beyond* community-based services. This was in contrast to the Hospital Plan, which simply defined 'care in the community' as all other alternative services *'outside* the hospitals' (my emphasis), thus regarding residential care as one community care option.[126]

The Community Care Plan envisaged 63,000 new residential places for older people by 1972 and the closure of all former workhouses 'within the next ten years'.[127] This was the first explicit official statement, but the Community Care Plan and its subsequent revisions offered no initiatives, specific service objectives or minimum standards based on assessment of the needs of older people. Local authorities were merely left to 'consider and revise their own intentions in the light of what others are doing' and 'the picture as a whole'.[128] Their proposals merely confirmed wide variations in existing and future policy and in local definitions of need.[129] According to some critics, 'the exercise appeared to deteriorate into an "average operation" both at the Ministry and local authority level', with each target 'simply an arbitrary number set a little ahead of the current average number of places in local authorities'.[130] But others saw this as 'a spur to doing something', setting national standards against which local authorities could be judged and stimulating overall provision.[131] Although loan sanctions for residential homes were maintained throughout the post-1964 Labour government's economy drive, revisions to the Community Care Plan were abandoned.

By 1970 there were nearly 100,000 local authority or local authority-supported residential places for older people in England, still short of the 133,000 places (20 per 1,000 of the over-65 population) envisaged in the Community Care Plan for 1972.[132] Some 13,000 places were in former workhouses or similar institutions, and joint-user arrangements were still in operation.[133] More than 40 per cent of 'small' home places were in reality in premises with more than fifty beds, testimony to the Ministry's quantitative-led and finance-first policies. The Hospital Plan limitations further disadvantaged frail or chronic sick older people: the net rise of 10,600 hospital beds for them in the 1960s compared unfavourably with the 50,000 increase of the 1950s.[134] This was significant given that underlying bed demand among the 75-plus, who used 'eight times more health and social service than the "normal equivalent adult"' and occupied roughly 80 per cent of residential places, had increased by nearly 50 per cent, compared to 11 per cent for the general population between 1951 and 1971.[135] There were also 40,000 self-funding older residents in voluntary and private residential and nursing homes by 1969.[136]

The aim to create a homely atmosphere was reaffirmed under new guidelines for 30–50-place smaller homes, offering more single and double rooms.[137] Former workhouses and larger premises were renovated, divided into 'units of more homely dimensions' or replaced by purpose-built homes.[138] Congenial groupings of residents were encouraged by the provision of 'small and numerous sitting-rooms', rather than the 'handsome main lounge'.[139] These guidelines remained unchanged, although the average beds per new home increased from twenty-seven before 1953 to forty-five by 1970.[140] The 1962–7 Williams inquiry concluded that increasing demand necessitated more money for extensive staff recruitment, training and enhanced working conditions to guarantee the amount and quality of care required.[141] By 1971 the Council for Training in Social Work was providing eight full-time one-year and fifty-two in-service training courses for residential staff.[142] The quality of care was thus slowly recognized, even if only in response to Townsend's *The Last Refuge* in 1962.

Townsend's primary concern – that all existing forms of residential care failed to provide a 'normal' living environment – demanded extensive changes to social policy.[143] Most old people entered residential homes not because they were frail or disabled, but as a result of poverty, homelessness or insufficient community-based services. If these issues were addressed, many might manage at home, leaving smaller numbers of 'sick' older people in fewer health-administered residential institutions. This contributed to a policy reorientation, reflected in the post-1962 reforms which were designed to support more frail or disabled older people at home. Thus amendments to the 1948 National Assistance Act enabled local authorities to provide a direct meals service; the 1968 Health Services and Public Health Act extended their powers to promote the welfare of older people and to provide mandatory home help services; and the 1970 Chronically Sick and Disabled Act confirmed the right of eligible older persons to apply for aids and adaptations.

Day care and short-stay services were also promoted. Similarly, subsidies for sheltered housing schemes were made available under the 1958 Local Government Act. Deficiencies in National Assistance income support and its low

uptake by older people were addressed under the revamped supplementary benefit system from 1966.[144] Potentially, statutory residential care provision for the
minority older population with no or little informal support had expanded into
'full community care', helping '*all* old people' in their own homes for as long as
possible.[145] Yet, 'the period from 1964–70 saw no great expansion of domiciliary
services.[146] Audrey Hunt's work, based on the 1967 government social survey, concluded that 'the home help service would need to be increased ... between two and
three times.[147] During the 1960s the number of sheltered housing units grew from
21,000 to almost 100,000, but Townsend's minimum target of fifty units per 1,000
elderly required some 400,000 by 1970.[148] David Thomson later drew attention
to the economic plight of older people, whose living standard 'falls further and
further behind that of the non-aged community': 'the declining true value of pensions ... is the cause of the rising numbers of the elderly in institutions.[149]

Such shortcomings partly reflected political and professional preoccupations
with residential care, encouraged by the availability of loans and the problem
of bed blocking in the NHS. Thus 'the homes have come to loom larger and
larger as things that are good in themselves rather than as practical solutions to
a pressing difficulty ... even if this means sacrifices in the community services.[150]
Indeed, despite revelations concerning the lack of opportunities for self-expres-
sion, absence of a homely atmosphere and a 'Literature of Dysfunction' focusing
more on 'what is wrong with institutions rather than how they can be well run',
residential care attracted a measure of 'complacency.[151] It was officially regarded
as an economic and humanitarian asset. For frail older persons, it was cheaper
than hospital or intensive domiciliary provision, which 'could not expand sufficiently ... without being so costly in manpower and finance as to be prohibitive',
while 'an employee in a residential home would be able to provide a similar service to a number of old people at the same time.[152] As for humanitarian grounds,
the 1967 Williams Report considered residential homes were homely places,
where the lonely could be brought to live out their lives in companionship and
friendship.[153] Similarly, the 1968 official survey claimed that:

> only three of over 500 residents interviewed complained about the staff. Indeed,
> many residents spontaneously remarked on the kindness and attention ... most resi-
> dents are quite content to be living in a home ... the gloomy picture of old people's
> homes ... is not supported by any evidence from this inquiry.[154]

Whether this illustrated 'the snare of gratitude' among undemanding older residents remained an open question.[155]

If such attitudes retarded the development of alternative services for older
people, their position on the policy agenda slipped further in relation to the
social priorities for post-1964 Labour governments. Earlier concerns over
alleged demographic crises and the burden of dependency associated with old
age and older people were now set on one side.[156]

The 1968 Seebohm Report heralded a major restructuring of local authority social services, with unified social services departments (SSDs) incorporating child and welfare services with some responsibilities for health, education and housing, to 'provide better services for those in need because it will ensure a more co-ordinated and comprehensive approach to the problems of individuals and families and the community in which they live'.[157] While D. V. Donnison saw this 'great State paper' as a springboard for action, for Townsend it was 'lacking in analysis, drive and vision and it gives an insufficient picture of the objectives that should be pursued'.[158] The Seebohm Report proposals featured in the 1970 Local Authority Social Services Act (effective from 1 April 1971), as new SSDs unified child, welfare and local health departments, bridging residential and community care provision for older people within generic 'personal social services' (PSS).

Measures under the 1973 National Health Service Reorganisation Act effectively meant that 'local health authority services were nationalized and brought under the same management as hospital services, while the administration of family practitioner services was aligned with the new authorities'.[159] The 1973 Act also stipulated that health and local authorities should collaborate and empowered each authority to make available to the other goods, services, staff and other facilities.[160] Accordingly, the new Area Health Authority boundaries were matched by those of local authorities responsible for PSS in the restructured system (operative from April 1974).

Initially, the Seebohm Report objectives seemed to be achieved. The PSS were seen 'as a distinctive innovation motivated by universalism', and the SSDs 'rapidly established themselves as much bigger actors on the local government scene than their predecessor departments'.[161] Whereas the 1960 equivalent of total PSS expenditure accounted for just 0.2 per cent of gross national product (GNP), this quadrupled to 0.8 per cent by 1974.[162] Between 1970 and 1974 total PSS expenditure (capital and current) grew on average almost 14 per cent annually, compared to 4 per cent in health, 3 per cent in social security and 5 per cent in overall social services spending.[163] Some 45 per cent of this was directed to older people, who benefited considerably from the expansion of both residential and community care.[164]

Assuming high employment rates and economic growth, post-Seebohm planning envisaged a 10 per cent growth rate on current account per annum by the early 1980s, reflected in the Local Authority Social Services Ten Year Development Plans for 1973–83. Guidelines specified twenty-five residential places, twelve home helps, 3–4 day centre places and 200 meals a week per 1,000 older population, for example.[165] Yet this was torpedoed by growing economic uncertainty. The Ten Year Development Plans were abandoned in 1974, and the 1976 white paper slashed capital expenditure and cut current annual PSS spending growth to a mere 2 per cent, ostensibly allowing for demographic change and other pressures.[166]

In response, PSS planning switched to 'needs-scarcity' based on priority.[167] Limited resources were reallocated to client groups and services considered most in need according to cost-effective criteria. Older people, the mentally ill and disabled, and children and families were recognized as priority groups, with community-based services promoted as a low-cost alternative to institutional arrangements. Joint planning measures between health and local authorities were reinforced by a combined financing programme in 1977, under which local authority SSDs were temporarily allowed to receive Area Health Authority funding to enable more old people to leave long-stay hospitals and so reduce reliance on hospital-based services.[168]

While annual PSS current expenditure grew on average over 2 per cent during 1974/5–1978/9, annual net capital spending fell by more than a third.[169] Older people fared badly among the priority groups, and the estimated shortfall of 46,000 residential places by 1979 represented almost 40 per cent of the current 117,000 local authority or local authority-supported places.[170] Aggregate places actually fell that year to 17.7 per 1,000 older population, well below the official 25 per 1,000 guideline.[171] In 1975 'about 100–150 homes were closed or left unoccupied as a result of financial stringency'.[172] The thirty-year workhouse closure programme was also incomplete, with 'perhaps seven thousand places still in use in old workhouses', leaving the association of residential care with the humiliation of the workhouse.[173]

In contrast, voluntary and private sector residential home places for self-funding residents increased by 25 per cent (to over 50,000) during the decade to 1979.[174] With a further 15,000 local authority-supported voluntary sector places, the non-public sector now accounted for 40 per cent of all places. Thus a mixed economy in provision was in place, and the 7,000 former workhouse places represented just 4 per cent of the total number of places.

As for the community care orientation, the proportion of older people receiving home help services doubled to 8.7 per cent between 1962 and 1976.[175] Yet the proportion of home help recipients with high care needs was static at roughly 20 per cent of the total in this period, suggesting that the service was more thinly spread and posing the question whether it could ever replace residential care or enable those with high care needs to continue living independently. One alternative was sheltered housing, with over 300,000 units provided by the early 1980s compared to below 100,000 units a decade earlier.[176] Yet 'sheltered housing predominantly satisfied *housing* need' rather than social or physical need, providing for some who might 'live perfectly adequately in ordinary housing' and, in that sense, offering 'too much for too few'.[177] Thus a Leeds study in 1979 revealed 'how alike Sheltered Housing tenants are to the rest of the elderly living at home', in contrast to Part III residents with greater dependency.[178] Their distribution varied widely, from just one to 278 units per 1,000 older population, with no guarantee of greatest needs taking priority.[179] As a result, 250,000 retired people remained on council waiting lists for sheltered accommodation in 1979.[180]

Community care had been affirmed since the 1950s, but its meaning fluctuated. A social care services focus led to reduced dependence on residential provision by expanding community care, but joint health and social care services implied expansion of community care *and* the maintenance of residential provision, as 'care and treatment *outside* the hospitals' (my emphasis) in the 1962 Hospital Plan confirmed.[181] Further, new concepts of 'care *by* the community' had emerged by the late 1970s.[182] All this compounds the difficulties of interpreting and evaluating the data, although residential care must be understood within the changing objectives of community care policy, rather than in isolation.

Nonetheless, the principal arguments in the late 1970s still focused on 'spending far more on keeping residents in homes than ... in the community ... and finding the resources for doing so by cutting down on the community services'.[183] This was the outcome of the need to manage the revenue effects of the earlier capital programme within tighter revenue budgets, which was not only more expensive but also contradicted the community-led policy. Tight budgets also threatened the quality of care: increases in residential care in 1976–9 spending lagged behind rising unit costs.[184] Overall, services for older people during the late 1970s showed reduced growth and an insignificant shift from residential to community care. This may have been the inevitable result of the number of older people as a client group, as the PSS total expenditure had roughly doubled to 1.1 per cent of gross domestic product (GDP) over the 1970s, with older people consuming 45 per cent of that.[185] Yet the needs of all frail older persons were still unmet. To make matters worse, Labour's expansionist PSS plans for the 1980s were halted by post-1979 Conservative governments.

Privatization and 'Unplanned' Expansion in the 1980s

The Conservative government sought to reorient welfare policy on the premise that the individual's needs should be met by the family and the free market, working '*with the grain* of human nature, helping people to help themselves – and others'.[186] The 1981 white paper *Growing Older* argued that 'the primary sources of support and care for elderly people are informal and voluntary'. This should be understood against a commitment to reduce state involvement and public expenditure, not least on the welfare programmes, which accounted for 40 per cent of the total in 1979–80.[187] Despite this, overall welfare expenditure actually increased by 11 per cent in real terms from 1979–80 to 1984–5, with spending on 'social security' and 'health and PSS' rising by 28 per cent and 17 per cent respectively.[188] These paradoxical outcomes need to be explained.

From the late 1970s direct state social security funding, in the form of supplementary benefit (later income support), was used to support older residents
in voluntary and private residential and nursing homes, subject to their financial
assets. In 1980 the policy was formalized with higher benefit limits; consequently, annual supplementary benefit expenditure soared from £10 million for
11,000 claimants to £2,400 million for 253,000 during 1979–91.[189] 'In no other
area has public sector spending escalated so dramatically'.[190] Tighter controls
squeezed local authority budgets to support residents in voluntary sector accommodation, the number assisted in England in this way falling to just 3,000 (2 per
cent of the total) by 1990.[191] In contrast, 63 per cent of residents in private and
voluntary sector homes were funded by supplementary benefit in 1991.[192] Thus
'public expenditure had been re-routed away from direct provision to private
sector providers through the social security budget [supplementary benefit]'.[193]
The typology of the home for older people also changed as the number of private
and voluntary sector residential and nursing home places almost doubled to 86.6
per cent of the total (just under 460,000) by 1997, compared to 44.3 per cent in
1980. At the same time local authority home places almost halved to 71,000.[194]

What drove this state-fuelled expansion? It is tempting to assume ideological
motives, with state funding *deliberately* routed to favour private sector homes.
But while the government sought to reduce local authority funding on care
provision, Ray Robinson argued that 'the pursuit of specific policy objectives
has led to the *unplanned* expansion of substitute programmes' (my emphasis).[195]
Roy Parker too saw private sector growth as 'incidental'.[196] Unlike cash-strapped
local authority funding, the supplementary benefit budget was not cash-limited
and required little or no assessment of applicants' care needs. Its availability for
the costs of residential and nursing home provision, but not of services for people living in their own homes, 'perversely' encouraged residential rather than
community care, according to the 1986 Audit Commission Report, *Making a
Reality of Community Care*.[197] The 1987 Firth and 1988 Griffiths Reports proposed revisions, endorsed in the 1989 white paper *Caring for People* and the
1990 National Health Service and Community Care Act (effective from April
1993). By then there was an '*over*-supply' of residential accommodation:

> Over the decade 1979–1989 the numbers of beds in the private residential sector
> trebled, to 31.1 places per 1000 people over 65. Yet it is estimated that only 11 places
> ... are required to support severely disabled older people ... as much as one-half, do
> not need to occupy residential places on the basis of disability.[198]

This is questionable, as other studies suggested that only a sixth of newer residents in private sector homes might cope at home, even with community-based
services.[199] The latter expansions were limited by rate-capped and squeezed local
authority expenditure on the PSS for older people, with only a 1.8 per cent real

term annual increase on average during the 1980s.[200] Community care and day care provision for very old people even declined during this period, as did net additions of local authority-subsidized sheltered housing units.[201] Compounding this was the increase in the ageing population: perhaps a quarter more older people were in long-term care establishments in 1992 than would have been the case if age-specific rates had remained unchanged during the 1980s, but the number of the 85-plus increased by 56 per cent and of the 75-plus by 24 per cent in this period.[202] More important were continuing NHS hospital bed closures, which particularly affected older patients. In 1981 there were 352,000 hospital beds, in 1991 255,000, while the average geriatric hospital patient stay was reduced from seventy-eight to forty-five days in 1979–86.[203] Consequently, many older patients had to be discharged, and typically a private residential (or care) home or a nursing home was the only option. This is important, since the surge in private sector homes from about 1980 involved a relocation of many discharged patients, as well as new applicants from their own homes.

Whether for ideological or personal reasons, more relatives of older people chose private sector homes for them. These were mostly run as small family businesses, unlike the large local authority 'institutions'. Their portrayal of 'family values' and a 'family atmosphere' may have eased the guilt of those placing older relatives in these homes, and the 'private' home retained some status, even if it did rely on state funding.[204] In this context, the unprecedented growth of private sector homes during the 1980s and early 1990s was not simply a matter of oversupply, but reflected shortfalls or restrictions on the alternatives, continued and increasing socio-demographic demand, and public perceptions linking local authority care homes with institutions, stigma and even the workhouse.

Conservative politicians claimed that free market principles enhanced choice and self-determination.[205] But there was little evidence to support this, with studies suggesting that 'the actual choices of residents, both public and private, were very limited'.[206] Restrictions included their physical or mental state; lack of time, mobility or energy to investigate the options; shortage of money; the patchy distribution of suitable homes; and waiting lists. Less predictably, there were few listings or guides to private homes, and many did not supply brochures describing their facilities. Contract arrangements dealt primarily with restrictions on residents, suggesting little choice here.[207] Moreover, private proprietors often turned away difficult, confused, very frail, aggressive or obese clients. An emerging two-tier system favoured 'the younger, fitter and wealthier elderly', whereas 'the growing numbers of severely disabled elderly people with multiple problems', dependent on public funding, had very little choice.[208]

Competition within the private sector and with the public sector, it was claimed, added to proprietors' incentives to make their homes more efficient and better value than their public equivalents. Simultaneously, consumer demand ostensibly drove client-led services and improved the quality of care for older residents. In practice, private sector homes were unevenly provided, and in 'areas where demand is so buoyant ... little competition exists'.[209] Yet larger companies acted as cartels, undercutting smaller, family-run rivals or raising prices, and financial incentives operated less effectively where proprietors themselves depended on the state funding given to eligible older residents.[210] Above all, the relationship between cost-effectiveness and quality was debatable: fewer staff, untrained or unqualified labour, inadequate equipment and lower maintenance costs represented savings to the home, but at what cost to the residents? As the average life of a private care home was three years, with bankruptcies running at 10 per cent, the homes were sometimes bought and sold without reference to the residents, while facilities or individual living arrangements were revised without consultation.[211] Market mechanism benefits were questionable or even 'against the interests of consumers'.[212]

Growing concern resulted in the 1984 Registered Homes Act and associated Codes of Practice, *Home Life*, for private residential homes; and the National Association of Health Authorities Guidelines for private nursing homes.[213] The new legislation aimed to ensure that 'required physical standard amenities are being provided ... the proprietor has no criminal record ... [and] to improve the quality of care'.[214] It also extended its coverage to small private homes, those with four or fewer residents, which previously had been exempted. *Home Life* asserted that:

> those who live in residential care should do so with dignity; that they should have the respect of those who support them; should live with no reduction of their rights as citizens ... as full and active a life as their physical and mental condition will allow.[215]

Unlike the 1984 Act, *Home Life* was not legally binding, merely officially endorsed, suggesting considerable ambiguity about the minimum level of care envisaged.[216] Local registration authorities and newly created tribunals were left to interpret and enforce standards of care in their area's private sector homes. The outcome was varied minimum borderlines, with some transgressors escaping deregulation or prosecution.[217] Local registration authorities were to scrutinize applications, conduct annual inspections, and suggest training or remedial measures where necessary, but this incurred direct costs on local authorities and so undermined their own services. The result was reluctance and even resentment.[218]

Meanwhile, cases of mistreatment and abuse of older residents in private sector homes were coming to light. *The Realities of Home Life*, an investigation into fourteen Birmingham private homes in 1987, exposed evidence of regimentation, dangerous medical practices, mistreatment, understaffing and low pay.[219] *Cold Comfort* similarly highlighted exorbitant charges and underspending on essentials in private homes.[220] Investigative journalism highlighted extensive abuse.[221] A television documentary, *The Granny Business*, showed neglect, filth and indignity in Kent's private homes, one reviewer deploring 'forgotten ones, left to rot ... defenceless old people don't have the legal protection against abuse or neglect'.[222]

Although the Opposition in parliamentary debates concentrated on private sector scandals, there were examples of abuse in local authority homes too.[223] An independent review of Camden's local authority homes, for example, revealed 'the persistence of workhouse conditions in a welfare society'.[224] Even more worryingly, 'if the same kind of independent investigation of the residential services were undertaken in Anywhereshire it would produce a broadly similar and equally depressing litany of criticisms'.[225] It called for a legal framework for local authority homes to be established under the 1990 NHS and Community Care Act. Yet contrary to public perceptions, the 1988 Wagner Report asserted that 'people who move into a residential establishment should do so by *positive* choice' (my emphasis) among various good quality alternatives, including intensive community care services, housing provision and availability of all sector residential provision.[226]

Reforms and a Tiered Care Market since the 1990s

Reforms under the 1989 *Caring for People* and the 1990 NHS and Community Care Act sought to 'stop the haemorrhage in the social security budgets' on private sector residential care by removing perverse incentives and boosting community care in line with individual need and enhanced choice.[227] Responsibility for funding devolved from central government to local authorities, which were also required to assess applicants' needs and financial eligibility. The new funding comprised a special transition grant and normal block grants attributable to the PSS. Each special transition grant was reserved solely for residential and community care services, but 85 per cent had to be spent in the private or voluntary sector. Such needs-led and collective features might favour community care, but the 85 per cent rule had the effect of forcing local authorities to continue spending more on residential care, because private sector community care provision was still in its infancy. It also limited investment in local authority residential and community care. Moreover, residents in private or voluntary sector homes were offered more state funding via a means-tested Department of Social Security Residential Care Allowance, paid as part of income support, but not those living in local authority homes or in their own homes, which discouraged *non*-residential care, even when this was preferred by older people and was less expensive.

The normal block grants for the PSS, excluding the special transition grant, actually fell by 5 per cent in real terms during 1992/3–1995/6, producing a 'quite horrendous' situation, in which the 'hardest hit were elderly people'.[228] These funding constraints froze local authority baseline residential fee rates for eligible claimants, thereby restricting their access to expensive (private) homes.

This in turn affected many care and nursing homes, since 72.5 per cent of their residents had their fees paid in full or in part by local authorities and/or the NHS in 1997.[229] This partly explains the decline in the total number of care and nursing home places across all sectors, with an annual average net reduction of 10,600 during 1997–2003 following the 1997 peak of 528,600, like long-stay geriatric and psycho-geriatric hospital beds halving to just 23,200 during 1995–2003.[230] As a result, more residents faced being transferred or a change of environment and fewer choices, particularly of nursing homes for mentally ill older people.[231] Many were left in inadequate facilities, for perhaps half of those in care homes required nursing home or hospital care, while a quarter of nursing home residents needed hospital care.[232]

Rationing and even withdrawal of services for older people in their own homes also occurred. Home help contract hours increased by 76 per cent during 1992–2002, even though the total number of recipients fell by 27 per cent, suggesting that fewer of the most dependent clients were helped by more intensive services.[233] Yet even if 'scarce resources are targeted more effectively than hitherto', the majority deemed at lower risk were left vulnerable or unsupported, while the increasing and inappropriate discharge of older patients from NHS hospitals arguably represented a 'form of abuse'.[234] Increasingly, notions of rights or choice were undermined by rationing and charges, as local authorities struggled to stay within their budget.[235] Yet replacing individual entitlement to open-ended state funding by local authority decision-making within capped budgets was applauded by some, as it curbed spending on care provision.[236]

Post-1997 Labour governments also endorsed the mixed economy of care and encouraged the non-public sector: 'it is no longer who provides the social care that matters. It is the quality of care that counts'.[237] By 2008, 92.1 per cent of care and nursing home places were in the voluntary and private sectors, and 39 per cent of all residents were self-funding, up from 27.5 per cent in 1996.[238] Individual fee contributions amounted to £3.28 billion in 2006, over half the total care home costs.[239]

The quality of residential care may have improved: in 2008, 88 per cent of private sector home places were in single rooms and 15 per cent of for-profit nursing home places were premium priced, with weekly fees exceeding £800, compared to the UK average of £675.[240] In contrast, 12 per cent (41,000 or more) of residents in for-profit homes were in shared bedrooms, with the average weekly charges of £578 for a nursing home and £415 for a care home.[241] Self-paying residents are sometimes charged £50–100 more than publicly funded residents, so that they are in effect subsidizing the latter, with perhaps one in five homes adopting this approach.[242] (One local example disclosed £785 weekly care home fees for self-payers compared to £566 for the publicly funded in part or in full in 2006.[243])

The introduction of the national minimum wage in 1999 further affected many private sector home providers, as their profitability depended on keeping costs down. This was compounded by an increase of the minimum paid holiday entitlement from twenty days to twenty-eight from 2009.[244] Those forced out of business were replaced by major for-profit providers who could benefit from economies of scale: the average newly registered for-profit nursing home in 2008 had forty-seven beds, compared with twenty-six in 1987.[245]

Within England's welfare pluralism, a two-tier market of residential care has emerged, polarizing around exclusive care with extra costs for the better-off at one end and minimal measures for many dependent on squeezed public funding or with straitened means at the other. The gap between the two is widening, with many of the (mainly female) poor, old and vulnerable suffering the legacy and stigma of the workhouse. Essentially, the lower-end homes 'become second class and those who use them and work in them feel second-class citizens'.[246] Disputes over blurred boundaries between free health care and means-tested social care remain unresolved, provoking 'a groundswell of public disquiet'.[247] Efforts to reduce discharges from NHS long-stay beds have shifted the responsibility for nursing care to local authorities. This has resulted in some older people having 'to sell their homes to pay for the [nursing] care, which had once been provided free'.[248] This effectively penalizes older people, who have to sell their possessions to pay for their care costs, thereby breaking the 1948 social contract. Worse still, self-funders are seemingly unprotected in the care system. The publicly funded have care managers to make the arrangements and provide an overview; they also have resort, if necessary, to the local authority complaints procedure.[249]

To address the lack of a regulatory framework for local authority homes, an independent local authority inspectorate with powers to protect and enforce the rights of residents in both local authority and private homes was established, alongside complaints procedures under the 1990 Act.[250] An updated Code of Practice, *A Better Home Life*, published in 1996, acknowledged the special needs of dementia sufferers and extended coverage to more long-term care facilities for older people provided by the NHS, local authorities and voluntary and private sectors.[251] The 2000 Care Standards Act, which replaced the 1984 Registered Homes Act, introduced new national minimum standards and the Care Homes Regulations 2001, which set out the all single-bedroom criterion for all new homes.[252] Accordingly, the National Care Standards Commission was established to regulate and inspect all adult residential and community care services in England. This was replaced by the Commission for Social Care Inspection the following year. In 2009 this was merged with two other regulatory bodies, the Healthcare Commission and the Mental Health Act Commission, to form the Care Quality Commission (CQC), a 'super-regulator' which took full responsibility for health and social care in England.[253] Care Trusts, established under the 2001 Health and Social Care Act, combine the powers of NHS primary care trusts and local authority SSDs to commission and be responsible for both health and social care, in an attempt to overcome divisions here.

Attempts to challenge the post-1948 means-tested and targeted care system were made by the 1999 Sutherland Commission, which recommended free and comprehensive care, but the government rejected this. Nevertheless, free personal and nursing care became available in Scotland from 2002, although domestic help and 'hotel' costs still have to be met by residents, subject to their financial means and exceeding half the total residential care fees.[254] The 2006 Wanless Report on funding for long-term social care recommended a universal entitlement based on need through a 'partnership model', the state funding a minimum level of care with co-financing to top up service users to a benchmark care level.[255] If implemented, this model would allow 450,000 more people in England to access social care. In 2006 that figure was one million.[256] The Wanless Report fed into the white paper *Building the National Care Service* in 2010 and the Dilnot Commission Report on Funding of Care and Support in 2011.[257] The latter recommended the capping of lifetime individual contributions to their social care costs (currently unlimited) at £35,000 and an increased £100,000 means-tested threshold (currently £23,250), above which people are liable for their full care costs. This would address unfair and potentially catastrophic care costs imposed on better-off older people, but would cost the state an additional £4.2 billion by 2025, a challenge which any implementation of the 2012 Social Care white paper will have to acknowledge.[258] Meanwhile the family has increasingly become the central pillar of care provision, saving the government an estimated £119 billion a year.[259]

Aspirations to empower all older people seeking social care have to be placed in the context of the projected doubling of the 85-plus population and 1.7 million more adults needing care by 2026.[260] Government commitment to provide universal, seamless and good quality care for all those in need will have to be assessed, with the cost of such care expected to rise from £14.6 billion (1.16 per cent of GDP) in 2010–11 to £31 billion (2 per cent) by 2025–6 if the reforms currently proposed are implemented, and to £23 billion if they are not.[261]

2 THE JAPANESE CONTEXT

This chapter reviews the development of Japan's residential care for older people, focusing on statutory residential provision under the 1929 Poor Law and post-war welfare arrangements. Alternatives and complementary care and the legacy and stigma associated with *obasuteyama* (granny-dump mountain) are also discussed.

Obasuteyama

In Japan institutional care can be traced to the late sixth century, when the aged, destitute and frail, without a family to care for them, were placed in poorhouses along with the sick, disabled, vagrants and orphans.[1] These were charitable facilities provided by the emperor, monks and philanthropists, inspired by Buddhism or Confucianism.[2] There were, however, very few, and specialized institutions did not appear until the 1870s.[3] The first charitable small almshouse exclusively for older people opened in 1895, but there was no official involvement in indoor (institutional) relief before the 1929 Poor Law.

As a result, the institutionalization of older people in Japan is less associated with Poor Law institutions than with *obasuteyama*, by which eldest sons left aged parents who had outlived their usefulness to die of starvation and exposure. While this suggests a lack of filial respect and family neglect, for older people '*obasuteyama* is a symbolic metaphor representing the pathos and unfulfilled expectations of their later years ... a harsh reality encapsulated and objectified by its transformation into a symbol of suffering and sacrifice'.[4] Elderly 'residents refer to the story to express their sense of shame, isolation, and abandonment ... they have been denied their rightful place among [the] family but ... others view them as objects of pity or scorn'.[5] Japanese literature and folklore have fostered the image in the public imagination, and it was confirmed by Shichiro Fukazawa's 1957 novel *Ballad of Oak Mountain*.[6]

Industrialization and modernization have undermined the Confucian ethic of filial piety and extended family living arrangements. Increasing longevity, the migration of young people to the cities, regional economic hardship and more women entering the workforce have all limited family care for older relatives. Nevertheless, 'Japanese families still feel obliged to provide welfare for their immediate members', obligations affirmed in the 1950 National Assistance Act, which made state support supplementary to family care.[7] Thus 'institutionalization ... highlights the disjuncture between the cultural norm of filial piety (and its expression in the ideal of co-residence) and a changing social reality'.[8]

Charitable Provision and Limited Poor Law Relief, 1868–1932

Throughout the nineteenth century, most needy older people were supported by their family, neighbours or the local community.[9] Confucian precepts demanded filial piety, honour and assistance for older people in general and for parents in particular. This was underlined in the Imperial Message on Education in 1889 and inscribed in law, notably under the Meiji Civil Code of 1898. The traditional *ie* (patriarchal family) system featured the eldest son, who was responsible for his aged parents, who would generally be cared for by his wife and other members of the extended family. In return, they would inherit the family's entire estate.[10] Although this was formally abolished under post-1945 constitutional reforms, 'surprisingly, this system has survived in some families of rural communities in contemporary Japan'.[11]

Following the 1868 Meiji Restoration, Japan emerged as an industrial nation under the slogan 'Enrich the Country and Strengthen the Military'.[12] By this date some Western nations were beginning to acknowledge concepts of citizenship and welfare, with limited state intervention and varying emphases on free competition and the role of the individual.[13] With gradual acknowledgement that people needed to be protected from exploitation, harsh working conditions, poverty wages and insecure employment, notions of state welfare developed. Although such social ideologies might seem paradoxical or even antagonistic, *laissez-faire* states intervened on behalf of the poor.

Japan's economy and culture were different, notably the 'partial rejection of the concept of *laissez-faire*', with initiatives concerning industrialization and its associated social problems.[14] Japan had a highly centralized, authoritarian and paternalistic government, emphasizing family-based nationalism centred on worship of the emperor as a living deity, with little state concern for needy individuals. An 'Emperor-first and absolute ideology' regarded 'all of Japanese society as a great family, stretching from the father figure Emperor at the top to the individual family below, weaving around all individuals a strong and unlimited sense of obligation to all above them'.[15] Traditional values were reinforced under 'supremacy of custom' and 'submission to authority'.[16] The family was deemed to be primarily responsible for the care of its needy members, while the state assumed no overall responsibility for social security and 'even boasted the absence of poor laws'.[17]

Nonetheless, the state might protect 'its children – the Japanese people' by offering aid on the basis of mercy, charity or a strong moral duty, but not from any welfare mentality.[18] From 1874 Japan's first poor relief legislation offered minimal outdoor relief to the needy aged 70 or over without family, alongside orphans and the severely disabled.[19] This represented at best 'discretionary and charitable assistance'. It was ostensibly 'mutual care and support, driven by compassion', but it deterred individuals from seeking relief and associated this with shame and stigma.[20] The legislation was more draconian than the English 1834 Poor Law, and the number of Japan's relief recipients remained nugatory – a mere 1,200 people in 1877 and 3,800 in 1909.[21] Meanwhile, perhaps 21 million people (nearly 60 per cent of the total population) struggled at or below the relief level in 1883.[22] Among those aged 70 or over, 16,000 were considered destitute in 1909, but just 1,021 were given outdoor relief, roughly the same as recorded suicides in that age group.[23] The relief was tightened further, with a mere 362 recipients aged 70 or over in 1918, and the relief level remained very low, usually based on the cost of a small quantity of rice for a limited period to prevent death from starvation. It was even less than the allowance given to prisoners.[24] Indoor relief was not provided until the 1929 Poor Law (effective from 1932). This left charitable organizations and concerned individuals to fill the gap.

In 1895 the first charitable 'old people's almshouse' was opened in Tokyo. This 'marked the beginning of charitable initiatives exclusively for older people'.[25] Indeed, these almshouses were significant in recognizing for the first time that the problems of old age and older people required specialist provision distinct from other groups. They would later raise standards and treatment in the old people's almshouse.[26] By 1911 sixteen charitable old people's almshouses had opened, caring for up to 430 residents, though this paled beside the 1.47 million over-70s by 1908.[27] This may be explained because 'with a strong sense of mutual support, there would be no need for the old people's almshouse and hence, no admissions, even if one builds a modest one'.[28] While a small minority did require some form of institutional care, 'because they associated the old people's almshouse with a grim waiting place for death and with failure and shame, most would have avoided entering it at all costs, while others even said they would rather die'.[29] Precisely because of this, old people's almshouses found that 'begging a small donation, even a handful of rice is extremely demanding'.[30] The founder of Osaka Yoroin, an old people's almshouse opened in 1902, recorded that 'In the first six years, there were no donations so I had to use all my private moneys to buy essentials for my residents. But as the resident number increased to 150, the problem loomed as my money was not enough'.[31]

In 1923, when the country was experiencing harsh economic conditions and social unrest, Japan suffered the Kanto earthquake. Severe famines ensued, compounded by the Great Depression, which led to soaring unemployment and widespread poverty. People who regarded themselves as hardworking then began to perceive poverty not in terms of beggars and the destitute, but recognized that 'the circumstances of the needy could not be regarded as just personal and family problems'.[32] To compensate for the lack of public relief institutions, from 1908 the government offered small grants to officially recognized, 'good' charitable facilities, including charitable old people's almshouses, the funding coming from government general budgets and the emperor. Local authorities soon adopted the practice.

In 1927, thanks to a large donation from the emperor, the first public old people's almshouse, Rakufuen, housing up to 500 people, opened in Tokyo, initially for earthquake victims. The main building, of 'super-modern appearance', included an infirmary with four twenty-five-bedded sick wards with a staff of thirty doctors and sixteen nurses, and a 'house' block consisting of 6–10-bedded dormitories and small rooms for couples and families.[33] On admission, all had health check-ups before being allocated to an appropriate accommodation block. Rakufuen thus reflected new standards of care and commitment to the vulnerable aged.

This contrasted with the first public 'mixed' poorhouse, Tokyo Borough Poorhouse, established in a rundown terraced house in 1872, 'to hide the shame of the capital prior to the imperial visit of Russia'.[34] An official 'vagrant hunt' found 240 beggars and vagrants of all ages, including nine aged over 65, increasing to 1,000 people by 1880.[35] Despite overcrowded and substandard conditions, no replacement facility was built until 1896 and official aid was withdrawn, since 'Borough-funded indoor relief would increase the idle citizenry and thus be a waste of money'.[36] Thus up to 133 people of all ages and conditions were squeezed into one large dormitory, classified only by sex.[37] Accommodation blocks exclusively for the aged were added, but continuing mixed arrangements were aggravated by more admissions and overcrowding. Given that its principal objective was to maintain social order, there were strict controls which resulted in frequent absconding.

Beginnings: The Poor Law Institution, 1932–45

With poverty and related social unrest increasing, the government introduced the 1929 Poor Law (enacted in 1932). Eligibility criteria were relaxed by lowering the age limit for relief from 70 to 65 years and for the first time including indoor relief. However, its implementation had to wait three years due to financial restraints, and the government made use of charitable facilities rather than building its own institutions, by authorizing these as 'publicly sanctioned Poor Law institutions', which entitled them to receive indoor relief for eligible residents (the 'indolent' or 'morally delinquent' were excluded, as were the able-bodied and those with families). Relief recipients were disenfranchised and had no right of application or appeal.[38] Relief levels barely improved. Nonetheless, the number of recipients increased over ten-fold, peaking at 237,000 in 1937.[39] Of these, some 85 per cent were given outdoor relief. Nearly a quarter of recipients were aged 65 or more, with 49,000 on outdoor relief and 5,000 on indoor relief in 1937.[40] Relief was given to only 41 per cent of older people who needed it, according to an official 1935 survey.[41]

By 1940 the 101 charitable and thirty public old people's almshouses had 4,600 residents, and Takiko Okamoto has suggested that regular Poor Law resources contributed to them being more systematically developed.[42] Yet the new resources were offset by smaller municipal subsidies and fewer charitable donations and membership fees. Thus central funding was counterproductive, since 'the consequent reduction of charity and local subsidies made the financial situation even worse'.[43] Many charitable old people's almshouses became publicly sanctioned Poor Law institutions under the 1929 Poor Law and received between 3 and 55 per cent of their revenues from state indoor relief by 1942, but most continued to accommodate large numbers of older residents ineligible for this sort of relief.[44]

In most charitable old people's almshouses, the diet consisted of only rice, soup and vegetables. Unpaid work by residents and their helping each other and the staff were also expected. The manager of the Beppu old people's almshouse in southern Japan recalled poor hygiene there during the 1930s: 'the sick and frail elderly were covered by ... lice and suffered appalling pain, unable to sleep at all. It seemed like these nearly killed them'.[45] Conditions in Japan's oldest and now biggest public mixed poorhouse, Tokyo Borough Poorhouse, were no better. One visiting officer considered 'a ratio of 56 inmates per room' as 'fairly spacious' in 1938, which suggested massive overcrowding.[46] High mortality also featured: 36 per cent of the 4,700 old people's almshouse residents in 1936 were categorized as 'able-bodied', but two-thirds of the rest died within six months of admission.[47]

Although Japan's charitable almshouses were often patronizing and traditionalist, according to Ogasawara many were founded by individuals sensitive to social problems and committed to meeting local need. They were humane and responsive to individuals' needs, rather than profit-focused or managerial in approach.[48] Accordingly, they looked beyond formal eligibility criteria and were more flexible and swift in making arrangements. Dedicated, often unpaid staff worked with older residents to maintain the almshouse and look after each other, and the communal living areas created domestic if regulated living units of typically 10–20 people, similar to a large extended Japanese household. Together they collected membership fees and donations and organized fund-raising events. Pre-war charitable old people's almshouses might be sociable, small facilities in adversity, featuring homely care and flexibility in meeting a variety of needs – precisely the successive post-war governments' policy objectives for residential care for older people. Ogasawara concluded that 'although pre-war old people's almshouses have attracted very little attention, and thereby been underestimated, one can learn no less from them'.[49] This, however, turned a blind eye to the stigma associated with the institutionalization of older people.

Parallel efforts to develop philanthropy followed the foundation in 1908 of the Central Charity Association, influenced by the English Charity Organisation Society (COS) created in 1869.[50] In the same vein, the first meeting of the National Association of Charitable Work for the Elderly in 1925 initiated the 'modernization of charitable initiatives for the elderly'.[51] Forty-two people from twenty-three old people's almshouses attended. The National Association of Elderly Institutions was established in 1932. It promoted residential care through regular meetings, staff training, publications, research and national surveys.[52] By then, a support system of elected, unpaid area commissioners had been instigated by the Osaka City municipal authority to identify and assist needy people in their own homes.[53] Other localities later adopted this system.

However, charitable initiatives and efforts were undermined in 1937 by the outbreak of the Sino-Japanese War, followed by the Second World War. They were then integrated into the war regime under the Ministry of Health, which was established in 1938 'to strengthen the nation's force and enhance its welfare', though the former objective took priority.[54] Under the 1938 Social Services Charities Act, the state exercised greater power over non-public social services organizations, ostensibly by offering small grants, seeking 'to incorporate charitable initiatives into the war regime, in which military forces and the full participation of the Japanese were emphasized'.[55] As the Second World War intensified, money was diverted from social welfare: the number receiving poor relief in 1942 was just 54 per cent of the 1937 total (237,000) – less than 0.1 per cent of national expenditure.[56]

Residents in old people's almshouses were badly affected. An official recalled that 'the Ministry of Health ... obviously placed a prime priority on winning the war ... the principle was that burdens on the nation should get only any unused resources'.[57] Starvation threatened, as food was strictly rationed and supplies were scarce: the manager of the Chiba old people's almshouse was concerned that his residents 'go out more often, probably because of lack of food in the almshouse, and some become sick since they eat whatever they can get, even mouldy stuff'.[58] Those barely able to work were forced to labour on the land or were given extra duties, with every open space utilized to grow sweet potatoes and vegetables, while all material and equipment that could be used as military supplies were removed. Air raids destroyed a quarter of all old people's almshouses, leaving just 102 with roughly 3,000 residents in 1945, one-third down on the 1940–1 averages.[59] Those evacuated to rural districts fared little better: half the 700 elderly evacuees from Tokyo Borough Poorhouse died of starvation.[60] In the words of a military officer:

> Only 900 mobile inpatients can be evacuated and, at the safe places, they are to engage in farming and stock farming ... there is no point to evacuating frail inpatients in Matsuzawa Mental Hospital ... Just bomb the hospital and kill the patients and then disguise this deliberate bombing as an accident.[61]

Overall, old people's almshouse mortality rates ranged from 40 to 60 per cent in the closing years of the war.[62]

Four Acts attempted to compensate for inadequate poor relief and wartime turmoil by providing more generous benefits, mainly for the military and their families.[63] Various local and regional social policy efforts also sought to help employees. The 1922 Health Insurance Act introduced national health insurance for employees of large firms. The 1938 National Health Insurance Act extended cover to the self-employed and agricultural workers, while the 1931 Industrial Injury Assistance Act provided limited and specific coverage for previously unemployed casual labourers working mainly on construction sites. By 1943 almost two-thirds of the population had health insurance cover.[64] A retirement pension scheme was introduced in 1941 in mining, manufacturing and other industries vital to the war effort. This was extended in 1944, although there was no unemployment insurance system until 1947.

Yet these insurance schemes were not comprehensive; they focused on 'improving people's health for long battles in the war', but neglected poor and frail older people.[65] Similarly, the pension scheme sought 'to finance the huge military expenses needed to continue the war' by raising insurance contributions.[66] Meanwhile, poor and frail older people without relatives to support them were restricted to outdoor relief and occasionally indoor relief under the 1929 Poor Law, subject to municipal discretion and any charitable aid, and outside stigma-free health and pension schemes operating in parallel to the 1929 Poor Law.

Thus claims that 'state welfare in Japan ... began to develop in the years between the two World Wars' can be supported only by ignoring the durability of the 1929 Poor Law and its strong underlying family-based nationalism.[67] In other words, the social reforms aimed 'to maintain and reproduce the health and physical strength of a military force' by focusing on employees essential to the war effort and economic growth.[68] In contrast, the rudimentary Poor Law targeted residual or unproductive groups, including the poor and frail elderly. Neither the reforms nor the Poor Law satisfied the criteria of universality, equity, civil rights and basic life protection. Rather, Japanese measures were 'welfare-like' or 'insufficient, traditional, and "pre-modern"', compared to those in England.[69]

Even then, the ideology underlying pre-1945 welfare schemes – national, goal-driven welfare overlaid with Japanese traditional values – did not disappear.[70] The post-war Japanese state finally acknowledged central responsibility for all citizens, but as the Ministry of Health and Welfare confirmed some fifty years later, 'the pre-war systems exerted a great influence on the design of post-war social security systems'.[71] This was reflected in the supplementary and restrictionist principle underlying the 1950 National Assistance Act, which superseded the 1929 Poor Law. Subsequently, this principle applied with developments in post-war statutory residential care provision for older people under the 1950 Act, as did the stigma attached to public welfare, particularly in its institutional forms. Moreover, philanthropic work and its underlying ethos were never officially endorsed, but at grassroots level it helped to shape post-war old people's institutions.

Post-War Measures, 1945–55

The war devastated Japan: some 1.85 million people were killed; one quarter of the national wealth was lost, excluding military resources; national income halved; almost half of the country was laid waste; and exacerbating it all, 6.25 million Japanese were repatriated from the former Asian colonies.[72] An official survey estimated that 8 million (11 per cent of the population) needed emergency relief by the end of 1945.[73]

Under instruction from the Allied Powers' general headquarters, the government endorsed the 'Old' National Assistance Act in 1946, which replaced the 1929 Poor Law. This was intended to address a modern welfare philosophy, yet retained conditional elements by excluding the 'indolent' and 'morally delinquent'.[74] Actual levels of public assistance were 'murderously' low, less than half the average urban working-class household income in 1948, for example.[75] Nonetheless, 2.81 million people received public assistance in 1947, far in excess of the 100,000 wartime relief recipients under the 1929 Poor Law, though still barely a third of the estimated needy.[76]

By 1950 some 9,200 older people were given public assistance in 'general public assistance institutions' (formerly Poor Law institutions), up from 3,000 in 1945.[77] But almost all institutions had insufficient food, daily necessities and equipment, although supplies from the Licensed Agencies for Relief in Asia (LARA) during 1946–8 and the charitable Community Chest Fund from 1948 enabled many residents to survive. With mortality rates at Rakufuen, in Tokyo, and Dowaen, in Kyoto, at 57 per cent and 50 per cent respectively in the immediate post-war years, institutional life was characterized as a 'struggle to obtain food and fuel and to maintain hygiene'.[78] Older residents and staff survived only by begging for food, farming and raising cattle in order to purchase necessities. In Dowaen in 1946:

> 14 January. 60 per cent of the rationed sweet potatoes were rotten, not fit to eat. 23 May ... all three meals consisted of just rice porridge ... 1 July. No rice at all. Vegetable soups for days and now even weeds are eaten ... 23 July. Due to severe shortages of food, people steal small offerings of food meant for ancestors in front of tombs in a nearby grave.[79]

In 1950 the revised ('New') National Assistance Act replaced the 1946 Act, providing the basis of current social security measures, in accordance with Article 25 of the new Constitution:

> All people shall have the right to maintain the minimum standards of wholesome and cultured living and in all spheres of life: the State shall use its endeavours for the promotion and extension of social welfare and security, and of public health.[80]

Conditional elements in the 1946 Act were repealed, and human rights were fully recognized under the 1950 Act: applicants could apply for public assistance and appeal to senior administrative officers and the courts if they wanted to contest the local welfare officer's assessment of their needs.[81]

Under the 1950 Act, eligible claimants of all ages were to be assisted in their own homes or in 'assessed institutions'. The latter included 'old people's institutions' (formerly 'general public assistance institutions') for 'those who cannot live independently because of the advancement of ageing'.[82] No age limit was specified, but those aged 60 or over were later identified in the 1957 Ministry Code of Practice, and Article 39 of the 1950 Act set minimum standards for these institutions for the first time. In order to be admitted to an old people's institution, the local welfare office first assessed the financial means and needs not only of the applicant but also of their family. This reflected the supplementary and restrictionist principle underlying Article 4 of the 1950 Act. This echoed the pre-war situation where only the destitute without any family support might, as a last resort, receive state poor relief. It seems that legal and customary or moral obligations, pressure on the family in the care of older relatives, and the stigma associated with public welfare (particularly in its institutional form) remained strong. Japan's eligibility criteria contrasted with those set out in the English 1948 National Assistance Act, which – in theory at least – were based solely on the needs of applicants, whatever their financial and family circumstances.

The chronic sick or frail who needed frequent or 24-hour care were effectively excluded from old people's institutions, as were the acute sick. In 1949 there were fewer than 18,000 beds in 133 psychiatric hospitals across the country. These targeted acute cases, though an estimated 1.3 million people (1.48 per cent of the total population) were considered mentally ill, including the elderly with dementia.[83] General hospital provision was also underdeveloped and expensive, and there were no statutory welfare services beyond the 'all-inclusive' institutional provision, ostensibly offering basic security for the needy destitute in society.

The 1951 Social Services Reform Act (which replaced the 1938 Social Services Charities Act) allowed non-profit organizations to establish 'social welfare corporations'. These were in effect quangos and came under strict central government control. They acted as subcontractors to the public sector by providing statutory services according to official guidelines, and in return received public funding and tax allowances.[84] Only local authorities (both prefectural and municipal) and social welfare corporations could establish and manage old people's institutions, subject to approval by the prefectural authorities. This maintained central government involvement and public funding (both capital and maintenance) of social welfare corporation old people's institutions, and helped to compensate for the shortage of direct local authority institutions in the immediate post-war years. It also perpetuated the pre-war publicly sanctioned yet charitably owned Poor Law institutions, roughly 40 per cent of which had closed between 1943 and 1951 as they were underfunded.[85] The 1951 Act also created 'local welfare offices' in the forty-seven prefectures and in 800 major municipal authorities to administer public welfare services, with separate non-profit social welfare councils (quangos) to oversee social welfare corporations and other non-profit enterprises and charities.

Between 1950 and 1955 the number of old people's institutions almost tripled to 460, with 86 per cent of the 290 new institutions established by local authorities and the rest by social welfare corporations. This reflected official acceptance of responsibility for needy older citizens.[86] Yet their 26,700 places accounted for just 0.54 per cent of people aged 65 or more, and catered for those with virtually no income or family help. Almost all the residents in 1953 were dependent on public assistance, and 82 per cent had no relatives to support them.[87] The stigma associated with *obasuteyama* was still strong: a 1953 official survey found that only 10 per cent of respondents had positive images of old people's institutions, while 15 per cent did not know there were any, and half expressed shame that they were ever resorted to.[88]

Institutional life offered little beyond basic provisions and care, supplemented by help from fellow residents and 'voluntary' or near-obligatory work. In 1953, 15 per cent of old people's institutions had no organized recreation, and 37 per cent did not subscribe to magazines.[89] The ratio of nursing and domestic staff to residents was 1:33 and 1:25 respectively.[90] Residents could undertake paid work to pay for the services they received. In some cases it was obligatory – in 1953 almost 60 per cent worked, half of them up to four hours a day and many doing considerably more.[91] With 12 per cent of institutions offering no recompense for work and 84 per cent paying a paltry wage of 500 yen or less a month, residents' chores undoubtedly contributed to the institutions' budget under continuing post-war austerity measures.[92]

At least 118,000 older people required statutory institutional care in 1955, but many were excluded under the 1950 Act.[93] They struggled because public health care and other social services were still rudimentary, and there were very few private and voluntary residential facilities. Even those living with their family could be victims of neglect or abuse from relatives, who were too poor or too busy to make ends meet. Professor Yuzo Okamoto noted:

the common practice in rural parts of Japan that the frail or sick elderly living with family were 'left' with just rice balls and water at home during the day ... it was only when family members came back home from the rice fields at night that they were changed and given something a bit more nutritious like an egg ... yet, once they became wholly bedridden, that was the 'end' by common consensus ... they were left unfed ... in order to hasten death and avoid long-term nursing care ... there was no history of nursing for the very dependent elderly for years ... the family was usually 'beside the frail elderly at death' ... nursing of elderly parents has to be understood as a myth surrounding Japanese care of the elderly.[94]

Obasuteyama seemed to have invaded the family home.

Nonetheless, such failings must be understood in the context of Japan's post-war stringencies and perceptions of state responsibility for the needs of its citizens. Faced with mass poverty, both the public and the government considered care of older people to be a family responsibility, and saw economic recovery as a national priority rather than expanding public welfare provision beyond public assistance for the neediest. Nor was demand for old people's institutions strong: only 30 per cent of Japanese people reached the age of 65, with average life expectancy 58 for men and 61 for women. Fully 80 per cent of older people lived with their offspring throughout the 1950s, and the need for family care was generally quite brief. Nor did it entail round-the-clock or intensive nursing. This can be explained by inadequate medical care and correspondingly low survival rates after an acute or critical illness, or survivors left with life-limiting disabilities or failing health. Thus shortages and deficiencies of statutory residential care provision, let alone its quality or alternative or supplementary services, were not a political priority.

However, it can reasonably be said that the 1946 and 1950 National Assistance Acts did support many of the needy, including older people. During 1945–55 on average two million people a year received public assistance either at home or in an assessed institution, consuming 46 per cent of the Ministry of Health and Welfare budget in 1950, with significant expansion in old people's institutions.[95] Without this legislation, the poorest 'would have suffered much more severely from social upheaval after the war', and 'it would be difficult to realize the present welfare services if these principles had not been instituted'.[96]

Delayed Responses, 1955–69

With Japan's economy recovering, the Ministry of Finance, in its 1956–7 white paper on the economy, announced that the post-war era had come to an end. In its wake would come the period of 'high-speed economic growth'. Prime Minister Hayato Ikeda (1960–4) anticipated a doubling of national income in the course of the 1960s, but it actually tripled by 1970, and Japan's GNP ranked second among the capitalist countries. Annual growth rates exceeded 10 per cent in real terms between 1955 and 1970, resulting in appreciable improvements in living standards. Even so, the government continued to prioritize economic growth over social welfare, with just 2.5 per cent of Ikeda's annual budgets apportioned to welfare-related programmes.[97] Until 1970 social security expenditure was less than 6 per cent of national income, though this was partly offset by family care and enhanced company welfare.[98] Nevertheless, 1956 was also the year when Japan's impending rapidly ageing population and its consequences were officially acknowledged for the first time, along with the needs of other vulnerable groups excluded from the post-war economic recovery.[99] Economic growth facilitated welfare expansion, with the newly amalgamated Liberal Democratic (Conservative) Party, in power from 1955 to 1994, affirming the 'construction of a welfare state along with anticommunism and world peace' in its 1955 constitution.[100] Deputy leader and later Prime Minister Nobusuke Kishi (1957–60) acknowledged the need for more provision for a greater proportion of the population in need, culminating in universal public pensions and health care schemes, which were implemented in 1961.

Until then Japan's public pensions schemes were selective: war veterans, war widows and pre-war public sector employees received generous non-contributory pensions, with post-war civil servants and employees of public organizations or large private firms also adequately covered, while the self-employed, agricultural workers and employees of small firms had none. Consequently, just 29 per cent of the working population were in a public pension scheme, and less than 6 per cent (450,000) of the 60-plus received any kind of pension in 1957.[101] The 1959 National Pension Act offered a basic state pension based on length of flat-rate contributions, along with a small, non-contributory yet means-tested 'welfare pension' for the poor aged 70 and over. Nor were Japan's public health care schemes universal: some 32 per cent of the total population were not covered in 1956, but all were under the 1958 National Health Insurance Act, which, along with the 1959 National Pension Act, became effective from 1961, so that this year arguably marked the beginning of a welfare state in Japan.[102]

In practice, however, pension reform was 'shaped to meet Japanese goals: the best deal for employees of large firms, to reward high productivity ... pension funds used for low-interest public loans to support infrastructure investment', while the health care scheme 'favoured younger workers ... rather than the higher-need elderly'.[103] For example, some 2.1 million (64 per cent) of the 70-plus received a part or full non-contributory 'welfare pension' of 1,000 yen a month in 1961, which compared unfavourably with an average monthly income of 13,000 yen for new graduates.[104] Similarly, the national health care scheme covered only half the total medical costs for most older people, whereas many workers in employment-based health care schemes enjoyed full coverage. In sum, the government retained a pre-war welfare philosophy, embedded in the national goal of rapid economic growth.

Shortfalls in public welfare for 'unproductive' groups had become more acute. In 1959, 85 per cent of old people (defined as aged 65 for men and 60 for women) living alone struggled at or below public assistance levels, and some 65 per cent of those living with their family were heavily dependent on them.[105] An estimated 39,000 older people eligible for public assistance urgently required admission to an old people's institution in 1960, but all the 37,500 places were already taken.[106] Given the thousands of older people ineligible for public assistance but requiring residential care, the actual shortage was much higher. Moreover, the distribution of old people's institutions was patchy – 44 per cent of the 869 local authorities had none in 1960 – with the proportion of older people receiving public assistance in old people's institutions rather than at home varying from 6 per cent in Iwate Prefecture to 38 per cent in Osaka City. (The national average was 17 per cent.[107]) Similarly, the ratio of residential places per 1,000 older population ranged from 1.7 in Iwate to 12.5 in Osaka (7.1 nationally).[108] By comparison, England offered seventeen residential places per 1,000 older population.

Improvements in old people's institutions came slowly. The 1957 Ministry Code of Practice set minimum guidelines for old people's institutions and other assessed institutions under the 1950 Act. This was made imperative after a fire in one old people's institution in 1955 killed ninety-eight elderly residents. Building regulations were crucial as most institutions were wooden constructions.[109] Although 'general public assistance institutions' under post-war emergency measures were upgraded into designated institutions for particular groups, their services and standards varied, and guidelines establishing a desirable level of standards were overdue. However, the guidelines lacked legal force and were far from satisfactory, as they permitted single-storey timber buildings. So, even in 1962 over 90 per cent of old people's institutions were timber-built, with many of them constructed as temporary expedients or for military purposes.[110] Only when full public subsidies for refurbishment or rebuilding became available were these replaced by concrete structures. Other recommendations set out an institution's size at 30–200 places; toilet provision of 1:13 for female and 1:20 for male residents; and a standard bedroom to include four residents with a floor area of 35 square feet each.[111]

Since 'minimum' guidelines were the basis for full if limited entitlement to public subsidies, they were regarded as the 'standard' by almost all old people's institutions, leaving little scope for innovation or enhanced provision. Unsurprisingly, institutional life barely changed, characterized by rigid timetabling, near-obligatory chores performed in rota, a monotonous daily routine and basic provisions and care. Moreover, there was little consideration for the specific needs of older residents.[112] Thus the recommended ratio of attendants to older residents remained at 1:25 for fifty-place older people's institutions and 1:30 for larger ones; many institutions employed no qualified nurses; and doctors typically visited only once a week.[113] Unsurprisingly, 'it was not uncommon that frail or sick old people quietly died in old people's institutions'.[114]

More dependent older people were excluded from old people's institutions because of financial and family ineligibility or due to severe disability or frailty. The 1957 guidelines allowed up to 20 per cent of the places in old people's institutions to be used for residents not fully on public assistance but on low incomes, but any place that became available was taken by the greater number of applicants eligible for public assistance. With hospital and private or voluntary sector residential care provision expensive and/or in short supply, they were left to fend for themselves or rely on their family. To address the problem, in 1961 the first of a new type of nursing home for frail older people requiring frequent or 24-hour care was opened and soon supported by government grants. The government then authorized another new type of facility for functionally independent older people with incomes somewhat above current public assistance limits, subsidizing capital and maintenance costs. Both facilities were formalized by the 1963 Elderly Welfare Act.

As an alternative to institutional care, home help services were instigated by a local social welfare council quango in Nagano Prefecture in 1956 and were soon taken up in other localities, attracting government funding in 1962. A year later, 132 local authorities were employing 530 home helps for the poorest elderly householders. They did the cooking, laundry and cleaning as well as providing personal help.[115] Arrangements were means-tested and restricted to those on public assistance and without family support, thereby perpetuating the stigma associated with public welfare. Nonetheless, home help services were welcomed as they meant that recipients could stay in their own home, and thus avoid or defer admission to the still more stigmatized old people's institution. A 1960 Ministry inquiry established that only 16 per cent of the 65–74-year-olds were prepared to consider entering an old people's institution, with 60 per cent expressing their determination to avoid being admitted to one at all costs.[116] A 1959 local survey produced similar results.[117] Thus *obasuteyama-* or institutionalization-related stigma and preference for privacy and family care remained strong.

From 1962, with government funding, local authorities and non-profit social welfare councils built 'community welfare centres' for more active older people. These offered advice, recreation and education. In 1963 government funding were also given to 'old people's clubs'. These were self-governing community groups, which expanded dramatically, with 35,000 clubs boasting 2.3 million members – a quarter of the over-60s population.[118] Cash allowances to compensate for the lack of a universal state pension were offered in fifteen prefectural and 315 municipal authorities by 1958, with free health care for people aged 65 or over first introduced in Sawanai Village municipal authority in northern

Akita Prefecture in 1960.[119] However, these arrangements were often arbitrary, varied from one authority to another, and lacked a systematic approach: 'service programs, whether institutional or in the community ... do not reflect any sort of comprehensive needs-analysis or program planning'.[120]

In 1962 the Central Social Welfare Advisory Council proposed comprehensive care packages for older people. It recognized that:

> public welfare provision exclusively for the elderly was restricted to public assistance and institutional care under the general 1950 National Assistance Act. Unlike children or physically handicapped people, who were provided welfare services systematically under the separate acts, those for the elderly lagged behind ... to promote welfare of the elderly was the responsibility of the state and local authorities.[121]

Subsequently, the 1963 Elderly Welfare Act offered a package of measures to regulate all health and social care services, including residential care, separate from the 1950 Act. Under the new 1963 Act the existing 664 old people's institutions, providing 45,500 places, became 'old people's homes' for those aged 65 and over who could not remain independent for financial, physical, mental or environmental reasons.[122] The foreign term 'home' implied modern, less institutional settings, and the eligibility criteria were relaxed, taking family circumstances into consideration, so that, for example, a needy older person living with the family could get a place in an old people's home if their living arrangements were unsuitable. Yet these were still assessed institutions so that the local welfare office compulsorily means-tested and needs-assessed applicants *and* their families.

The 1963 Act regulated two other existing facilities, authorized by the government as 'nursing homes' and 'low-fee homes', both again using the adopted term. The former, similar to the English model, provided nursing and personal care for people aged 65 or over, who, because of severe physical or mental impairment, required frequent or constant help that could not be supplied in their own home. Nursing homes were regulated as assessed institutions, in that admissions required the local welfare office's needs- and means-tested assessments, although the emphasis here was on needs and there were no financial limits since a sliding scale of fees applied. Like the pre-1963 old people's institutions, providers of old people's homes and nursing homes were restricted to local authorities and social welfare corporations (quangos).

In contrast, low-fee homes, similar to sheltered housing in England, were not assessed institutions and applicants made their own contracts with them, although an applicant's household income had to be within a specified threshold. Designed for functionally independent people aged 60 and over who lacked adequate housing for financial and environmental reasons, low-fee homes generally offered single rooms and aimed 'to provide a bright and comfortable life with modest fees for the moderate-income elderly'.[123] They proved very popular and were later categorized as the original 'type-A homes', with 'type-B homes' added in 1972 and 'care houses' introduced much later in 1989. Type-A homes served meals, while type-B homes required their tenants to cook for themselves. Care houses provided meals and interim care via home help services, with residents unable to cope being required to seek an alternative. Given their housing focus, low-fee homes are excluded from residential care provision here, though they were categorized under the 1963 Act. Other arrangements under the 1963 Act included free health check-ups, home help and well-being promotion services. To supervise and promote these services and the new Act, an Elderly Welfare Division was created within the Social Affairs Bureau of the Ministry of Health and Welfare in 1964.

The new Act looked beyond minimum means-tested institutional provision; service packages became less restricted, finance-centred and stigmatized and more needs-led, exemplified in the nursing home provision.[124] Yet critics argued that it was supplementary rather than innovatory and its impact should not be exaggerated. They saw 'only a compilation of existing services' and 'a lofty rhetorical preamble with a potpourri of tiny programs designed to pique the interest of one group or another'.[125] One Ministry official recalled that 'the Elderly Welfare Act ... in practice was the Act for old people's homes'.[126] Professor Soji Tanaka too noted that 'despite the broad scope of the Act, the focus was on institutional provision reflecting the long history of dominant institutional care'.[127] Continuation of the assessed institution status meant that the legal right of admission to an old people's home or nursing home was not automatic.[128] Nor could applicants choose their home; they were simply assigned a place. Moreover, the Act set no compulsory standards, using the word 'can' rather than 'must', and could neither ensure continuing development nor resolve shortages in residential care provision. In the face of growing demand, those at or below public assistance levels were prioritized, so applicants' financial and family circumstances remained critical in the admission procedure.[129] With residential care provision expanding and few central or local initiatives, it appeared that 'throughout the 1960s, there was little interest in developing programs for the unproductive elderly'.[130]

Others saw the 1963 Act as a catalyst in the development of social services for older people, as it contributed to reforms and an expansion of services for older people.[131] Thus the 1968 National Council of Social Welfare Report, which investigated bedridden older people at home, found that about 200,000 of all over-70s were bedridden, one-half having no medical treatment and only 8,000 receiving support from anyone but the family.[132] The public health physician N. Maeda recalled experts being 'shocked by the high rate of 4 per cent of all elderly bed-ridden, about twice the European rate'.[133] Revelation of this *obasuteyama* in the home challenged the myth of dedicated Japanese family care. Acknowledging this, the 1968 Ministry's Report on the growing old age problem admitted that there were shortages and that services for bedridden older people living at home were badly distributed. It called for expansion in home-based and residential care provision.[134] This was reflected first in the 1969 Welfare Plan and later in post-1970 reforms, resulting in a significant expansion of services.[135] By then, forward-looking local authorities had set up their own programmes. Among these, Tokyo's free health care for most over-70s stands out. This was started in 1969 by its governor, Ryokichi Minobe, and was soon taken up in many other localities. By 1973 it was available across the whole country.

Hospital Expansion and Quality Care Issues in the 1970s

The expansion of welfare services was made possible in part because attitudes to an economy-focused public policy were changing, brought about by the undesirable side-effects of rapid economic growth – pollution, urban overcrowding and intractable inequalities in wealth. Welfare programmes were called for to help those adversely affected by or excluded from economic growth; yet economic growth made public investment in welfare developments possible. Equally important was an increasing awareness of the crisis of Japan's rapidly ageing population.[136] In 1970 Japan became an 'ageing society' according to the United Nations' definition, with people aged 65 or more exceeding 7 per cent of the total population, and with average life expectancy in 1973 reaching 70.5 for men and 75.9 for women. Acknowledging that Japan would experience the highest rate of population ageing of any nation in the coming decades, in 1970 the Ministry proposed further systematic development of services for the burgeoning older population.[137]

Accordingly, public welfare expenditure for the aged almost doubled from 1971 to 1972. Overall social security expenditure increased by 28 per cent in 1973, that year also seeing Prime Minister Kakuei Tanaka's announcement of the 'Economy and Society Plan: A Vital Welfare Society', with the catchphrase 'Pollution Halved and Welfare Doubled'.[138] New initiatives included free health care for most over-70s; health care charges for family members reduced from 50 per cent to 30 per cent under employment-based health insurance schemes; expensive medical treatment subsidized; and an increase in the old age pension. The Branch of Policy for the Elderly was established within the Cabinet Office to promote programmes for older people, as well as research and legislation. Total social security expenditure as a percentage of national income more than doubled by 1979, by then exceeding 12 per cent.[139]

As principal consumers of health care and pensions, older people were the main beneficiaries. Health care expenditure for this age group increased by 55 per cent in 1973–4 and by 30 per cent the following year.[140] Some 53 per cent more over-70s received hospital treatment in 1973 than in 1970, and by 1979 they consumed 17 per cent of all health care spending, although they comprised only 5 per cent of the total health care service users.[141] Pensions expenditure (rising from 1.6 billion to 8.8 billion yen during 1973–9) amounted to 40 per cent of the total social security budget.[142] It was the better-off 10 per cent or so on earnings-related pensions who benefited most, whereas 40 per cent of 65–9-year-olds had no pensions at all, and many over-70s received only the meagre, non-contributory, means-tested 'welfare pension', derisively named the 'sweets pension', since it was only enough to buy sweets for grandchildren.[143]

Acknowledging *obasuteyama* in the family home and insufficient residential care provision, the government set targets under the 1970 Emergency Five Year Plan for Residential Facilities, and 17,000 old people's home places, 37,000 nursing home places and 540 community welfare centres were completed by 1975–6.[144] With more frail and bedridden older people, the government encouraged the expansion of nursing homes, places in which outnumbered old people's home places by 1979.[145] This was largely attributable to a significant expansion in social welfare corporation (quango) nursing homes, then making up three-quarters of the total. From the late 1970s these old people's institutions were increasingly taken over by quangos, which strictly followed central guidelines for certified residents. In return they received public money for 75 per cent of the capital costs and full maintenance fees. The total number of 142,000 places, with 4,800 more places in private care homes by 1979, compared well with 67,000 a decade earlier, although the 1979 figures represented just 13.8 per 1,000 of the older population.[146]

The ideology of 'normalization' emerged late. This emphasized 'de-institutionalization' and community care. Attempts at community integration of the homes were dubbed 'socialization of the homes'. Accordingly, from 1978 nursing homes offered short-stay and respite care for bedridden older people living at home. From 1979 day care services, which were often attached to nursing homes, offered frail older people living at home weekly or twice-weekly services, including baths, meals, rehabilitation and consultations. The flagship home help services employed more than 10,000 staff by 1976, compared to just 800 a decade earlier, yet this represented just nine per 100,000 population, compared to 138 in the UK and 825 in Sweden.[147] Moreover, these services were restricted to those on low incomes and without supporting relatives, so less than a third (30 per cent) of households with at least one older person were eligible in the late 1970s.[148] Other community-based services included hiring adapted beds for bedridden older people from 1969; rehabilitation for the disabled at home and those discharged from hospitals in 1971; and nurse visits for frail older people and meals services for those living alone, both in 1972. These, however, were insignificant and varied from one locality to another.

Overall, neither residential nor community care provision kept pace with a growing frail older population. By 1975 an estimated 360,000 older people living at home were bedridden, compared to the 40,000 nursing home places then available.[149] Most were wholly dependent on family carers, but the quality of family care was increasingly questioned. Japan's bestselling novel *Man in Rapture* by Sawako Ariyoshi explored the problem, depicting the struggle of a woman obliged to care for her confused father-in-law and the fragility of family bonds.[150] In 1975 Japanese older people had the second highest suicide rate in the world, averaging sixteen deaths a day due to loneliness, family conflicts, illness or financial worries, but 'the most proper reason is to eliminate the self when it has become a drag on others (family above all)'.[151] At *Pokkuri-dera* (literally, 'sudden-death without suffering temple') near Kyoto, every year more than 40,000 elderly visitors placed underclothing before the Buddha, praying, 'Please let me die peacefully before I am no longer able to change my underclothing and have to face shame and burden my family'.[152]

Fortunately there was an institutional alternative: the hospital. Until 1973 Japan had no geriatric or psycho-geriatric hospitals as such, although some general hospitals admitted older patients. Their subsequent expansion followed provision of free health care for most over-70s in 1973 and a surge in elderly admissions: 91,000 over-70s hospital patients in 1970 and 188,000 by 1980, with 171,000 more aged 65–9, making 432,000 65-plus inpatients, or 4 per cent of all those over 65.[153] Their average hospital stay was 103 days, compared to fifty-six days for all ages.[154] Some acute and general hospital beds doubtless substituted for nursing home places: of an estimated 362,000 bedridden older people in 1978, 69 per cent were cared for at home, with 18 per cent in nursing homes and 13 per cent in hospitals.[155] Effectively, 'enormous numbers of older people were living in hospitals, most with little or no need of intensive medical care'.[156] 'Social hospitalization' was for older patients who needed social care but little or no medical treatment, but whose families could no longer cope.

How did this come about? First, statutory nursing homes, then the only alternative to 24-hour family care for bedridden or frail older people, offered only 80,000 places in 1980, compared to the 432,000 hospital beds then occupied by 65-plus inpatients. Second, hospital provision was free for most over-70s, although per capita costs were two to three times those in nursing homes. Third, unlike nursing home provision, hospital admission involved no means-testing and little needs assessment, and thus incurred no welfare stigma or lengthy and often degrading assessment procedures. Hospitals offered medical *and* social assistance and so masked the shifting of social care arrangements. Families could say that the admission was 'a necessary hospitalization' and so avoid the stigma associated with *obasuteyama*.[157]

Yet another *obasuteyama* was arguably created in hospitals, for places were 'less comfortable for the non-acute bedridden elderly requiring little medical treatment ... [who] ... can be much better cared for in nursing homes'.[158] 'Many elderly patients were unnecessarily made and left bedridden with nappies and bedsores and lived their last years in an inappropriate environment'.[159] Nonetheless, hospital care was free, non-means-tested and less stigmatized, and relieved the family of the responsibility of care. Families usually could not or would not take older relatives back home, since there was hardly any public or affordable community support for them. Ironically, belief in a robust tradition of family care and few institutionalized elderly in Japan continued, for hospital statistics concealed socially hospitalized older patients who were effectively residents for much of the time, while household surveys included them within extended families.

Turning to qualitative aspects of residential care, in 1966 the Ministry issued new guidelines on standards and the administration of old people's homes and nursing homes. However, these hardly differed from the 1957 guidelines for old people's institutions. The 1972 Social Welfare Advisory Council's Report depicted the homes as 'places for living' rather than 'shelters'.[160] Although this was not officially endorsed until 1986, the Report led to revisions of the 1966 guidelines in 1973. The new guidelines recommended no more than two persons per bedroom in old people's homes (previously four) or four in nursing homes (previously eight), with improved staff to resident ratios. These specifications applied only to post-1973 new homes and were not legally binding. The result was greater variations in provision: the 1975 average size for nursing homes was seventy-seven places, but sixty-two nursing homes (nearly 9 per cent of the total) had in excess of 100 beds.[161] Almost all nursing home rooms were multi-bedded, with 60 per cent having six or more beds.[162] Admittedly, 'hardly any elderly people living with family had their own rooms', and Japanese houses typically featured communal but limited space, though whether this justified the nursing home provision is debatable.[163] Official attitudes varied, and older residents' views were rarely considered. No literature reflected residential life and experiences from the residents' perspectives before 1979, though recent accounts are considered elsewhere.[164]

Modest efforts to promote a homely atmosphere were made in some local old people's and nursing homes. These included allowing residents to wear their own clothing, and on-site shops and cafeterias supplemented by regular trolley visits, buffet-style dinners and a choice of meals on special occasions. These initiatives gradually influenced other homes, and the first five-year national survey of elderly homes in 1977 noted improvements in quality and standards. Moreover, the first guidebook for residential care staff that year sought to improve standards, reinforced by the introduction of training courses for staff in 1979, followed by official qualifications in care and social work in 1987.[165]

'Life guidance' measures, ostensibly promoting residents' well-being, took the form of near-compulsory physical exercises or bans on watching daytime television, even though Ministry officials acknowledged that the home 'should not provide morale-driven services and must restrict its role to non-morale provision such as good food and care'.[166] This implied the continuity of the patronizing and managerial practices seen in pre-war old people's almshouses or Poor Law institutions, In the late 1970s older residents still called their attendants 'Teacher' or 'Miss'.[167] Staff shortages and increasing care requirements also undermined care standards and quality. In 1977 nearly 90 per cent of nursing homes finished serving meals before 5 pm to fit working patterns, while a third gave baths only once or twice a week.[168] A fixed number of incontinence pad changes rather than 'anytime in need' featured in three-quarters of nursing homes.[169] With insufficient rehabilitation and stimulation, and a questionable 60 per cent of nursing home populations bedridden, 'I don't want anything', 'I have no expectations' or 'I have lived too long' were frequently heard remarks.[170] A third of residents were suffering from dementia, but clear guidelines and specially trained staff were absent due to lack of consensus.[171]

As for stigmatization, even a nursing home attendant admitted, 'I feel ashamed and don't let on where I work because people still don't know the difference between the nursing home for ordinary frail older people and the means-tested old people's home for the solitary poor'.[172] The Minister of Labour Kenzaburo Hara stated explicitly in 1972 that 'those elderly in old people's homes were below those who already are subhuman'.[173] This occasioned a public outcry, but the poor residents' shame and submission were only made worse. Typically, 'old people superficially welcome "comfort" visits by voluntary groups and the locals but actually detest them deep down ... they "pity" their own circumstances and dread it to be known that they are here by the neighbourhood'.[174]

Growing Needs: Government Responses in the 1980s–90s

Japan's economic slowdown led the government to 'reconsider welfare' and to champion a 'Japanese-style welfare state' and 'vibrant welfare society'. Thus Prime Minister Masayoshi Ohira (1978–80) proposed public welfare, 'while retaining a traditional Japanese spirit of self-respect and self-reliance, human relations which are based on the spirit of tolerance and the traditional social system of mutual assistance'.[175] The primacy of the family was reasserted, with recourse to public assistance seen as a last resort. According to Michio Watanabe, a former Minister of Health and Welfare, 'those who put elderly parents in nursing homes are guilty of impiety', while increases in public health care expenditure reflected 'rising numbers of families who don't take their hospitalized parents back to their homes'.[176] Unsurprisingly, the government reacted to the 'social hospitalization' of older inpatients because of the rocketing increase in public health care spending, by focusing on allegedly irresponsible and indifferent families.[177] Similarly, it castigated the hospitals for colluding with 'bad' families and profiting from social hospitalization, though it did not provide appropriate alternatives.

In 1982 the Elderly Health Care Act targeted social hospitalization. Free health care for most over-70s ceased, user fees were introduced as a disincentive, and flat-rate monthly fees for non-acute inpatients replaced pay-as-you-go charges to stop unnecessary treatment and medication. The government also introduced 'specially authorized geriatric hospitals' for longer-term chronic sick older patients. These employed fewer medical personnel and gave less treatment than did general hospitals, thereby reducing health care spending. General hospitals where beds were predominantly occupied by older patients were designated as specially authorized geriatric hospitals, and their health care spending were subsequently reduced. More disturbing were efforts to make hospitals identify older patients deemed to be socially hospitalized and discharge them to their families or to local authorities. Meanwhile the government retained supplementary and means-tested measures in flagship nursing home provision, the number of nursing home places more than doubling to 161,000 during the decade to 1990 to represent 10.8 per 1,000 older population, compared to 7.5 a decade earlier.[178] These increases were offset by a reduction in the number of old people's home places. As a result, the amount of residential provision proportionate to the older population barely changed during that decade.[179]

In contrast, hospital provision continued to expand. By 1990 there were 1.68 million beds (fourteen per 1,000 general population), the world's highest ratio.[180] The 65-plus occupied 694,000 of these – 41 per cent compared to 35 per cent in 1980 – and their average stay was seventy-nine days, with one-third hospitalized for over a year.[181] Overall, 922,000 older people in Japan were in statutory institutional accommodation of some kind in 1990, 61.9 per 1,000 older people compared to 13 per 1,000 in 1960, and higher than many other developed countries.[182] Continuing 'social hospitalization' of older patients thus replaced other less supported and/or inadequate 24-hour care alternatives.

Meanwhile, the problem of the health/social care divide became more acute, particularly between hospitals and nursing homes. According to a 1985 official report, although hospitals and nursing homes were meant to target different clienteles, hospital patients and nursing home residents differed very little in terms of their physical and mental condition and the health and care services they received.[183] Yet the administration of the two, including admission procedures and financial arrangements, were very different. To address this problem, the government sought new intermediate facilities somewhere between medical and social care, but tending towards the latter. This partly reflected the unpopularity of nursing homes because of their assessed institution status. For this reason many hospital patients, potential users in the community and their families still preferred hospitals to nursing homes. Thus in 1988 the government authorized a new health care facility within the health care system for the chronic sick or frail elderly requiring medical assistance but not hospitalization, with the aim of returning them to the community within three months by providing rehabilitation and support for independent living.

This new measure appeared to address not only the health/social care divide, particularly the lack of social care in hospitals and health care in nursing homes, but also 'social hospitalization' and the lack of and shortcomings in nursing homes. Above all, fewer medical staff and less medical treatment, as well as the short-term stay in such facilities, would curtail health care expenditure on older people, which had risen 12 per cent a year during the 1980s – twice the overall public health care spending rate.[184] By 1995 the new health care facilities were providing over 100,000 beds, but 'despite the emphasis on rehabilitation and on returning people to the community, most patients were entering from *home* rather than from hospitals, and were staying for extended periods' (my emphasis).[185] Indeed, with an average stay of 147 days in 1993 and half of patients unable to return to the community owing to the absence of alternative provision, social hospitalization now featured in health care facilities, arguably creating yet another *obasuteyama*.[186]

A further attempt to tackle health care expenditure on older inpatients was the introduction, in 1992, of new 'designated long-stay beds' for chronic sick patients within authorized hospitals, in effect extending post-1982 'specially authorized geriatric hospitals' to wards or sections of non-geriatric hospitals. Like the post-1982 specially authorized geriatric hospitals, the new long-stay beds offered more nursing but less medical care. The scheme was extended in 1997 to clinics with twenty or fewer beds. It did little, however, to reduce the social hospitalization of older inpatients, but arguably concealed this by giving these patients a legitimate label – 'long-stay' inpatients – thereby securing them longer-term, if reduced, hospital care. The long-stay beds were later categorized as 'medical-led long-stay beds' under the existing health care system, or 'nursing-led long-stay beds' which were transferred to the new long-term care insurance system. In short, the government's response to the social hospitalization of older inpatients remained firmly focused on cost-cutting measures through the makeshift changeover or designation of beds occupied allegedly by socially hospitalized older patients from medical-focused, expensive beds to more care-led, cheaper ones in 'specially authorized geriatric hospitals' (1982–), intermediate 'health care facilities' (1988–) and 'designated long-stay beds' in authorized hospitals (1992–). This barely improved life for older inpatients in multi-bedded wards, though it did secure free or affordable 24-hour institutional care in a familiar setting.

With the population continuing to age, it was predicted that the estimated 700,000 bedridden older people and 1 million living with dementia in 1991 would rise to 1 million and 1.5 million respectively by 2000.[187] Meanwhile, changing patterns of family care and a shrinking pool of family carers as women entered the workforce presented further problems. Nearly 80 per cent of carers were themselves aged 50 or more, and the periods of care were becoming longer, with half the carers having nursed for over three years, adding to their burden.[188]

Some 80 per cent of respondents to a 1989 poll expressed anxiety about their own or their spouse's old age care.[189] Thus the 'Japanese-style welfare state', which was trying to avoid 'profligate', Western levels of spending, appeared unsustainable and demanded policy changes.[190]

In 1989 the government launched the Gold Plan, a 'ten-year strategy for health and welfare promotion for older people'. This emphasized community care, although residential care was also envisaged, with improved targets from 1994. The Gold Plan appeared to offer universal help, 'not just for those unfortunate enough to be poor and to get left out of the traditional family', but also for 'ordinary' older people with families.[191] Its supporters concluded that 'endowed with a huge budget, it emphasizes development of home-based welfare services, and it re-examines the relationship between a state and its municipalities'.[192] Indeed, most targets were achieved, with 80 per cent of facilities and amenities in operation by 1997, and all residential and community care programmes, except for care houses, had sufficient funds to meet their 1999 targets.

However, critics argued that this 'implicitly redefined the family role, shifting the responsibility of care back to the family to take advantage of Japan's high co-residency rates', and to cheaper and *temporary* health care facilities than permanent nursing homes.[193] Japan's home help provision was only 40 per cent of Sweden's, even in 1999. Similarly, the 570,000 statutory residential places, including 280,000 *temporary* beds in health care facilities and 67,000 *means-tested* places in old people's homes, represented just twenty-seven per 1,000 of the elderly older population, far below that in many Western countries.[194] Meanwhile, nursing home waiting lists increased from 29,000 in 1990 to 105,000 by 1999.[195] Increases in nursing home and health care facility places did not outstrip expected decreases in hospital beds: at least 300,000 older patients remained socially hospitalized for longer than six months in 1994.[196] Nor did the intermediate health care facilities resolve 'the old divide between the social welfare care services [nursing homes] ... and the medical services [health care facilities] for the aged'.[197] Health care facilities were often occupied by older people waiting for a place in a nursing home well beyond the intended three months, while frail older people with few medical requirements remained in general hospitals. Indeed, it was claimed that 'some hospitals are therefore *de facto* nursing homes'.[198]

Qualitative improvements were limited despite the change of the official definition of a home from 'a shelter' to 'a residence' in 1986. A 1988 national survey of elderly homes found that half the nursing homes did not allow residents to keep religious relics, and that while a third of residents had personal effects, other homes typically permitted a 'maximum of three boxes'.[199] Privacy suffered: only 3.5 per cent of nursing home rooms were single, without keys even for women's bedrooms. And just 2.9 per cent offered a choice of meals, and only 4.9 per cent served dinner after 6 pm.[200] Under the assessed institution status, residents' rights were rarely considered or were undermined by patronizing staff, regulations and proscriptions: one resident seeking a room change was told, 'If you say such nonsense again, I will throw you out'.[201] Over three-quarters of old people's homes lacked amenities, such as a newsagent or tea shop, but strict curfews prevented residents from going out at night or at weekends when there were fewer staff.[202] Most nursing homes now changed residents' incontinence pads at 'any time in need' but subject to staff availability, and 74 per cent acknowledged that residents developed bedsores.[203] Moreover, whereas 90 per cent offered rehabilitation, just 9 per cent employed specialists, which added to staff workloads.[204] Most nursing homes still had multi-bedded rooms, reflecting the official minimum standards of 'four people per room', with the '53 square feet per capita living space' guideline unchanged since 1973.

In order to achieve good quality and person-centred care geared to independent living and recognizing individual dignity and diversity, in 1989 the Ministry published the comprehensive Code of Practice for statutory residential facilities of all kinds, derived partly from the English 1984 equivalent *Home Life*, which was revised in 1994.[205] Even so, improvements were slow to take effect. The Ministry Home Inspection Reports in 1995 revealed disturbing cases, including incontinence pads changed in public, no meals served after 5 pm, and 'sloppy' management of residents' accounts.[206] In short, institutionalization rather than normalization was the hallmark of many homes well into the 1990s. Worse still, residents of old people's homes and nursing homes faced higher fees for their services in 1980, something that affected poorer residents, while user fees for domiciliary services were also introduced in 1982, again negatively impacting poorer households.

Socialization of Care and Inequalities since 2000

An economic slump during the 1990s led to falling tax revenues and constraints on social expenditure.[207] The national health care system faced huge debts, caused not least by the continuing social hospitalization of older inpatients. These problems were compounded when Japan became the world's fastest ageing society, with its over-65s population doubling from 7 to 14 per cent of the general population in just twenty-four years in 1994.[208] An estimated 2 million older people required some nursing, yet the proportion living with their children declined from 70 to 54 per cent during 1980–95, and those living alone increasing from 8.5 to 12.6 per cent.[209] In the mid-1990s over 60 per cent of older people were looked after by their families, but 65 per cent of carers were themselves elderly, and the average period of caring was six years.[210] A 1994 national survey found that half of all family carers had subjected their elderly relative to some form of abuse, and one in three acknowledged feeling 'hatred' for the elderly relative.[211] This was attributable partly to fewer carers and the heavier burden placed on them, reflecting changes in demographic and residence patterns, gender roles and employment practices. Persistent social pressures on family obligations compounded these difficulties, in extreme cases resulting in the murder of the whole family. Attitudes to family care also changed, with less than half the respondents to a 1994 poll regarding the care of frail older relatives as a family responsibility.[212] In short, the limitations of and deficiencies in family care, featuring domestic *obasuteyama*, were magnified and led to a call for expansion of public care provision and additional funding to achieve this.

This was the context in which the government introduced its comprehensive Long-Term Care Insurance (LTCI) Act in December 1997. The insurance-based approach was regarded as 'more acceptable than a hike in taxes', since it was targeted, and while half of LTCI funding came from general taxation, insurance premiums, which were less vulnerable to economic downturns, accounted for the rest.[213] Above all, the insurance mechanism guaranteed entitlement, which was considered better than the means-tested and targeted tax-based system, which had 'stigmatized long-term care and produced little competition between providers'.[214]

On 1 April 2000 the Act came into operation with the slogans 'From Care by the Family to Care by Society' and 'Socialization of Care'.[215] The care of older people was no longer 'expected' to come from families or 'allocated' by the state, but now became part of a social contract, featuring mandatory contributions, universal entitlement and some consumer choice. LTCI arguably marked a decisive shift towards a greater mix in care delivery. It was celebrated as 'the biggest reform in Japan's welfare history'.[216]

In brief, LTCI is a compulsory, insurance-based national social care system, with everyone aged 40 and over paying insurance premiums. Under the new system, any older person can apply for a standard national assessment. This was originally based strictly on care needs and ignored financial means or family support, but from 2005 family support was taken into account. The eligible are assigned to one of six (seven from 2005) categories according to need, the category determining the maximum benefits they can receive, which are paid in kind. People can use home-based and residential care services from any provider, their decision helped by a care manager with a care plan. Service users pay a 10 per cent user fee, although those on benefits or low income are subsidized according to their means. Central government plays an essential role in financing half of the LTCI funding and regulating the prices, content and scope of the services. But the municipal authorities are the insurers, and are responsible for setting premiums, planning and overseeing services, and managing finances, which allows some autonomy and flexibility to meet local needs within central government guidelines.[217]

LTCI residential arrangements include existing nursing homes (1963–), intermediate health care facilities (1988–) and new 'nursing-led' designated long-stay beds in authorized hospitals (1992–), distinct from new 'medical-led' ones which remain within the health care system. In 2000 the combined bed capacity of the three was 650,000, or twenty-nine per 1,000 older population.[218] At least a further 600,000 long-term places were provided outside LTCI, including over 500,000 long-stay beds in hospital settings, some 60,000 post-1950 means-tested old people's homes, 30,000 private care home places and 13,000 'group home' places. This highlights the difficulties in obtaining a comprehensive picture and data.

The LTCI proved very popular and expanded much faster than official projections. According to a 2005 poll, 61 per cent of respondents made 'high' to 'moderate' appraisals of LTCI, compared to 44 per cent in a similar poll in 2000, suggesting that 'within a short period, LTCI has been widely accepted in Japanese society'.[219] Total LTCI expenditure rose by 27 per cent in the first year and 13 per cent in the second year, compared to the planned annual 4 per cent increase. This was largely attributable to revision of the 1951 Social Services Reform Act and allied legislation in 2000, which promoted devolution, privatization and deregulation of social services, allowing for-profit and non-profit agencies to provide most LTCI care services.[220] Excluded were the three pillar residential facilities, their providers still restricted to local authorities and social welfare and health corporations (quangos). For-profit and non-profit LTCI providers increased hugely compared to local authorities and quangos, which suggests that expansion was significant in community care but not in residential care. Overall, the number of service users increased from 1.49 million (6.8 per cent of the older population) in 2000 to 3.29 million (13 per cent) in 2005, with the LTCI total expenditure doubling to 6 billion yen in the same period.[221]

However, these positive outcomes masked important changes, particularly in the balance between community and residential care. Arguably, LTCI has promoted community care as a cheaper option, helping 65 per cent of all beneficiaries at just a quarter of the total costs.[222] Moreover, its recipients were largely those certified as having light care needs (the lightest and second lightest), comprising nearly a half of all certified people by 2005. The number of home-based service users rose from 970,000 to 2.51 million during 2000–5, while residential care users increased only moderately, from 520,000 to 780,000 during the same period. This suggests unequal service distribution, and the burden of family carers looking after severely disabled older relatives barely changed after LTCI. In theory LTCI services cover a maximum of two hours' home help three times a day, but subject to the care needs levels of an eligible person and his or her (and the family's) ability to pay. Indeed, a 2002 study reported that the burden on family carers increased after LTCI, compared with 1996.[223] Demand for residential care remained high, with nursing home waiting lists alone standing at 233,000 in 2002.[224] Certified older people eligible for both community and residential care often chose the latter, a decision prompted by subsidized 'hotel costs'. Ironically, one survey in 2001 revealed that 56 per cent of certified older people applying for nursing homes did not actually require residential care.[225] By 2005 the three pillar LTCI facilities accommodated 780,000 residents, including 41 per cent of those with light or moderate care needs.[226] Arguably, 'the increased institutionalization observed in Japan was not an inevitable consequence ... Rather, it resulted from the specific design of LTCI'.[227]

By then LTCI expenditure had reached alarming levels, and the government's response focused on cost-cutting through stricter eligibility criteria and needs assessment, increased insurance premiums and top-up user fees. With a policy focus on community care, despite acute shortages of nursing homes, the government capped new residential places at 3 per cent of the older population and withdrew capital investment subsidies which had covered 75 per cent of the construction costs of new nursing homes. These changes were integrated into the first major revision of the LTCI in 2005.[228] As a result, total expenditure dropped for the first time in 2006.

With a 40 per cent decrease in the total home help hours, home help services are now restricted to older people with severe disabilities living alone.[229] The care need categories of many existing service users were reassessed, and users had to accept reduced services or pay more. Similarly, nursing home residents now have to pay 'hotel charges' in addition to the 10 per cent user fee. This makes older people reluctant to seek residential care, while producing no reorientation towards community care, which also increased its fees, reflected in the low take-up rate of LTCI community care users: in 2010–11 almost 5 million older people (16 per cent of all over-65s) qualified for LTCI services, but over 1 million used no services whatsoever, and 3 million choosing home-based care took only 40–60 per cent of their entitlement.[230] This reflected what they could afford as well as the lack of available or suitable services, particularly short-stay (respite care) provision. Although subsidies are given to people on benefits or low income, these cover only part of the costs and meet the minimum standards only. Thus only the better-off can afford full user fees for all certified LTCI services as an alternative to family care.

Quality care concerns in residential care provision have attracted more attention. In 2001 the government prescribed zero restraint in all LTCI residential facilities, except 'under emergency circumstances in order to protect residents from risk'.[231] Only 11 per cent of facilities adopted zero restraint, the rest practising restraint 'in order to prevent residents from accidents', 'owing to staff shortages' or 'in response to requests from residents or their families'.[232] So, in 2006 the government banned all types of restraint. For those with dementia, many nursing homes used government subsidies to convert up to 20 per cent of their places into single or double rooms designated mainly for them, not from concern about residents' privacy or quality of life, but to avoid upsetting other residents.[233] Meanwhile the 'four people per room' guideline for the remainder remains in place – even in 2006 only 12 per cent of all rooms in the three pillar LTCI residential facilities were single rooms.[234]

In 2003 the government formalized another type of LTCI nursing home, comprising units of around ten single rooms and semi-private communal space, offering a more homely environment – 'a Home from home'.[235] This was extended to 'group homes' for people with mild to moderate dementia, offering 'normal life' through mutual help among residents and a few staff. This is important since 90 per cent of residents in LTCI facilities reportedly suffered some degree of dementia.[236] Positive outcomes include residents having more privacy and keeping personal belongings; greater interaction with other residents in semi-private communal rooms; and improving appetites, mobility and sleep patterns.[237] Yet such accommodation is a supplement rather than a replacement, because it can be accessed only with higher hotel charges, suggesting economic rather than social priorities. In contrast, with the retention of the 'four people per room' standard in the pillar LTCI facilities, many on minimum pensions or limited private means have found that 'the single room option is almost non-applicable', since even subsidized and reduced hotel charges amount to almost their entire pension.[238] They may fare even worse than less frail but poorer residents on public assistance in means-tested old people's homes, where under the revised minimum 'all double-bedroom' guideline, over 90 per cent of bedrooms are now single or double, although these homes may carry a strong welfare stigma as assessed institutions.

This new approach has thus created a dual system, with new, high-quality homes for better-off residents paying extra, and basic, old-fashioned homes for the worse-off, echoing the developments seen in England. Thus, while LTCI has successfully 'socialized' care, it 'has also played a part in creating social inequalities amongst old people … to benefit middle- to high-income households'.[239] LTCI shifted the focus of eligibility criteria of applicants away from their *financial* means towards their care needs, yet this has added to financial pressure on lower-income households. It deters them from accessing services they are entitled to, forcing them to ration their take-up of qualified services or reduce their pre-existing services.[240] Ironically, they are the group for whom 'targeted' services had been 'allocated' free of charge or with small charges under the pre-2000 tax-based, means-tested system, although the latter featured rationing and was associated with welfare stigma.

Financial burdens on older individuals were also extended to the insurance-based health care system, where small, flat-rate user fees for health care costs were replaced by 10 per cent user fees in 2001 (20 per cent in 2004 and 30 per cent from 2005). 'Hotel costs' for older patients in hospitals, introduced in 1994, increased substantially in 2005, ostensibly to reduce inequality between hospital patients and LTCI residents, with thresholds for a subsidy for expensive medical treatment also being raised in 2006.[241] User fees help restrict overuse or misuse of services, but they also sever the social contract, with the majority of older people who have contributed during their entire working lives and still continue to contribute in order to be entitled to *all* the health and social care services in their old age. Instead, they now have to use a large part of their pension or private savings to get even *some* of the eligible services. Significantly, 'voluntary' discharges from hospitals and LTCI facilities, or relocation to cheaper yet inappropriate and poorer quality accommodation of worse-off older people unable to afford hotel costs, have increased. How they cope in the community is unknown. Worst of all, in 2006 the government announced the closure by 2012 of 280,000 long-stay hospital beds, occupied mainly by chronically sick older patients. This produced a tremendous public outcry and fears that thousands of 'refugees' would be thrown into the community without 24-hour care alternatives.[242] The government response has been no more than a 'provisional' delay of the closures.

Prospects for long-term care for Japan's frail older population are further affected by continued population ageing and changes in the structure and function of family care. In 2010, 23 per cent of Japanese people were aged 65 or more, the highest level in the world. It is predicted to reach 30 per cent by 2025.[243] Seventy-seven rural municipal authorities already had more than 40 per cent of over-65s in their populations in 2000, and the numbers are expected to increase rapidly as younger people migrate to the cities.[244] Some 2.8 million older people required some form of care in 2000 (expected to reach 5.3 million in 2025), with 48 per cent of these aged 80 or over.[245] In 2000, 3.03 million older people lived alone; this was expected to rise to over 6.8 million by 2025.[246] By 2025 LTCI expenditure will rise sharply from 7.9 billion yen in 2010 to 21 billion yen, requiring higher insurance premiums or taxation or both, and retrenchment in expenditure.[247] Opting for increasing insurance premiums and user fees will compound social inequality among older people. Thus the government and other agencies face a daunting task if LTCI services for *all* older people in need are to be secured in the current economic downturn and continued population ageing. This problem also confronts the British government, but Japan's situation may be more urgent and serious since its 2025 LTCI expenditure will represent 3.5 per cent of GDP, compared to an estimated 2 per cent for England.

3 THE NORFOLK EXPERIENCE

This chapter considers regional residential care arrangements for older people in England. It examines how national legislation and policies were interpreted and implemented by the local authorities or councils after the 1920s according to their individual contexts, rather than attempting to fit them within broad or assumed national trends. Focusing on statutory residential care provision, the chapter examines whether regional experiences have any relevance to the national context. Features peculiar to the region are noted, while stressing the interaction of national and regional priorities, influences and practices. The county of Norfolk is the English example, and the chapter looks at Norfolk county and Norwich county borough councils separately until the 1974 local government reform in England and Wales created the enlarged unitary Norfolk County Council.

In the early twentieth century, indoor long-term care for the aged poor, sick or frail in Norfolk was provided mainly in twenty-two union workhouses under the 1834 Poor Law, each administered by an elected board of guardians.[1] Under the 1929 Local Government Act, county and county borough councils took over Poor Law services and workhouses, which were subsequently administered by their Public Assistance Committees. Norfolk comprised three councils: Norfolk county itself and the more urban Norwich and Great Yarmouth county boroughs.

Norfolk is England's fifth largest county and covers 2,074 square miles of mainly rural and low-lying country. It was dominated by Conservative councils throughout the period studied.[2] Its sparse, largely homogeneous population increased from 505,000 in 1931 to 742,000 by 1991, people aged 65-plus then constituting 19.2 per cent, compared to the national average of 16.1 per cent.[3]

As an independent county borough until 1974, Norwich offered many contrasts to Norfolk county. It consisted of the principal city and the fourth most densely populated district in eastern England. Norwich had several major manufacturing industries, some of them in decline, and a long history of political radicalism.[4] Its population expanded slowly from 115,000 to 127,000 between 1931 and 1991, with its inhabitants aged 65-plus doubling from 8.6 to 17.1 per cent, again above the national average.

Different Starting Points, 1929–48

Norwich Workhouse: War Damage

Under the 1929 Act, Norwich county borough council established separate Public Assistance and Health Committees, with cooperation between the two encouraged.[5] It had one large general workhouse, built in 1859, which could house more than 1,000 paupers. It was described as 'a handsome red-brick building in the Tudor style', 'quite imposing' but 'very like that of a prison ... the only building in Norfolk to conform to the stereotype of the Victorian workhouse'.[6] There were fewer than 700 inmates, including quite a few 'casuals' and 160–70 sick patients in its infirmary, extended in 1911 to treat over 300 acute sick patients. This reflected a shift towards more specialized, medical-oriented care.[7] In contrast the 'house' contained almost exclusively aged or frail inmates – 141 of the 176 in 1926 were aged 65 or over, and the other thirty-five were frail.[8]

On 1 April 1930, the appointed day for the 1929 Act, the Norwich workhouse was renamed the Norwich Public Assistance Institution (PAI), catering for 730 inmates, half of them in the infirmary and a quarter classified as frail, although accommodated in the house.[9] Under the 1929 Act, local authorities could appropriate PAIs as public hospitals, thereby raising the prospects of improved health care, integrated services with other medical institutions and treatment untainted by stigma. However, the Norwich Public Assistance Committee initially considered that 'it was not practical from an administrative point of view for the buildings to be severed from the remainder of the Institution and run as a separate unit ... [with] some doubt whether the existing Infirmary was satisfactory and suitable for modern requirements'.[10]

The house featured a forty-bedded male dormitory and the women's infirmary wards with 110 beds, 'causing inevitable overcrowding'.[11] Amenities barely improved, and residents were allowed out on Saturday afternoons, subject to the master's permission.[12] A monotonous diet included a breakfast and supper of bread and margarine, with 'a bonus of cake' with Sunday supper, and those over 60 were allowed tea, butter and sugar instead of broth, if it was 'deemed expedient to make the change'.[13] Lunch featured meat pie or roast meat, vegetables and occasional puddings.[14] A twelve-year-old girl, who regularly visited with others to sing carols to residents during the 1930s, recalled:

> I shall never forget the stark surroundings – the smell of carbolic soap – the long skirts and aprons of the women and the grisly appearance of the men ... No smell of roast turkey and I can't remember seeing a Christmas tree but the high lofty ceilings and windows lent a brightness ... but it still feels grim[15]

Older able-bodied residents worked: men grew vegetables to supplement their meagre diet, with some taken on as casual workers by local farmers; women's duties included scrubbing the stone floors, sweeping and cleaning. Disciplinary measures, including a bread-only diet for one day, were imposed for the least offence. The pre-1929 classification of elderly 'inmates' persisted: Class I enjoyed the best conditions and privileges, whereas Class IV had the most basic conditions and had to work.[16] With the workhouse mentality as well as its physical legacy, local people resisted transfers to the infirmary wards at Norwich PAI (renamed Woodlands Hospital in 1941) and insisted on the voluntary Norfolk & Norwich Hospital.

The outbreak of the Second World War brought considerable hardship and disruption, with some sick wards adapted as an emergency medical service (EMS) section auxiliary to the main Norfolk & Norwich Hospital and 320 infirmary inpatients discharged.[17] Overcrowding was aggravated by casualty admissions and transfers from the Norfolk & Norwich and other EMS hospitals as well as the arrival of 191 London evacuees in October 1939.[18] The opening of the 105-bed male infirmary block in January 1940 helped, but did nothing for the women's side or the house.[19] Nursing shortages did not augur well for standards of care. Four additional nurses assisted 160 more infirmary inpatients by February 1940, but the reduction of four attendants in the house meant a falling attendant to patient ratio of 1:13.[20] Norwich PAI was bombed in air raids on 27 and 29 April 1942. A direct hit on the male house block, then accommodating 150 men, killed twelve 'old and feeble' residents and injured twenty others.[21] While 157 casualty cases were admitted, 601 existing patients/residents had to be evacuated to ten Norfolk PAIs (324 people) accompanied by sixteen female staff, to three mental hospitals (93) and to the nearby ancillary White Lodge Hospital (184, including casualties).[22] These emergency arrangements were made by the new Social Welfare Committee, which replaced the Public Assistance Committee in September 1941.[23]

The Committee also looked for suitable longer-term accommodation elsewhere, since reconstruction of the bombed block was impractical.[24] Provision for large numbers could not be found within Norwich, although temporary accommodation for 25–30 bedridden female cases was found at Crown Point, a large home just outside the area.[25] The Shipmeadow PAI near Beccles in east Suffolk, some eighteen miles from Norwich, was adapted as wartime accommodation. This was a former House of Industry built in 1767 and closed in the 1930s.[26] From September 1942 evacuees billeted in various Norfolk PAIs were transferred to Shipmeadow PAI (now renamed St James's Hospital), with a maximum capacity of 175 residents.[27] Sudden, traumatic events thus triggered 'temporary' arrangements that would last for more than a decade. By then the Norwich PAI accommodated some 300 patients/residents, including evacuees from various Norfolk PAIs, in undamaged blocks.[28]

For more permanent accommodation, the Committee envisaged a complex of buildings with 415 beds on a 16-acre site adjoining Earlham Green Lane, near Norwich PAI.[29] Proposals for specialist facilities for the bedridden, the less frail elderly, mental patients and twenty 'mother and baby' cases were frustrated by cost and planning issues, so the search resumed for existing premises that could be converted. The first Holmwood home for thirty frail female cases was approved in 1943, with twenty-two female patients moving from Norwich PAI later that year (see Table 3.1).[30] The Lawns, a former short-stay nursery under the Government Evacuation Scheme, was obtained in 1945 for thirty-five bedridden or frail female patients from Norwich PAI and Crown Point.[31] Mulburton Hall was added next, taking twenty-five female residents from Shipmeadow PAI, with The Oaks, a fourth home for thirty-five female cases, also approved.[32] However, there were no alternatives for males in Norwich PAI or Shipmeadow PAI, where overcrowding was severe, with 'as many as 58 patients in the attics'.[33] Nor was good quality care maintained in the newly opened small homes: incidents at The Lawns involved 'careless treatment and unkind remarks from matron and the younger nurses'.[34]

Norfolk Workhouses: Survival

A joint Public Health and Assistance Committee was established for Norfolk under the 1929 Act to coordinate services and maximize economic resources without duplication.[35] Its Public Assistance Sub-Committee (PASC) supervised the thirteen new local Areas, which succeeded the Poor Law Unions.[36] On the appointed day for the 1929 Act, the PASC took over fourteen former union workhouses, with a combined bed capacity of almost 2,000, and renamed these PAIs (see Map 3.1).[37] With the exception of Attleborough PAI, all were very old. Three were built before 1780 and the rest during the 1830s and 1840s. They were long overdue for structural alterations and improvements. At least six were considered 'all bad and not really adaptable in any scheme for the chronic sick'.[38] They were also large, averaging 150 beds each (King's Lynn PAI exceeded 300), with wards or dormitories of 10–15 beds, though some wards housed more than forty. Most did not satisfy local needs: as Map 3.1 shows, Area 5 had a population of 36,000 and two PAIs, whereas Areas 4 and 6 covered 38,000 people, but had none.[39]

In 1930 Norfolk's fourteen PAIs catered for an average of almost 1,300 residents, who largely 'approximate to one single class, i.e. the aged chronic – half of whom are ill enough to be in the sick wards'.[40] The County Medical Officer's annual report that year suggested that 985 PAI beds were designated for the sick, 830 of them for chronic mostly elderly cases, with others reserved for mental patients (45), sick children (50), maternity cases (30), tuberculosis sufferers (10) and others (20).[41] Most PAIs distinguished between sick/frail wards and 'house' resident accommodation, although only two had infirmaries.[42] Among the sick, chronic elderly patients sometimes mixed with the mentally ill or senile, sick children or even tuberculosis sufferers.[43] Similarly, in 'house' dormitories, frail elderly residents were often placed with casuals. The predominance of sick or frail elderly people meant that the PAIs were 'really homes for the aged with the concurrent diseases'.[44] There were perhaps 1,000 older residents altogether in Norfolk PAIs in 1931, 2.8 per cent of the county's older population. Other needy groups were housed separately.[45]

Using local authority appropriations under the 1929 Act, the PASC earmarked Swainsthorpe PAI, on the outskirts of Norwich, for non-violent senile patients. They were transferred from nearby St Andrew's, a county mental hospital, where more than 100 such cases were inappropriately accommodated, with 'distinct overcrowding'.[46] Swainsthorpe was adapted for 176 patients, and thirty-five residents were moved to neighbouring PAIs as senile patients began to arrive, followed by other PAI 'troublesome patients'.[47] Heckingham PAI was appropriated as a 'low-grade defectives' institution, ancillary to the county mental deficiency colony at Little Plumstead Hall, opened in 1930.[48] When Heckingham PAI was transferred to the Mental Deficiency Acts Committee in 1932, its fifty-eight residents had to move to nearby PAIs.[49] Both measures eased overcrowding and made better classification and location of patients possible. They also saved Norfolk county council considerable expenditure on additional hospital or colony accommodation – Swainsthorpe's economies alone exceeded £71,000.[50]

Following an extensive survey of Norfolk PAIs in 1933, the Ministry of Health recommended the appropriation of Attleborough PAI as a public hospital. Yet the PASC felt that 'the present two-fold service (Poor Law Institution [*sic*] and Voluntary Hospital) adequately meets the needs of the sick in a county such as Norfolk'. It concluded that 'it does not appear necessary to adopt any further classification beyond that of senile dementia and epilepsy'.[51] The location of PAIs was also considered, as 'persons admitted to ... Institutions should be as near as possible to their homes'.[52] Plans to adapt Gayton PAI for dementia cases were discussed but not implemented, while rationalization proposals led to the closure of Great Snoring PAI in 1934, as it was underused.[53]

Unlike Norwich PAI, Norfolk PAIs suffered only minor or temporary wartime disruption, although conversion of Attleborough PAI to an EMS hospital in September 1939 resulted in the dispersal of its residents among three neighbouring PAIs.[54] EMS arrangements in King's Lynn PAI increased its bed occupancy rates from 38 to 72 per cent by 1942.[55] Similarly, the 324 evacuees from Norwich PAI in 1942 briefly raised bed occupancy rates. Various wartime arrangements, involving EMS civilian inpatient transfers, London evacuees and even prisoners of war or refugees from Europe, featured in some Norfolk PAIs, but caused no major disruption.[56] Most Norfolk PAIs escaped bombing and were able to maintain more than 1,700 beds, with occupancy rates averaging 75 per cent.[57]

For this reason, developments in alternative or supplementary accommodation for older people were limited. Norfolk's only hostel for the aged, The Lodge in Mulbarton, was used by ten homeless Norwich elders and was run by the Forehoe and Henstead Rural District Council under the Government Evacuation Scheme. In 1944 visiting Norfolk PASC representatives 'were very much impressed with the Hostel ... The rooms are light and airy and they [the residents] appeared to be very happy'.[58] Such accommodation might 'give as good an imitation of home life with the accompanying freedom of action together with the amenities'.[59] Nevertheless, 'the question of old people's homes must necessarily be left for the time being', whereas 'accommodation for poor law children could ... be put in hand straight away'.[60]

Renewed interest followed the Ministry's 1947 Circular 49/47, 'The Care of the Aged in Public Assistance Homes and Institutions', which urged local authorities to improve their institutional provision for older people.[61] Accordingly, the PASC looked for suitable premises: small homes for 30–5 people of both sexes, in or on the outskirts of towns, and well away from PAIs. Its first successful negotiation involved Catton Hall, just north of Norwich, in September 1947.[62] Ironically, Norfolk's only hostel, The Lodge, was closed in 1947, as it had just four residents due to 'the condition of the property and particularly ... its isolated position'.[63] Like Norwich PAI, life in Norfolk PAIs barely improved: starting in 1931 residents might have 'books delivered ... through the County Library, daily papers and periodicals', but installation of a wireless came late, and only Gressenhall PAI had a shop where small luxuries could be purchased.[64] Basic improvements here included some windows 'lowered by two feet to allow patients in bed to see out' and benches replaced by chairs in 1947.[65]

To summarize: over the decade preceding 5 July 1948 (the appointed day for the 1948 National Assistance Act), Norwich and Norfolk developed contrasting forms of accommodation for sick and infirm older people. External factors played a major role in Norwich. Its only workhouse/PAI was part-adapted as an EMS section; the male house accommodation was severely bombed; and it was finally appropriated in 1948 as a hospital under the 1946 NHS Act. All this forced the new Social Welfare Committee to seek alternative accommodation, acquiring and converting old premises to clear temporary beds at Norwich PAI and Shipmeadow PAI as rapidly as possible. Proposals for three small homes for female cases were drawn up by 1948, with a fourth for another thirty-five in its final stages. Provision for male patients was less advanced as plans for Earlham Green Lane were frustrated, but accommodation searches were in progress, and given the record for female patients, the prospects were promising.

In contrast, Norfolk PAIs were largely untouched by the war, and the only hostel for the aged closed. Only in 1947 did the PASC finally start looking for small homes. None had opened, although six properties were in the process of being acquired. It is reasonable to assume that the very different starting points of the two authorities would affect regional residential care developments and policies in the post-1948 era. Similarities are found between the two, however. Neither Norwich nor Norfolk PAIs experienced major improvements during 1929–48 because both authorities were reluctant to invest in them, particularly if there was any likelihood that they would be transferred to the respective Health Committees or be closed. Yet new appropriations were slow to take effect. Meanwhile, more than 100, mainly elderly, Norfolk PAI residents were transferred from local PAIs to others under the limited rationalization measures in response to cost criteria.

Contrasting Developments, 1948–63

Norwich Hostels: Transition to Hostels

Post-war welfare legislation categorized the former workhouse/PAI resident population, the 1948 National Assistance Act requiring local authorities to provide residential or Part III accommodation for those 'in need of care and attention', with the 'sick' transferred to hospitals managed by Regional Hospital Boards (RHBs) under the 1946 NHS Act. In Norwich the RHB took over the former Norwich workhouse/PAI (renamed the West Norwich Hospital), with its 125, mainly aged, chronic sick patients.[66] A new Welfare Committee succeeded the Social Welfare Committee, with a Hostels Sub-Committee responsible for former Shipmeadow PAI (renamed St James's Home), with its 135, mostly aged, male residents and the three small hostels with ninety older women. This suggested comparatively good local provision, although there were few local authority-supported residents in voluntary homes.[67]

In 1949 the opening of The Oaks, a fourth hostel for thirty women from St James's Home, marked the end of former PAI accommodation for women, and the Hostels Sub-Committee declared 'the acquisition of four or five additional hostels' for men as its next priority, since St James's Home was 'a temporary establishment ... remotely situated and in a very poor state of repair', according to the Ministry of Health inspection report.[68] Two small hostels for men, Hill House and Drayton Wood, opened in 1951, followed in 1954 by the first mixed hostel, Eaton Hall, and a sixty-two-place male hostel, The Grove, after which St James's Home was closed. Meanwhile, the first purpose-built voluntary home for older people, Corton House, opened in 1952. It provided thirty beds, including ten designated for Norwich or Norfolk local authority-supported residents.[69] Thus by 1954 the Hostels Sub-Committee had established a creditable 270 places – 'Norwich a Pioneer with Home for the Elderly' and 'Eaton Hall ... Clear Example of 20th Century Social Progress'.[70] In contrast, the former Norwich workhouse, West Norwich Hospital, had no major alterations or renovation, but was accommodating 100 or so mainly aged chronic sick patients, alongside 170 acute sick cases in 1955.[71]

The Norwich hostels ranged from urban dwellings with tiny gardens on main roads to isolated country houses in spacious grounds.[72] Each (barring The Grove) provided around thirty places and was segregated by sex (apart from Eaton Hall). Most hostels had an informal atmosphere and offered various recreations, including handicrafts (from 1953), film shows (1954) and television (1955).[73] But they suffered the disadvantages of dated, converted properties: three were at least five miles from central Norwich, and most were obsolete – Mulbarton Hall dated from 1750 and several others were nineteenth-century buildings. They were all demolished or rebuilt from the mid-1960s.

Overcrowding was common, with high ratios of shared rooms and packed communal spaces. Of the 285 available beds, 89.1 per cent were in 3–8-bedded rooms, leaving just five in singles and twenty-six in doubles. The thirty-place Holmwood offered only 3–6-bedded rooms, and the matron of the thirty-place Eaton Hall reported that at mealtimes it was 'quite impossible to sit them all comfortably ... There was no room at all to pass the food and attend to their wants'.[74] The problems worsened as waiting lists grew in the late 1950s, and some hostels put extra beds in existing bedrooms.[75] Furthermore, the layout of the hostels was unsuitable for growing numbers of very elderly, frail or disabled occupants. In 1960 the average age of residents was 78 years, with twenty-three over 90 and some 150 requiring considerable nursing care.[76] Yet only seventy residents had ground-floor accommodation, and without lifts, the rest had restricted access to the grounds, dining hall or dayrooms.

Staff shortages reflected difficulties with recruitment and the remoteness of some hostels. None had designated night attendants even in 1957, and during the day as well as at weekends in the early 1960s, just one attendant might be on hand.[77] Nursing staff to resident ratios averaged 1:6 in 1960 (1:9 at The Grove), which limited care standards: roughly half its residents had only one bath a fortnight, the matron reporting that 'she will need 42 hours more staff time if all [69] residents are to be bathed weekly'.[78] An increase in part-time nursing staff followed the reduced staff working hours from the late 1950s, and five of the eight Norwich hostels still had no full-time day or night attendants by 1962.[79] Yet problems in the converted homes could not necessarily have been anticipated and were a somewhat unkind penalty on early and prompt local efforts to follow ministerial directions, rather than await the outcome of measures taken elsewhere.

Nevertheless, in prioritizing the closure of St James's Home, the Hostel Sub-Committee focused on existing residents rather than new applicants or patients transferred from geriatric and psychiatric hospitals. Indeed, once St James's final female residents had transferred to The Oaks in 1949, it had assumed that 'no additional residential accommodation would be required for female residents'.[80] The first five-year local plan, submitted in 1949, envisaged just nineteen additional places to meet new demand up to 1954, promptly increased to ninety by the Ministry.[81] The Committee also appeared oblivious to accelerated demand for residential accommodation, as smaller, more attractive and conveniently located replacement hostels became available. Whereas the 1950 waiting list for St James's Home was negligible, twenty people were waiting for small hostels in 1950, rising to eighty by 1959.[82] Meanwhile, twelve more beds were squeezed into existing homes and five frail women were admitted to newly designated local authority-supported wards in the voluntary Great Hospital, with five more on its waiting list.[83] In 1955 a short-stay scheme was introduced for frail older people living at home to ease the care burden on their relatives.[84]

By then the Committee had acknowledged that more residential provision was needed. This was seen in the establishment of a Joint Sub-Committee of the Health, Housing and Welfare Committees to consider an 'old people's community' on a 1.5-acre site at the Midland Street Clearance Area.[85] Within this complex was the first purpose-built home, Alderman Clarke House, a two-storey building offering thirty-two places, including fourteen ground-floor beds for frail residents.[86] A similar home, Bishop Herbert House, provided for thirty younger physically handicapped people, followed in 1962 by Heartsease Hostel, which duplicated Alderman Clarke House.[87] Northfields House was completed in 1963 and replaced Hill House.[88]

By 1962 Norwich had ten small hostels, two of them purpose-built, with 360 Part III places representing 21.1 beds per 1,000 of its older population, well above the national average of 16.1.[89] There were also thirty-nine local authority-supported residents in voluntary homes, but forty remained on waiting lists, with projected increases to 100 in 1970 and 147 by 1975.[90] To address their needs, the ten-year local plan for 1962–72 included a thirty-five-place home at Ber Street in 1963, a thirty-place home for dementia cases in 1966 and two sixty-place homes after 1967. It was assumed that these new places would be sufficient for the next decade.[91] The plan was submitted to the Ministry and incorporated into *Health and Welfare: The Development of Community Care*, published in 1963. Overall, Norwich's planned 545 places by 1972 represented 27.4 places per 1,000 older population, again ahead of the estimated national average of 20.0 per 1,000.[92]

Norfolk: Two-Tier Development

A 1948 survey confirmed high levels of physical or mental disability among the 1,100 residents in Norfolk PAIs: nearly a quarter suffered from senile dementia, a similar number were bedridden and almost a third required some nursing and could no longer live at home.[93] This usefully demarcated them into the chronic sick group requiring health care in NHS hospitals and the non-sick, frail group requiring care in residential or Part III homes. On the appointed day for the 1946 NHS and 1948 National Assistance Acts, the twelve Norfolk PAIs became seven Part III homes and five NHS hospitals, though all (other than two of the hospitals) were under joint-user arrangements, and so had both Part III and NHS beds (see Map 3.2).[94] The new Welfare Committee assumed responsibility for 315 non-sick Part III residents, but joint-user arrangements meant 111 of these were accommodated in NHS hospitals, while two-thirds (388) of the beds in the Part III homes were occupied by NHS patients.[95] This blurring of the demarcation between Part III homes and NHS hospitals would continue for two decades. To avoid any association with the workhouse, the Welfare Committee classified its new Part III homes as 'county homes' and renamed them: for example, Gayton PAI became Eastgate House.[96] Yet the buildings physically expressed the Poor Law legacy as they were former workhouses/PAIs.

When preparing for its first five-year local plan in 1949, Norfolk provided neither small hostels nor local authority-supported voluntary home places.[97] Its plan addressed this by adopting a two-tier approach. Thus it proposed six small converted hostels offering 170–80 beds for 'normal old people', and suggested that 'infirm and handicapped persons' would be provided for 'by improving and effectively modernizing the whole or portions of three of the existing county homes'.[98] These were Homelea (formerly Lingwood PAI), Howdale Home (formerly Downham Market PAI) and Hill House (formerly Pulham Market PAI), which together were accommodating ninety-seven Part III residents and 204 NHS patients.[99] Beech House (formerly Gressenhall PAI) would provide 'supplementary accommodation', with St Barnabas's (formerly Thetford PAI), Eastgate House (formerly Gayton PAI) and Beckham House (formerly West Beckham PAI) closing, as alternative accommodation and other circumstances permitted. By offering small hostel places for more active residents and county home places for the frail, 'the Council will meet the total estimated needs of their area'.[100] But this underestimated residential accommodation needs, restricting suggested 'homely' hostel-type provision to more active residents, and retained at least four former workhouses/PAIs. Nevertheless, ministerial approval was obtained.

The number of Part III residents rose from 300 in 1948 to 550 in 1951, mainly because the RHB, faced with severe bed shortages and long waiting lists, transferred its elderly chronic sick cases to the Welfare Committee.[101] The RHB also had to deal with a growing number of chronic sick or very frail patients who were unsuitable for transfer to Part III accommodation. While retaining 260 beds in Part III county homes, the RHB 'felt unable to promise to evacuate any particular number of beds by any particular date'.[102] For its part, the Welfare Committee was deterred from reducing its joint-user beds or 'proceeding with the modernization of the three county homes'.[103] For this reason, revised estimates suggested that only 100 county home residents (18 per cent of the total) were fit enough for transfer to hostels, implying that the six planned hostels were sufficient.[104] They accordingly noted that some 450–500 frail residents would remain in the three county homes, with Beech House used as a fourth 'on a more or less permanent basis' for 'anti-social and dirty types'.[105] By substituting yet another former PAI for new hostels, they confirmed that Norfolk was 'in the fortunate position of having sufficient accommodation in their retained county homes to meet their probable needs'.[106] Evidently, obsolete former PAIs were considered good enough for frail older residents, since 'experience has made it clear that there will always be a need for larger establishments'.[107]

Between 1951 and 1953 the six planned hostels opened across Norfolk, while ex-PAI St Barnabas's closed and its residents moved to a new hostel nearby (see Map 3.3 and Table 3.2).[108] These offered 200 places for more active male and female residents and were 'up to a standard which provides the maximum comfort for the residents'.[109] They featured more private arrangements: almost half the twenty-seven places at Keys Hill were in single or double rooms, and the thirty-eight-place Burnham Westgate Hall provided separate cubicles, some with their own lavatory facilities, for thirty single persons and four married couples.[110] This necessitated construction or adaptation costs per bed of £691 compared to the £593 national average.[111] Other accommodation was more variable: former voluntary premises near Attleborough were converted into the eighteen-place Lord Kitchener hostel, but this 'small ... uneconomic and poorly sited' residence was earmarked for closure under the ten-year local plan for 1962–72.[112] Sea Marge, an Edwardian, mansion-style house, opened for fifty-five frail residents in 1955, taking residents from the nearby ex-PAI Beckham House which then closed, an exercise in upgrading from 'poor accommodation' to an 'Excellent Home'.[113]

As in Norwich, smaller, more homely and conveniently located hostels attracted 'a new type of resident':[114] 'the large majority of hostel residents are admitted direct from their own homes and a fair proportion are people who would not consider admission into a county home'.[115] Consequently, the number of Part III residents in county homes was unchanged at around 550 during 1951–7, even though 250 or so hostel places had been created by 1955.[116] Many hostel residents were much older and less mobile, but the converted hostels had no lifts and only about one in seven of their places were in ground-floor accommodation.[117] Yet very few premises were capable of conversion into thirty-place hostels for such a clientele, whether near existing county homes or where demand for residential accommodation was high, reflecting Norfolk's size and scattered population.

Early in 1954 Great Yarmouth borough council opened its own purpose-built home, The Lawns. It was described as 'the most up-to-date and well equipped establishment ... in the country' and offered thirty-five single ground-floor bedrooms with 'none of the "institution atmosphere"'.[118] Suitably impressed, the

Norfolk Committee turned its attention to purpose-built homes, first seen in King's Lynn where demand for residential accommodation was high and where the nearby ex-PAI Eastgate House was scheduled for closure. In 1957 the 'more suitably and conveniently situated' Sydney Dye House opened, providing thirty single and three double rooms, half of them on the ground floor.[119] It had two relatively separate wings, with 'domestic properties ... to avoid institutional appearance'.[120] Furthermore, 'there are no irksome rules or regulations'.[121] This led the Committee Chair, Sydney Dye MP, to claim that Norfolk '[is] probably now one of the most advanced counties in England'.[122] Significantly, its residents were neither from the 60-plus cohort at the top of Norfolk's general hostels waiting list for urgent help nor from ex-PAI Eastgate House, but 'new applicants mainly from King's Lynn itself'.[123]

Recognizing areas of higher demand, the Committee obtained ministerial approval for more homes in 1958.[124] To cover central and western districts, St Nicholas's House opened at East Dereham in 1960, followed by Westfields at Swaffham in 1961.[125] Quebec Hall, a voluntary residential home, also opened at East Dereham in 1960, providing twenty places with forty-eight adjoining purpose-built bungalows for more active people, but benefiting mainly the better-off.[126] The two council homes closely resembled Sydney Dye House, but introduced four-bedded rooms.[127] This suggested greater economies, although the Committee Chair, Mrs Ethel Tipple, argued that 'while a number of people preferred a single bedroom, quite a large proportion did not ... a companion in their room ... gave them a feeling of security'.[128] This is questionable, but it is noteworthy that 'there was no question of paying a little more to secure a special type of accommodation in any of the Committee's homes. Everyone was treated the same whatever their financial provision'.[129] Serving north-east Norfolk, Aegel House opened at Aylsham in 1962, the first of the larger sixty-place homes, twenty of these in four-bedded rooms facilitating efficient and economic use of staff to care for frail residents.[130] This 'splendid achievement ... well designed and well situated in quiet surroundings' was an improvement on the converted hostels.[131] Woodlands, a similar sixty-place home at King's Lynn, was included in the ten-year local plan for 1962–72, primarily to replace Eastgate House.[132]

These new homes increased the stock of places and addressed the poor distribution of accommodation.[133] Moreover, it became possible to find and approve sites well in advance of construction, allowing time for investigation into current demand and projected needs in particular districts. This was also an advantage in the struggle for loan sanction for capital projects, since in the event of ministerial surpluses, the Norfolk Committee had sites earmarked and plans ready for approval.

At the time of submitting its ten-year local plan in 1962, Norfolk provided some 950 residential places, 465 in twelve small hostels (three of them purpose-built) and 485 in five former PAI county homes (See Map 3.3 and Table 3.2).[134] This represented 17.0 places per 1,000 county older population, marginally above the 16.1 national average, although 51 per cent remained in former PAIs. Joint-user arrangements were retained with seventy NHS patients in Howdale Home. The ten-year local plan envisaged replacing all five ex-PAIs with ten homes (490 places), along with five additional homes (220 places) to meet demand. A thirty-six-place home, partly to replace Lord Kitchener hostel, and two fifty-place homes specifically for dementia cases were also planned. With 340 new places by 1972, Norfolk would have twenty-nine 'small' homes, offering 1,290 places (19.8 per 1,000 county elderly population). If just short of national recommended averages of 20.0 per 1,000, these plans represented significant progress, not least in reducing the average home size from 100 to forty-four places. Given its inheritance of poor accommodation, the patchy distribution of places and the complexity of joint-user arrangements, the Norfolk Welfare Committee had made real progress, with the ten-year local plan to erase the imprint of former PAIs now a plausible objective.

The Consequences of Ministerial Priorities, 1963–73

Norwich: Modernization Halted

Only months after its ten-year local plan was published, Norwich Welfare Committee revised its capital programme, postponing the Ber Street home and dropping plans for a thirty-place home for dementia cases.[135] The following year, proposals to develop the Ber Street home jointly with thirty flats for independent older people were frustrated by the Ministry, which expressed concern 'that as the occupants of the flats became older ... the building would tend to become a large hostel for about 80 people' and that 'the space standards and estimated building costs were high'.[136] It therefore deferred sanctioning grant loans until 1966.[137] By then, the waiting list for Part III places had increased more than three-fold, with over half the 160 applicants 'in very urgent need' and 'between 15 and 20 people ... a real cause for anxiety'.[138] Alternative services offered little relief, with just forty older people in special housing in 1963, far below national guidelines.[139] Future projects were unpromising: the planned number of hospital beds for 1975 was barely higher than in 1962 and represented the lowest ratio to its older population in the East Anglia region.[140]

Inspections in 1965–6 of the seven converted hostels revealed 'unsatisfactory' conditions: lack of lifts, ground-floor beds and basic amenities; uneven flooring; many steps; and 'a great deal of overcrowding'.[141] Yet the Ministry sanctioned only £5,000 for a meals-on-wheels kitchen from the Committee's £264,000 capital programme for 1966–9. Essentially, Norwich was caught between ministerial priorities, which favoured 'projects which materially assist in the early closure of former Public Assistance Institutions' and those 'local authorities whose scale of provision is below the national average'.[142]

Quality issues were recognized, with the 1965 information booklet emphasizing that 'a homely and happy atmosphere shall prevail in the home and you and your fellow residents shall have the fullest possible independence and freedom'.[143] The revised modernization programme for converted hostels in 1964 included the appointment of an additional welfare officer to undertake routine visiting of older residents, and regular meetings of the chief welfare officer, matrons and superintendents of hostels to discuss general management issues.[144] A four-day refresher course for matrons and hostel superintendents in 1965 was followed by short courses for attendants. The Committee subsequently intended 'to give all residential staff the opportunity eventually of attending such a course'.[145]

Other innovations included respite care in some Norwich homes, giving family and informal carers short breaks, and day care for frail or house-bound older people.[146] This, however, was restricted by lack of space, staff and transport, so that only a handful of people were benefiting as late as 1971.[147] Day care provision for confused older people was introduced at the Bethel Hospital in 1972, which was soon supporting about twelve people every day.[148] A one-week 'holiday exchange' between Norwich and Great Yarmouth hostels offered a change of scene and hospitality from 1962. Other Norfolk hostels were soon attracted.[149] The scheme was restricted to better-off residents as it had to be paid for in full.

Early in 1968 Foulgers House in Ber Street opened. This was Norwich's first post-1963 home and the last to have associated dwellings for independent older people.[150] But this failed to ease the growing waiting list or satisfy ministerial priorities. Squeezing more beds into existing homes statistically had a perverse effect, 'because the overcrowding of existing hostel accommodation produces figures which, in comparison with other local authorities, suggest that we are better off than is the case'.[151] Consequently, in 1969 the Committee turned to the quality of existing hostels in the hope that its revised policy would be 'less likely to conflict with Department of Health and Social Security attitudes to loan sanction'.[152] As a result, there were no new residential places and fewer beds for its older population, but 'a far better quality' of existing hostels could, it was claimed, be achieved.[153] Accordingly, the 1964 modernization programme for converted hostels was revised in 1970 to provide 'single rooms which allow for privacy and a sense of identity'.[154] Just five residents (less than 2 per cent) in earlier converted hostels had single rooms, compared with 42 per cent in post-1957 purpose-built hostels or almost 90 per cent at the proposed thirty-seven-place home at Philadelphia Lane.[155] Finally, the Department of Health and Social Security (DHSS) relaxed loan sanction, allowing the new Social Service Committee (which replaced the Welfare Committee under the 1970 Local Social

Services Act) to build six forty-five-place homes during 1971–4 to replace its seven converted hostels.[156] Even so, in 1972, 'as yet, no beds have been replaced under the modernization scheme'.[157]

The new Committee started with the first replacement home at Unthank Road. This was based on a model constructed at Fulbourn, near Cambridge, designed for forty-eight residents in three two-storey wings.[158] Small-group living arrangements facilitated 'group identity and flexibility in management, and … [a] move from single sex to mixed homes'.[159] Moreover, they addressed the needs of 100 or so confused residents, who made up more than a quarter of the total Part III resident population by 1971. They remained in ordinary Part III homes under the Committee's policy 'not to segregate the elderly mentally frail and confused residents but to integrate them in all the homes'.[160] Meanwhile, geriatric and psycho-geriatric hospital beds were being phased out, and the reduction of beds at the Vale Hospital (formerly Swainthorpe PAI, designated for dementia cases) meant more confused people were in need of Part III accommodation. Within the new-style home, one or two units were designated for such cases 'to minimize the impact they may make on the other residents in the hostel'.[161] The new design and approach were later adopted at other replacement homes.

By 1972 the Committee had eleven homes offering 390 places (20.7 beds per 1,000 county elderly population), a bare improvement on 360 places in 1963 and considerably fewer than the 545 places envisaged under its 1962 ten-year local plan.[162] Anticipating more generous DHSS investment budgets, the Committee hoped to meet demand, end the waiting list of 120 and complete its modernization scheme.[163] Accordingly, its capital programme under its 1973 ten-year local plan included four additional homes (190 places) and five replacement homes (240 places), all based on the Unthank Road home design. In all, there would be 600 places in fourteen purpose-built homes by 1983, with some fifty local authority-supported voluntary home places.

This fulfilled the 1962 ten-year local plan one decade late, which raises the question whether the 1973 plan was sufficiently innovative. Indeed, Norwich's residential care arrangements by 1973 were no longer in advance of other local authorities. Worse was to come when the DHSS announced cuts and asked local authorities to revise and defer their capital programmes. The Committee consequently postponed work on its four additional homes, though all the five replacement homes were already under construction and deemed 'irrevocably committed' projects.[164]

Norfolk: The Survival of the Workhouse

The Norfolk Welfare Committee focused on the early closure and replacement of former PAI facilities under its ten-year local plan for 1962–72. In 1963 Woodlands in King's Lynn was completed, finally replacing Eastgate House, and in 1965 replacement homes at Stalham and Brundall allowed the closure of Homelea (see Map 3.4 and Table 3.2). The first stage of the Beech House closure scheme was instigated with the construction of replacement homes at Fakenham and Watton. However, there were still 295 people on the Part III accommodation waiting list, some of whom were 'in dire straits and in more need than some people already in hospital'.[165] This was compounded by the reclassification of NHS inpatients to Part III status and the reduction of geriatric and psychiatric hospital beds envisaged under the 1962 Hospital Plan.[166] One response was to encourage private home arrangements, with almost half (100) of the 1964 applicants admitted to such facilities, suggesting an emerging mixed economy in residential care.[167] Home help services were also promoted and in seventy cases 'specifically prevented the need for admission to Part III accommodation'.[168] Meanwhile, the first post-1963 home to address growing local demand opened at Rose Meadow in North Walsham in 1965. Nevertheless, Norfolk's Part III accommodation waiting list exceeded 500 by 1966, with sixty-two cases regarded as 'very urgent'.[169] Joint-user arrangements posed a particular problem at Howdale Home, which still had seventy NHS patients in 1965, since their retention blocked beds designated for Part III residents and delayed the second phase, a thirty-place wing addition.[170] Consequently, the Committee proposed a new sixty-place home at Heacham to replace Howdale Home and meet new demand in the area. This escaped the 1965 Ministry 'six-month deferment' on capital projects, although the home's capacity was reduced to forty-five places.[171]

However, the four additional homes in the ten-year local plan for 1962–72 were deferred, as was the closure programme for former PAIs, leaving the Committee with 'no alternative but to continue to use these establishments for a much longer period of time than ... anticipated'.[172] Deferrals delayed the ten-year local plan 'by 2.5 years', contradicting the priority of making 'two-thirds of the capital investment available to local authorities whose scale of provision is below the national average, the remaining one-third ... for projects which materially assist in the earlier closure of former public assistance institutions'.[173] Ironically, Norfolk had 'slightly above the national average' of Part III places per 1,000 older population, precisely because delayed closure of former PAIs retained some 400 beds or 40 per cent of the County's Part III residential stocks in 1966.[174] The Committee felt 'handicapped' by this, particularly since the county's 1969 65-plus population at 65,500 already exceeded the 1965 Registrar General's prediction of 64,400 by 1976.[175] Although the Committee replaced roughly 230 former PAI places between 1964 and 1970 and provided about 200 more to meet new demand, it was forced to keep open Hill House (108 places) and Beech House (117 places).[176] By 1970 there were 950 applicants for Part III places annually, with 700 on the waiting list. In addition, 350 self-funded residents were in private and voluntary homes.[177]

Alternatives to avoid or delay admissions to residential homes emerged and developed: the Committee's home help services assisted 3,100 older people in 1970, compared to 950 in 1965.[178] Some ninety meals-on-wheels schemes were in operation following a trial in the early 1960s, providing meals for over 1,000 older people. In addition, the housing needs of some 1,000 very elderly and frail people were addressed by forty-five sheltered housing schemes. As in Norwich, local authority Part III homes offered short-term amenities for up to two weeks, giving relatives of frail older people 'a well-earned rest'.[179] Between 1965 and 1970 the number assisted increased from sixty-five to 150 each year, and the first separate short-stay home opened at Acle in late 1975.[180] Day care provision offered 'relief to relatives [and] ... the house-bound elderly a new interest'.[181] Regarded as 'preventative ... less expensive alternative forms of care', the first day centre for thirty people opened in a building adjacent to Woodlands in 1972.[182] Collectively, such measures were useful, if limited, substitutes for 'full' residential home provision.

A further 'temporary expedient' was the deferred closure of Beech House until 1975, allowing 'the whole of the beds at the new [replacement] home at Watton to accommodate cases on the urgent waiting list'.[183] Similarly, a new home earmarked for growing demand in the Loddon area was integrated into the Hill House closure programme in 1971, while the forty-one-place St Edmund's home in Attleborough amalgamated with the nearby eighteen-place Lord Kitchener home rather than replacing it. A more radical plan involved the Committee building residential homes from moneys raised by selling land and former PAIs, obviating the need to borrow from or comply with central government. This envisaged six or so 'smaller homes (village homes) in conjunction with the provision of grouped dwellings for the elderly by the District Councils'.[184] Accordingly, a twenty-one-place home, Munhaven, with twenty adjoining bungalows opened in Mundesley in 1970, administered jointly with Erpingham Rural District Council.

This was a single-storey, purpose-built facility, featuring 'bedrooms grouped around a central "garden area"', with shared amenities, sitting rooms, a dining room and a 'general purpose room ... used for hairdressing, chiropody, etc. ... [which] ... proved most convenient'.[185] Similar designs were adopted in smaller homes, while small living units featured within larger ones.[186] The thirty-five-place Ketts Lodge in Wymondham, built in 1971, was a single-storey building, 'cruciform in shape ... The north, west and south wings will contain bedroom, sitting and toilet accommodation, and each wing is more-or-less self-contained'.[187] Similarly, the sixty-six-place Sydney House in Stalham (1964) and the forty-one-place Rose Meadow in North Walsham (1965) were designed with single-storey wings 'domestic in character and small in size', 'to encourage a homely atmosphere'.[188] Privacy and quality of care for residents were emphasized, with 'fewer double bedrooms and more singles'.[189] Thus, the second wing of High Haven, which replaced

Howdale in 1969, comprised fourteen singles and five doubles, compared to the four-bedded room arrangements in the 1958-built wing.[190] Similarly, twenty-one of the thirty-five places in Ketts Lodge were in single rooms, while a proposed home at Hellesdon comprised twenty-one singles and just two doubles.[191] These later homes also addressed the needs of more elderly and frailer residents by providing larger lifts, staircases with handrails on both sides, bedrooms connected to an internal call system and doors wide enough to accommodate wheelchairs. Day-time attendant staff to resident ratios were reduced from 1:9 in 1965 to 1:7.5 in 1967 and 1:6 by 1970, with an ambitious 1:4 proposed under the 1973 ten-year local plan, accompanied by increased staff training.[192]

The particular needs of some 200 confused residents, who made up 20 per cent of the total Norfolk Part III population in 1969, also had to be considered, as were the additional sixty mental hospital elderly inpatients waiting for transfers.[193] Ketts Lodge was the first home for those who 'would be a source of difficulty if they were in ordinary homes for the elderly'.[194] They required 'a very demanding degree of attention'; even so, thirty-six deaths were reported there during an eighteen-month period in 1972–3.[195] Accordingly, the staff establishment was revised, with the ratio of attendant staff to residents reduced from 1:6 to 1:4 and two additional night attendants from 1974. Contrasting with the policy of integration of confused people with other residents adopted in Norwich, the Norfolk Committee saw Ketts Lodge as its model for later homes, though none was built.

With the relaxation of loan sanction, the DHSS approved nine homes during 1971–3, including replacements for the last two ex-PAIs.[196] In 1972 homes at Harker House (Long Stratton) and Beauchamp House (Chedgrave) replaced Hill House, and the second phase of the closure of Beech House was underway the following year, with one replacement home opened at Glaven Hale (Holt) and two more at Diss and Costessey approved.[197] In preparing the ten-year local plan in 1973, the Committee sought to embody the requirement of 'at least two new homes every year' for the first time since 1964 and to 'preserve the present ratio of 19 places per 1,000 of the elderly'.[198] Accordingly, the ten-year local plan envisaged 280 additional places in ten new homes, including two to replace Beech House.[199] It also included a forty-place holiday home, a forty-place day centre and a trebling to 190 of local authority-supported places in voluntary homes, underpinned by substantial grant increases to voluntary organizations. Expansion of community care services was also envisaged, including a '90% increase in home help services [and a] 148% increase in meals-on-wheels'.[200] Yet financial constraints soon led to the deferral of the Beech House replacement homes by a further year. Proposed new homes at Acle and Hellesdon, already approved by the DHSS, narrowly escaped cancellation, although both were delayed and used as short-stay homes. Ominously, the revised 1974–7 capital programme included no new homes.[201]

To summarize: the Norwich and Norfolk committees were both frustrated by ministerial priorities, which severely restricted central government loan sanctions to their capital projects. Inevitably, the modernization programme (Norwich) and the former PAI closure project (Norfolk) under the 1962 ten-year local plans were delayed, leaving little scope to relieve their growing Part III home waiting lists. On the other hand, quality care issues were recognized, particularly in the post-1960 homes with their small living units and higher proportion of single rooms. The needs of very elderly or frail residents were addressed by single-storey buildings and additional facilities, while dementia cases were assisted by designated units within ordinary, purpose-built homes (Norwich) or the specialized Ketts Lodge (Norfolk). There were also improving ratios of nursing staff to residents, yet given growing numbers of very frail or disabled people, it remains questionable whether care standards improved for everyone. For those with severe physical or mental disabilities, resident-centred arrangements barely featured, with no choice of meals and little flexibility in daily routines. Above all, the optimism of the 1973 ten-year local plans was almost immediately quashed, with deferrals and cancellations of key capital projects. With both committees' plans curtailed by central government policy directives (1963–73) and financial constraints (1973–), more residents turned to voluntary or private sector homes, many self-funding and some local authority-supported, suggesting a mixed economy of residential care.

The End of Local Authority Part III Homes, 1974–80

Following the 1974 local government reorganization, an enlarged unitary Norfolk county council replaced the existing three councils: Norfolk county, Norwich county borough and Great Yarmouth county borough. Its new Social Services Committee (SSC) assumed responsibility for all forty-six local authority homes across Norfolk.[202] Early in 1975 two replacement homes opened for the last Beech House residents, so ending the physical association with the workhouse.[203] A year later the five Norwich replacement homes were completed or almost ready, so that at least 85 per cent of the total 1,900 places in Norfolk homes were now in purpose-built homes.[204] Lord Kitchener (in Attleborough), a home acknowledged as having 'disadvantages for the care of the elderly', was converted into a hostel for mentally ill adults.[205] In 1975 Herondale (in Acle) opened as the first short-stay home for those requiring temporary or respite care or rehabilitation. It 'proved to be extremely valuable' for over 500 older clients in that year.[206] A specialist day centre for confused residents was relocated from the obsolete Bethel Hospital to a new twenty-five-place centre at Gildencroft, on the outskirts of Norwich. It had 'greatly improved facilities and furnishing'.[207]

But none of this could satisfy the growing demand for permanent Part III accommodation. The older population comprised 16.4 per cent of Norfolk's general population by 1979, compared with the 14.9 per cent national average.[208] This required at least sixty extra residential places a year, on top of the 1977 waiting list of 360, including over 150 'urgent or critical cases'.[209] Whereas the ambitious DHSS 1983 target of 25 places per 1,000 older population required ninety places or two homes per annum, the new SSC ran into DHSS financial restrictions from the outset.[210] Moreover, with priority given to 'providing accommodation for the rapidly growing number of children in the local authority's care', budgets for the elderly were further squeezed.[211] With 'woefully inadequate' plans for just two homes for 1976–8 abandoned, the SSC acknowledged that 'it would not be possible to provide any new homes for several years'.[212] Nationally, 'about 100–150 homes were closed or left unoccupied as a result of financial stringency' in 1975.[213] Locally, the new Hellesdon home, completed in 1976, was mothballed for eighteen months, with all Norfolk's services for the elderly 'to be maintained at existing levels not even growing at the same rate as the population'.[214]

Economies in nursing and domestic hours in residential homes were disturbing, as 'the service is the staff, and it is not possible for needs to be met on an increasing basis'.[215] Most homes had only one 'night watchman' who was expected to supervise a resident population 'very much frailer than was formerly the case'.[216] The SSC agreed in principle to a minimum of two night staff in all local authority homes, yet supplied this only in twenty-two larger (46–66-place) homes.[217] Cuts to the standard working week for residential staff to forty hours by 1976 further reduced staffing levels.[218] Some homes received qualified nurses from the Norfolk Area Health Authority, but its staffing position was below national standards and was the weakest in the East Anglia region.[219] Not surprisingly, staff protested at cases such as the twenty-five-place home, with 'often only one care assistant on duty between 2.00 p.m. and 10.00 p.m. and at night between 10.00 p.m. and 8.00 a.m.'.[220] Following the 1979 'Local Survey on Night Staffing in Homes for the Elderly' recommendations, the SSC resolved to provide two night staff in all homes 'by transferring certain domestic work from day staff to night staff', rather than spending an estimated £140,000 on twenty-eight additional posts.[221] This expedient employed domestic staff with few qualifications and involved reductions in nursing staff training.[222] In such circumstances, staff in all homes at the current best practice ratio of one attendant per 4.5 residents would require 'an additional 85 whole-time equivalent staff' and still more to attain the 1:4 ratio envisaged under the 1973 ten-year local plan.[223] Thus services for older people were 'constrained by financial and manpower limitations, by the virtual absence of a capital building programme and by increasing costs'.[224] With an increasing ageing population, it was admitted in 1978 that Norfolk's 'population-related level of provision has "dropped" to its 1963 level'.[225]

The SSC now focused on community care 'to enable elderly persons to remain in a home of their own for as long as possible', something reflected in the 'People before Building' slogan in the 1976 DHSS consultative document.[226] Resources were reallocated to domiciliary and day care services and, within residential provision, 'from permanent long-term care towards short-term care'.[227] This coincided with unexpected additional joint finance funds with the Norfolk Area Health Authority, which became available in 1977.[228] Early joint funding schemes proposed bringing the 'mothballed' Hellesdon home into use, yet in July 1977 the SSC attempted to sell it, resulting in a four-day occupation of the home by local socialists and trade unionists.[229] In response to public pressure, the SSC made special financial arrangements with the Norfolk Area Health Authority and the voluntary Norfolk Old People's Welfare Association, which took over management of the home.[230] Renamed Ethel Tipple Court, it opened as a twenty-five-place short-stay home early in 1978, assisting some 500 people a year.[231] Even then, 'a former LA [local authority] home for the elderly [Drayton Wood], situated no more than a mile away ... was *at the same time* being converted into ... a first-class private hotel', after the SSC had sold it.[232] Other joint funding schemes included day care provision, meals-on-wheels facilities, intensive home care, night-sitting services, and vehicles and drivers to support home help services.[233] Although these measures helped to compensate for the SSC's severely restricted provision, government financial constraints undermined these efforts.[234] Such constraints also hit the hospital provision for older people, despite the fact that Norfolk already fell below national hospital guidelines and Norwich health district had 'the greatest shortfall in the Region of 223 beds' by 1979.[235]

Dogged by demand and spending reductions, the SSC introduced flat-rate weekly charges for home help and meals-on-wheels services and increased the minimum weekly charges to residents in local authority homes 'to preserve the viability of the service[s]'.[236] Meanwhile, the role of voluntary organizations was underscored in larger grants, 'aided by the careful "pump priming" provided by joint funding money'.[237] The number of voluntary schemes supported in this way increased five-fold between 1977 and 1979 under the Labour government, but possibly reflected its strong local Conservatism.[238]

Contrasting with the pessimism surrounding local authority Part III provision, 'the private and voluntary sector has been an area of growth ... shows no sign of decreasing', with four new home proposals being submitted every month in 1978.[239] There were 480 residential places in private and voluntary sector homes across Norfolk in 1975, rising to almost 1,000 by 1979.[240] At the same time, the 'permanent' Part III places gradually decreased to 1,820, reflecting some 120 appropriations for day or short-term care use. Local authority-supported beds in voluntary homes levelled off at 189 in 1980, which meant that 80 per cent of private or voluntary sector places were occupied by fully self-funded residents.[241]

Other individuals in local authority or local authority-supported voluntary home places also contributed to their maintenance costs. Meanwhile, significant numbers of chronically ill and/or frail older people remained in geriatric and psycho-geriatric long-stay hospital beds in the 1970s.

Despite its reduced ability to support those in private and voluntary sector homes, the SSC was responsible for the registration and inspection of these facilities and protection of their residents. This was certainly necessary, as the 1974 Ministry survey of forty-two private homes in England and Wales concluded that 'a third of the homes ... could be said to be seriously deficient in their amenities and/or in the qualities possessed by their proprietors'.[242] The SSC intended to inspect private or voluntary sector premises twice a year, but owing to a lack of personnel, many were uninspected in 1975.[243] Its 1977–8 budget accordingly included £5,390 for a full-time homes registration officer 'to improve the supervision and registration of 44 private and voluntary homes', although the sixty-five homes by then were too many for one person to deal with.[244]

Overall, residential provision for older people under the Norfolk SSC was slow, its 1,940 Part III places representing just 16.5 per 1,000 Norfolk older population in 1979, compared to 18.3 in 1974 and the '25.0 per 1,000' DHSS guideline, for which at least 1,000 new places would be required.[245] In contrast the private and voluntary sector expanded rapidly, and with their 960 places taken into account, there were 24.6 beds per 1,000 Norfolk older population, almost the DHSS guideline. These changes mirrored post-1974 national trends in residential provision for older people, the transition to 'mixed economy' arrangements increasingly reflecting private and voluntary effort *without* public subsidy. Greater emphasis on day or short-term residential care also featured more informal input, again reflecting the national trends towards 'care *by* the community'. These trends continued. The SSC had 'no new major projects ... in the Capital Programme' for 1980–4, whereas private sector places more than doubled, 67 per cent of them self-funded, with a further 280 voluntary sector places.[246] Successive Conservative governments expanded private sector provision by using central subsidies via state social security funding (supplementary benefit) available from 1980, with 38 per cent of private home admissions in Norfolk fully financed in this way by 1984.[247] Consequently, the next decade witnessed unprecedented growth in private homes in Norfolk, with local authority provision stagnating and later declining.

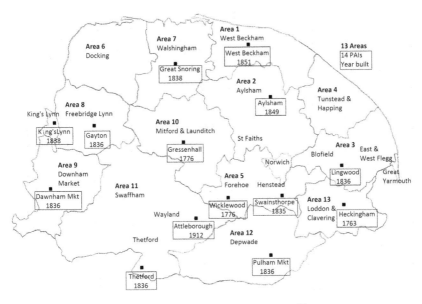

**Map 3.1: Post-1929 public assistance areas and location
of public assistance institutions (PAIs) in Norfolk.**

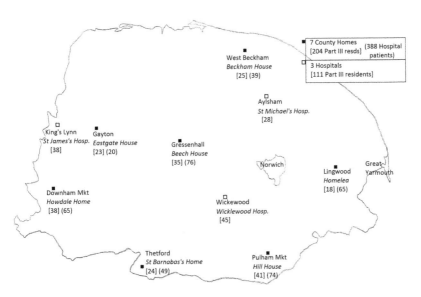

Map 3.2: Distribution of Part III (local authority) residents in Norfolk, 1948.

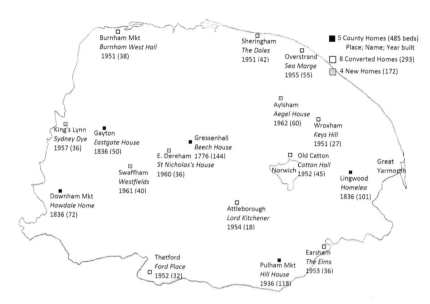

Map 3.3: Part III homes in Norfolk, 1962.

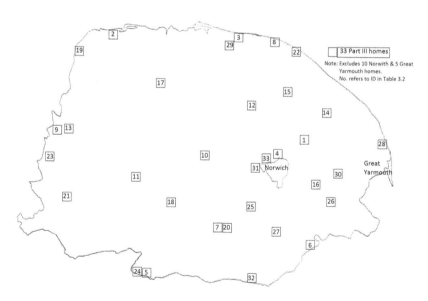

Map 3.4: Part III homes in Norfolk, 1979.

Table 3.1: List of Part III homes in Norwich, 1948–79.

ID	County homes (ex-PAIs)	Location	Opened	Beds	Notes
1	St James's Hostel	Shipmeadow	1767	135	Closed in 1954

ID	'Small' hostels	Location	Opened	Beds	Notes
1	Holmwood	Harvey Lane (Norwich)	1943	30	Converted (hostel); female only
2	The Lawns	Christchurch Road (N)	1945	35	Converted; female only
3	Mulburton Hall	Mulburton	1947	25	Converted; female only
4	The Oaks	Harvey Lane (N)	1949	35	Converted; female only
5	Hill House	Hethersett	1951	37	Converted; male only; closed in 1963
6	Drayton Wood	Drayton	1951	27	Converted; male only; sold in 1978
7	Eaton Hall	Pettis Road (N)	1954	30	Converted; mixed
8	The Grove	Catton	1954	62	Converted; male only; closed in 1971
9	Alderman Clarke	Midland Street (N)	1960	32	New mixed home with adjoining dwellings
10	Heartsease Hostel	Heartsease	1962	32	New mixed home with adjoining dwellings
11	Northfields House	North Park Avenue (N)	1963	30	Replacement for Hill House
12	Foulgers House	Ber Street (N)	1968	35	New mixed home with adjoining dwellings
13	Philadelphia House	Philadelphia Lane (N)	1971	37	Replacement; mixed
14	Somerly	Unthank Road (N)	1975	48	Replacement; mixed
15	Heathfield	Cannell Green (N)	1975	48	Replacement; mixed
16	Beechcroft	Blackhorse Road (N)	1976	48	Replacement; mixed
17	Mountfield	Chamberlain Road (N)	1976	48	Replacement; mixed
18	Ellacombe	Ella Road (N)	1976	48	Replacement; mixed

Table 3.2: List of Part III homes in Norfolk, 1948–79.

ID	County homes (ex-PAIs)	Location	Built	Beds	Notes
A	St Barnabas's Home	Thetford	1836	73	Closed in 1953
B	Beckham House	West Beckham	1851	64	Closed in 1955
C	Eastgate House	Gayton	1836	50	Closed in 1963
D	Homelea	Lingwood	1836	101	Closed in 1965
E	Howdale Home	Downham Market	1836	72	Closed in 1969
F	Hill House	Pulham Market	1836	118	Closed in 1973
G	Beech House	Gressenhall	1777	144	Closed in 1975

ID	'Small' hostels	Location	Opened	Beds	Notes
1	Keys Hill	Wroxham	1951	27	Converted (hostel)
2	Burnham Westgate	Burnham Market	1951	38	Converted
3	The Dales	Sheringham	1951	42	Converted
4	Catton Hall	Old Catton	1952	45	Converted

5	Ford Place	Thetford	1952	32	Converted; replaced St Barnabas's
6	The Elms	Earsham	1953	36	Converted
7	Lord Kitchener	Attleborough	1954	18	Converted
8	Sea Marge	Overstrand	1955	55	Converted; replaced West Beckham
9	Sidney Dye House	King's Lynn	1957	36	New (home)
10	St Nicholas's House	East Dereham	1960	36	New
11	Westfields	Swaffham	1961	40	Replacement for Eastgate House
12	Aegel House	Aylsham	1962	60	New
13	Woodlands	King's Lynn	1963	60	Replacement for Eastgate House
14	Sydney House	Stalham	1964	66	Replacement for Homelea
15	Rose Meadow	North Walsham	1965	41	New
16	Springdale	Brundall	1965	46	Replacement for Homelea
17	Cranmer House	Fakenham	1966	65	Replacement for Beech House
18	Linden Court	Watton	1967	45	Replacement for Beech House
19	Rebecca Court	Heacham	1967	46	Replacement for Howdale Home
20	St Edmunds	Attleborough	1968	41	Amalgamated with Lord Kitchener
21	High Haven	Downham Market	1969	61	Rebuilt on the same site
22	Munhaven	Mundesley	1970	21	With adjoining bungalows
23	Burman House	Terrington	1970	40	New
24	Priormead	Thetford	1971	20	With adjoining bungalows
25	Ketts Lodge	Wymondham	1971	35	Designated for the confused
26	Beauchamp House	Chedgrave	1972	45	Replacement for Hill House
27	Harker House	Long Stratton	1972	47	Replacement for Hill House
28	Clere House	Ormesby	1973	25	With adjoining bungalows
29	Glaven Hale	Holt	1973	45	Replacement for Beech House
30	Herondale	Acle	1975	35	Short stay home
31	Huntingfields	Costessey	1975	45	Replacement for Beech House
32	Dennyholse	Diss	1975	25	Replacement for Beech House
33	Ethel Tipple Court	Hellesdon	1978	25	Short stay home; sold in 1978

4 THE GIFU EXPERIENCE

In this chapter Gifu Prefecture is taken as Japan's regional case example. The period examined takes us into the 1990s, as statutory residential care provision for older people came later here. Drawing on official records and local publications, this chapter examines how the prefecture interpreted and implemented central legislation and policy goals according to its regional context. Under the 1951 Social Services Reform Act, Japan had a two-tier administrative structure in residential care provision for older people, with forty-seven upper prefectural (regional) authorities responsible for overall provision and some 800 lower municipal authorities running everyday administration. These arrangements were essentially unchanged during the period examined in this chapter.

Gifu Prefecture in central Japan (see Map 4.1 inset) is divided into twenty-six lower municipal authorities. It covers 4,173 square miles, with more than 80 per cent of the area forest or woodland and 25 per cent at least 3,000 feet above sea level.[1] The people are predominantly homogeneous and generally conservative in outlook. The population almost doubled from 1.07 to 2.12 million between 1920 and 1999, with the proportion of over-65s more than trebling from 5.2 per cent to 17.5 per cent, which is above the national average.[2] Since the municipal authorities were small, varied too much in size to be representative, and have few official records available to the public, the focus here is on upper Gifu Prefecture.

Charitable Pioneers: Almshouses, 1908–45

Gifu Prefecture had no direct prefectural or municipal authority Poor Law institutions for needy individuals throughout the 1929 Poor Law period (1932–45). Three small charitable old people's almshouses in the cities of Gifu, Takayama and Ogaki were founded in 1908, 1925 and 1926 respectively, helping an average of no more than fifty people altogether throughout the 1930s (Map 4.1) at a time when more than 71,000 prefecture inhabitants were aged 65 or over.[3] Although the rural elderly were unable to access almshouses, very few sought this type of care or were considered sufficiently needy, as a strong tradition of family care and community orientation prevailed.

Other types of institutional assistance were insignificant. One tiny charitable facility for the insane dated from 1840. It was attached to a Buddhist temple in Tarui, west of Ogaki City.[4] Here the Yamamoto family cared for between seven and fifteen patients, although none stayed more than a year or was aged over 60.[5] The prefecture's first General Hospital opened in 1875 at a Buddhist temple site in Gifu City, followed in 1878 by the Red Cross Hospital in the northern city of Takayama.[6] By the mid-1920s the two hospitals offered a total of 200 beds, and sixteen private small clinics across the prefecture provided some 400 more.[7] This represented just five beds per 10,000 prefecture population, but less than half were occupied, and then mainly by acute sick and wealthier patients.[8] Free or subsidized medical care developed slowly, but most of the chronic sick and poor elderly failed to benefit. In 1927 the prefecture's first tuberculosis sanatorium for thirty cases opened at a Buddhist temple in Gifu City, followed in 1939 by a 100-bedded sanatorium in the nearby hill town of Hino. With 2,700 TB deaths reported annually, this clearly was inadequate.[9] The same was true of provision for the mentally ill: although the 1919 Asylum Act encouraged asylum provision in every prefecture, Gifu Prefecture's first private asylum did not open until 1928. This asylum (later renamed Gifu Brain Hospital) initially had sixty-five beds, increasing to 137 by 1930, but there were by then more than 1,000 certified persons and still more uncertified in the prefecture.[10] As violent, dangerous or emergency cases were prioritized, moderate or chronic cases, including the senile elderly, were cared for at home by their families. In short, although institutional provision developed slowly prior to the 1929 Poor Law, there seemed to be no provision in the prefecture for needy older people other than the small charitable old people's almshouses in three cities.

Gifu Prefecture had three of Japan's first forty-eight old people's almshouses in 1926, but by 1940 Japan's 131 almshouses had nearly 4,600 residents, and Gifu's total of fifty almshouse residents was below the national prefecture average of almost seventy (excluding 1,500 residents in Tokyo).[11] By comparison, neighbouring Ishikawa, Toyama and Mie, each with similar or smaller older populations than Gifu's, accommodated an average of ninety residents. Moreover, none of the thirty direct public old people's almshouses was in Gifu.

Politics and rural conservatism partly explain this.[12] Despite the 1874 poor relief legislation, at least half of Gifu's rural population struggled at or below poor relief levels in 1879, simply because prefecture officials did not authorize any.[13] Between 1881 and 1889 Gifu had just 256 poor relief recipients in total, compared with over 1,000 each in neighbouring Shiga, Aichi and Mie and more than 10,000 in western prefectures like Okayama and Hiroshima.[14] Such local variations can probably be attributed to the local official attitude to central policy directives, which stressed restrictionist and minimalist measures. Thus Gifu Prefecture 'was one of the few prefectures, utterly loyal to the state principle of reducing its poor relief expenditure as much as possible'.[15] Even after the 1891 Nobi earthquake left 'over 400,000 persons ... homeless and almost without clothing', a mere thirty-nine people were given poor relief.[16] In 1895 the governor of Gifu Prefecture, Michio Sogabe, commended the prefecture's municipal authorities' vigilance in restricting relief recipients to just seventy-five during his two-year administration.[17] This official stance persisted, as reflected in a local newspaper article in 1917 on 'Prefecture's Pride, Japan's No.1 for Control of Poor Relief', which reported further reductions.[18]

The prefecture's needy older population therefore depended on informal help within the family or community.[19] For a tiny minority lacking any support, charitable aid assumed institutional form. In 1908 the social activist Kakutaro Kato provided Gifu Old People's Almshouse (Gifu Almshouse), a modest, one-storey, timber-built property, solely from his private funds.[20] He lived in and nursed Ms Go Nagata and two other elderly residents, just four admissions during 1914–22 reflecting his limited ability to combine nursing, fundraising and other responsibilities. Collaborating with a Buddhist priest, he established the Buddhist Old People's Association in 1918, which took over the management of Gifu Almshouse. Over time its finances were boosted by contributions from its members and public donations. With state recognition as a 'good' charitable facility, the Association also received regular central and local government grants, including the emperor's 'blessing moneys'.[21] Gifu Almshouse's resident population expanded from three in 1922 to more than twenty by 1930, with considerable overcrowding before a larger replacement facility opened on a nearby site in 1933 at a cost of 34,700 yen.[22]

Under the 1929 Poor Law, Gifu Almshouse was authorized as a 'publicly sanctioned Poor Law institution' and entitled to receive subsidies for eligible residents. Consequently, its charitable funds shrank and by 1940 comprised just 8 per cent of its annual income.[23] But the occupancy rate was only 60 per cent of the sixty-four-place capacity. Again, this may have reflected family orientation in the care of older people, reinforced by the prefecture's conservative outlook. Nevertheless, one initiative was instigated in 1921 by Governor Mumpei Ueda. He adopted the pioneer support system in Osaka under which unpaid area commissioners addressed local social problems by facilitating access to support for the poorest citizens.[24] By 1925 Gifu Prefecture had 100 commissioners helping over 4,000 cases, including the needy elderly.[25]

In Takayama district, sixty miles north of Gifu City, a 900-member Social Service Association was founded in 1922 'to promote provision for local poor citizens'.[26] A modest, wooden, one-storey old people's almshouse was built in the city centre in 1925, its cost coming from the Association fund. The Takayama Old People's Almshouse was also officially approved as a publicly sanctioned Poor Law institution under the 1929 Poor Law and so became entitled to state subsidies for eligible residents, although there were very few of these. It was replaced in 1937 by a two-storey, thirty-place facility on a larger site adjoining the Takayama Red Cross Hospital, its costs again funded by the Association.[27] The occupancy rate here was even lower than Gifu Almshouse, with only a handful of residents during the 1930s, even though Takayama City had the largest population in the prefecture at that time.[28] The almshouse was intended for the entire northern Hida region (40 per cent of the prefecture), but the family and neighbourhood orientation in informal care was even stronger here.

This was also true of a third almshouse in Ogaki City, eight miles west of Gifu City. The Ogaki Old People's Almshouse (Ogaki Almshouse), Yorokaen, originated in 1920 with the foundation of a Relief Club of five dedicated individuals who undertook charitable work, but the Club did not build the Ogaki Almshouse until 1926.[29] Their private moneys accounted for almost 80 per cent of its funds in 1923, although the Club did have local government support, with successive mayors of Ogaki City appointed as its president, and it received regular city grants. This enabled the Club to establish various welfare services, including a hygiene consultant centre and relief accommodation for those in custodial care. A donation of 10,000 yen from a local philanthropist, Hiro Yoshioka, enabled the Club to build a single-storey timber house on the southern edge of the city centre later in 1926, with construction and the site costing 13,000 yen (the 3,000 yen balance was met by other benefactors). The Club thus remained debt-free and received further donations, including land valued at 15,700 yen from Ms Yoshioka. It was reorganized in 1928 as the Ogaki Relief Foundation and provided a free medical centre in the former Ogaki City Hall (1930–3), free accommodation for casuals and vagrants at the almshouse site from 1931 and a nursery from 1940.

As with Gifu Almshouse, official approval and larger public subsidies were followed by a reduction in charitable donations: endowments stopped in 1933 and large donations effectively ceased in 1931.[30] Public money represented two-thirds of the Foundation's annual income in 1938, compared to a quarter in 1925, but its total income decreased slightly, mainly because there were no state relief subsidies and so no publicly funded eligible residents.[31] Money spent on provisions averaged just 1,700 yen a year during 1927–39, suggesting there were few residents; low costs in 1930 were 'due to the lack of residents'.[32] Proposals for new office accommodation and a workshop were dropped in 1933, and in 1936 there were just nine residents at a time when there was capacity for twenty-two.[33] Again, the inference is that the culture of informal care still prevailed in Ogaki, which, while more urbanized than Takayama, was rural in comparison to Gifu City.

The Second World War brought considerable hardship and disruption, particularly to the sick elderly, since their sons – who conventionally supported them financially – were conscripted. Starvation, lack of essentials and air raids made matters worse. Ogaki Almshouse began to accommodate eligible relief recipients under the 1929 Act for the first time in 1940, its numbers increasing as the war intensified. This increased state relief subsidies, which reached 4,200 yen by 1945 and undoubtedly helped the almshouse's expenses, which exceeded 3,500 yen by 1945.[34] Since Gifu Prefecture lacked direct prefectural or municipal authority Poor Law institutions during the war, Ogaki Almshouse was a significant provider for some, who would not otherwise have survived. However, conditions were harsh, with twenty deaths in the closing two years of the war, compared to five in the preceding two years.[35] Ogaki City was heavily bombed on 29 July 1945, with half the population wounded or killed and over half the buildings and houses, including the almshouse, destroyed.[36] There are no surviving wartime records from Gifu and Takayama Almshouses, but it is reasonable to assume that they also accommodated increasing numbers of publicly funded needy elderly persons.

Life inside the Almshouses

Fragmentary surviving records allow only glimpses of residential life in Gifu's three old people's almshouses. In 1936 forty-one of the total fifty residents were aged 60 or over and nearly half were able-bodied, although a quarter died that year and three were discharged.[37] Gifu Almshouse had eighty-one admissions, fifty-seven deaths and six discharges in the decade to 1933, suggesting a considerable turnover and short residence periods: 60 per cent lived there for less than three years.[38] Between 1914 and 1933, 80 per cent of admissions came from within the prefecture, while almost all who died in Ogaki Almshouse between 1927 and 1945 were from Ogaki City or nearby villages.[39] However, some Gifu Almshouse occupants were from Tokyo or Osaka, and the homeless in Ogaki Almshouse included a repatriate from Manchuria. Most residents had few relatives or friends, so the almshouses were their last resort. No one in Ogaki Almshouse contributed to their maintenance costs, and none received money or any type of payment for their help or work, which was probably offset against their maintenance costs or used to supplement almshouse provisions.[40]

Gifu's almshouses were modest wooden buildings with pleasant Japanese gardens, blending in with adjacent houses in urban residential areas. The Gifu Almshouse (redeveloped in 1933) featured two two-storey buildings, accommodating up to sixty-four people in twelve *tatami* (straw-matted) rooms, each with shared storage for bedding and personal effects.[41] It had a large dining hall, communal bathroom and lavatories on the ground floor, with first-floor rooms for Buddhist services and staff accommodation. Bedrooms nominally for six residents were shared by three or four. Takayama Almshouse (rebuilt in 1937) was smaller, with nine bedrooms for up to thirty people, but before the war it had just six residents.[42] The 1925-built original Ogaki Almshouse for up to twenty-two people was similarly underused before the war, with no more than a dozen residents. Thus all three almshouses had a domestic appearance and even a family atmosphere, offering some private space and adequate communal facilities.

Yet the low bed capacity and occupancy rates also reflected the strong stigma attached to almshouse provision. Only as a last resort might 'wretched' solitary and needy older persons ask for assistance in the shameful knowledge that such help was provided by the state on behalf of the emperor. Even after they were officially sanctioned as Poor Law institutions, almshouses were similarly regarded. Rather than being seen as a matter of welfare or right, residents were expected to be subservient and humbled, because their failure to achieve self-reliance or to have a supporting family placed a burden on the emperor and the state. This was especially true in traditionalist Gifu Prefecture, where even within 'charitable' almshouses, deterring all but the neediest solitary elderly remained an objective.

Nationally, almost 70 per cent of old people's almshouses were religious foundations, either Buddhist (as in Gifu Prefecture) or mainly Christian, but even these typically embodied familistic nationalism.[43] Thus Gifu Almshouse, which had a Buddhist ethos, also reflected the values of Shinto by emphasizing the paternal and benevolent role of the emperor. The foreword to the 1933 Annual Report of Gifu Almshouse included a poem dedicated to older people by the Meiji emperor, along with a list of 'blessing moneys' and 'imperial awards' given during 1924–33.[44] Similarly, at Takayama Almshouse, 69-year-old Shirakawa 'was awarded an honourable recognition from the Empress for his dedicated social work and management of the Almshouse' in 1936.[45]

How such principles operated within Gifu's three old people's almshouses is uncertain, for there are few surviving sources. The almshouses seemingly featured more discretionary and individual styles, and were probably more like a large family unit featuring mutual aid. Yet they also featured paternalistic, hierarchical and ordered regimes, in which familistic nationalism and traditional values were stressed. Frail older residents were nursed by more able residents, who were expected to look after themselves and assist others whenever possible. Nursing was supplemented by a skeleton resident staff, who were paternalistic in outlook but dedicated and often worked voluntarily (there were just three paid attendants in Gifu's three almshouses in 1936).[46] In contrast, public old people's almshouses in neighbouring Nagano and Shizuoka prefectures averaged one attendant to every three or four residents, which partly explains the spending per almshouse resident that year: 155 yen in Gifu compared to 409 yen in Nagano (the national average was 297 yen).[47]

There was no evidence of systematic cruelty or humiliation: the almshouses were generally homely. Each provided free and discretionary relief for needy older people, regardless of their physical or mental state, or social or financial background, although the numbers helped were minuscule. After the enactment of the 1929 Poor Law the charitable almshouses assumed more public functions, but these pioneers helped to shape post-war mainstream residential provision and so arguably perpetuated the social stigma.

All three almshouses survived or were rebuilt, though they were renamed or changed their management bodies. This allows them to be examined over time; however, as their records are fragmentary, sketchy and deal principally with the amount and description of provisions, this results in a rather quantitative approach.

Emergency Measures: Public Institutions, 1946–50

Following post-war welfare legislation, statutory national residential care provision for older people expanded steadily. Under emergency measures, Gifu City authority built a modest fifteen-place facility at Hino Town in 1947. This was used as a 'general public assistance institution' for the eligible needy of all ages under the 1946 National Assistance Act. In that year Ogaki City authority subsidized a forty-place facility to replace the charitable Ogaki Almshouse, which had suffered bomb damage, and authorized it as a 'publicly sanctioned general public assistance institution'.[48] Charitable Gifu and Takayama Almshouses were both authorized and utilized as publicly sanctioned general public assistance institutions. Such institutions were officially defined as 'assessed institutions', so applicants and their families were required to undergo means-testing and needs assessments by local welfare officers. All told, Gifu Prefecture had just four general public assistance institutions, including three publicly sanctioned ones which had started as charitable almshouses, prior to the 1950 'New' National Assistance Act. These accommodated some 140 people altogether, 115 of them aged over 65, at a time when the prefecture's older population exceeded 90,000 (5.8 per cent of its general population).[49] Inevitably, there was overcrowding: seventy-six residents were living in the sixty-four-place Gifu Institution in 1948 compared to thirty-two in 1940, and those in Ogaki Institution shared dormitories with at least nine others.[50]

In the immediate post-war years, the country experienced extreme hardship. Gifu Prefecture had 90,000 war victims (more than 7 per cent of its population) and 97,500 repatriates returning from the war fronts and former colonized regions.[51] A further 170,000 evacuees from urban prefectures were followed by thousands of victims from other devastated areas.[52] In 1948 at least 450,000 people (40 per cent of the total population) were living in substandard or unacceptable accommodation, including 10,000 in military barracks in the ruins of Gifu and Ogaki cities and 208,000 taken in by relatives or neighbours in overcrowded conditions.[53] Hundreds more were living on the streets or sheltering in wrecked vehicles. By 1950 about 4,500 homeless – 2,000 repatriates, 250 orphans, 250 single mothers and their children and 2,000 unemployed and their families – had been accommodated in publicly subsidized 'emergency relief institutions', which had been appropriated for each group.[54] With public assistance budgets severely constrained, the focus was on emergency cases and the poorest with no informal support. As elsewhere, supplies from the Licensed Agencies for Relief in Asia (LARA) and post-1948 charitable Community Chest Fund eased the lives of residents in these institutions.[55] Similarly, minimal-level public assistance helped over 32,000 destitute citizens living at home, including some 4,000 over-60s.[56] Using pre-war almshouses also saved the prefecture from capital expenditure in post-war austerity.

Low Demand and Low Bed Capacity, 1950–62

Under the 1950 Act, Gifu's four general public assistance institutions refocused exclusively on older people and were officially renamed 'old people's institutions'. However, they were assessed institutions within the terms of public assistance measures, so applicants and their families had to undergo compulsory means-testing and needs assessment. The next few years saw a major expansion in this sort of provision throughout Japan, beginning in Gifu Prefecture with the conversion or adaptation of suitable premises coincident with local charitable effort. Hence in 1949 a Buddhist priest, Mr Fukami, donated the Daisen-ji Buddhist temple properties and land in Tajimi City, 23 miles east of Gifu City, to its municipal authority. The authority then converted them into a thirty-place institution with a workshop for residents, two single-storey, timber-built houses for staff accommodation and a dining hall (see Map 4.2 and Table 4.1).[57] Its ten 2–4-bedded rooms represented a significant improvement on large dormitories. Lavatory accommodation was limited, the bathroom was outside and there were no covered walkways connecting the buildings. Even so, this was preferable to the lives of an estimated 410,000 people still in substandard accommodation, as even in 1954 only 40,000 people had been re-homed and 'housing shortages still remain the most serious problem'.[58]

In 1950 two local philanthropists, Ms Kozaka and Mr Yamada, funded the conversion by Seki City authority of a wartime military detention centre into a sixty-place institution, which was described as 'a paradise for the unfortunate elderly'.[59] It featured five wooden terraced houses, two of which were two storeys high, but, with upstairs accommodation ruled out for fire precaution reasons under the 1957 Ministry Code of Practice, the institution was limited to forty beds.[60] Gujo Town authority converted an emergency relief institution for repatriates near the Taga-Jinja Shinto shrine in 1952, but this was obsolete and was replaced within two years.[61]

Acknowledging the shortcomings of converted facilities, the municipal authorities looked for suitable sites where purpose-built institutions could be constructed, with rural Ibigawa Town authority earmarking a site within Taiko-

Ji Buddhist temple in 1951.[62] Ibigawa Institution was a modest thirty-place facility, costing less than 2 million yen and consisting of two rows of wooden, single-storey terraced houses.[63] Yet this institution set new standards, with indoor lavatory and bathroom amenities, covered walkways connecting the buildings and parallel rows of bedrooms, equipped with storage space and anticipating the 1957 official 'four people per room' guideline. Two more municipal authorities followed in 1952, building thirty-place institutions in Tarui Town and Nakatsugawa City to improved specifications.[64] It is worth emphasizing the continued association of prefecture public welfare provision with charity, whether based on religion (Buddhism) or the emperor (Shinto), reflected in the institutions' sites or buildings within or near Buddhist temples or Shinto shrines.

A larger, purpose-built facility for fifty people also opened in Takayama City in 1952, replacing the former Takayama Almshouse and admitting its thirty-three residents.[65] Another timber-built facility, it had separate dining and recreational rooms, medical services and relatively spacious 2–4-bedded rooms – its 48 square feet per capita sleeping space was more generous than the 1957 official 35 square feet per capita guideline, found in most other prefecture institutions.[66] This 'most elegant and modern old people's institution with plenty of sunshine and fresh air overlooking the North Alps' soon received 'visits from all over Japan, including Ministry officials, Gifu Prefecture Governor Mr Muto and welfare officers in Tokyo Council'.[67] Meanwhile, in response to overcrowding and greater urban demand, the combined capacity of the Gifu, Hino and Ogaki institutions was increased from 120 to 210 beds, through extensions and alterations.

In all, by 1952 Gifu Prefecture had ten old people's institutions (eight direct authority-run and two subcontracted to non-profit social welfare corporations), with 460 places (5.7 beds per 1,000 prefecture older population, slightly above the national average). Yet they were underused, with average occupancy rates of 72 per cent, well below the 90 per cent national average.[68] Proportionately there were more vacancies in rural institutions: the thirty-place Tarui, Nakatsugawa and Gujo institutions had thirteen, seventeen and seventeen residents respectively in 1952, whereas the urban seventy-place Gifu Institution was full, the sixty-place Hino had forty-three residents and the eighty-place Ogaki had sixty-two.[69] According to the 1953 national survey, this was because half the 365 institutions across the country were new and 'have not yet reached their full bed capacity'.[70] Gifu's rural institutions were indeed new, but so were those in adjoining rural Fukui Prefecture, which were almost full.[71] Fukui was only half the size of Gifu Prefecture, and its purpose-built institutions were better distributed and therefore accessible to the majority of its older population, whereas distribution of Gifu's institutions across its expansive territory and dispersed older population was poor: seven were in cities and three in nearby towns, leaving some 60 per cent (55,000) of its older population in rural areas with no access.[72] 'At least

4,000 eligible elderly people across the Prefecture required residential accommodation', but relied on informal help, as there were just 400 beds in existing institutions.[73] It is unknown whether eligible older persons would have entered an institution if one was available, given the stigma attached to them and the strong local tradition of family and community care.

Alternative institutional provision also remained underdeveloped. Although Gifu's hospital bed numbers increased from 2,600 to 5,700 between 1948 and 1953, almost 60 per cent were appropriated for TB or other infectious patients (3,400), with the remainder mostly for acute cases (2,000) or psychiatric patients (300).[74] There was no specialized provision for geriatric, dementia or chronic cases; nor were there any private or voluntary residential homes. Thus the means-tested old people's institutions dealt with relatively mobile cases without means, shelter and family support, but also frail or chronic sick cases. New demand also arose as 'the opening of new institutions, free from the gloomy image associated with "*obasuteyama*", attracted those who would not have considered admission to pre-war old people's almshouses'.[75] In these circumstances, the need for expansion was acknowledged and local plans in 1953 looked to ten new institutions or 600 new places, resulting in twenty institutions or 1,000 places in total by 1960.[76] Moreover, although modest wooden buildings were acceptable during post-war austerity, now it was felt that 'efforts should be made to create a brighter and comfortable atmosphere for elderly residents, for example, by providing recreational facilities'.[77]

Increasing demand for new types of residential accommodation for those excluded from existing institutions, notably the moderately well-off elderly without family support or those living with families but experiencing family friction, was made. Accordingly, residential homes for those non-eligible people were planned in Gifu and Ogaki in 1955.[78] The Gifu City authority plan involved a 15 million yen facility for 100 self-funded elderly people, with 'all single rooms and recreational, cultural and medical facilities'.[79] Similarly, Ogaki Relief Foundation, a subcontractor of Ogaki Institution (formerly Ogaki Almshouse), envisaged a private residential home, a 'paradise for the elderly ... with full facilities in a quiet residential area overlooking nice views'.[80] Yet neither plan was realized because both bodies failed to secure local government subsidies. Gifu Prefecture prioritized statutory provision instead, adding seven thirty-place institutions and 130 more beds to existing institutions between 1955 and 1962.

Old People's Homes: Stagnation, 1963–74

On the eve of the 1963 Elderly Welfare Act, Gifu Prefecture was able to offer 800 places in seventeen institutions (fifteen direct authority-run and two subcontracted to non-profit social welfare corporations), renamed 'old people's homes', still some 200 places short of the 1960 target.[81] This equated to 7.3 beds per 1,000 prefecture older population, no longer ahead of the national average, although Gifu's average bed occupancy rate of 96 per cent was better than an overcrowded 101 per cent nationally in 1960.[82] If the uneven distribution of homes in Gifu Prefecture was a feature, the prefecture also had the second lowest ratio of the over-60s receiving non-institutional public assistance. Just 14 per 1,000 of the over-60s (2,000 people) were assisted in Gifu, compared to 27 per 1,000 nationally or 44 per 1,000 in the western Kochi and Kagoshima Prefectures, which were also very rural, large and sparsely populated, but lacked family carers partly because its younger people tended to migrate to the cities.[83]

Once again, Gifu Prefecture was ignoring needy older people with limited family support, helping only the few who were completely alone and destitute. Such official restrictionism was generally accepted by the largely traditionalist population, who acknowledged their duty to care for older relatives and so were hostile to public welfare provision. The image of 'grim' old people's homes and *obasuteyama* associations were reflected in newspaper headlines as late as the 1970s: 'Elderly people living alone detest old people's homes'; '"Old people's homes, No way" voiced by older people living alone'; and 'Solitary old folks reluctant to enter old people's homes'.[84] Official restrictions and local antipathy left prefecture residential provision below demand and national averages: just three more authority homes, the last of their kind, were added during 1963–74.

Nevertheless, demand for residential accommodation increased, reflected in near-full occupancy rates in existing homes.[85] To ease the situation, Gifu Prefecture encouraged 'social welfare corporations'. These were non-profit organizations (technically quangos), which acted as subcontractors of the public sector. Subsequently, these corporations opened their homes in Miwa Town near Gifu City and Sakahogi Town, ten miles to the east, instigating moves away from direct authority-run to subcontracted and publicly funded social welfare corporation homes within the mixed economy of welfare. Yet both faced immediate financial difficulties as only 75 per cent of building costs were covered by public subsidies and general inflation was exacerbated by the 1973 oil crisis. Miwa Town Home soon went bankrupt, and Sakahogi Town Home was unfinished even after its delayed opening in 1974.[86] Thus the prefecture's provision peaked with 1,200 places in twenty-two homes, including four subcontracted to social welfare corporations, around 1975, well below the 2,000 places envisaged in Gifu's first ten-year plan (1966).[87]

To address growing demand, existing homes were replaced by larger facilities. These offered improved standards and eased overcrowding. Thus the 1933-built Gifu Home made way for a 'modern, glazed facility with plenty of sunlight and fresh air', described as a 'paradise for the elderly', in a quiet suburb, ten miles north of Gifu City in 1957.[88] This provided ninety places (increasing to 110 by

1966) and was the largest prefecture home. It too was a timber construction. A more robust replacement was built in 1975.[89] In contrast, the replacement Tajimi Home, constructed in 1959, was 'concrete-built, colourfully decorated and bright and modern'. It was called Tayoso, a Confucian association with a 'paradise for the elderly', a frequently used expression at the time for an ideal home.[90] However, its thirty-place capacity soon fell below the revised 1966 official 'minimum 50-place home' guideline, leading to construction of a fifty-place replacement facility on a different site in 1977.

Reflecting the growing rural older population and the 1966 official guidelines, other rural thirty-place homes were expanded, initially through extensions but later with new buildings at different sites. Thus Ena City authority replaced its thirty-place building with a fifty-place home in the hills outside the city in 1969; Tarui Town authority followed suit in 1972; and to cover more of the rural population, new fifty-place homes opened in Miyama and Mitaka.[91] Meanwhile, the 'makeshift and decrepit' Ogaki and Hino Homes were replaced by still larger 100-place facilities, which survived well into the 1990s.[92] Thus by 1972 the average prefecture home had fifty-seven beds compared to forty-seven a decade earlier.[93] Urban homes typically offered 100 or more places, while rural homes provided fifty or so beds.

These changes suggested a *less* 'homely' atmosphere, contrary to the official reclassification of homes under the 1963 Act. Although the post-1960 homes were fire-resistant concrete buildings, internally they were essentially the same. Larger homes simply provided more four-bedded rooms and scaled up communal facilities. However, living space per capita was cramped and unimpressive: a mere '26 square feet per capita' in Gifu Home in 1972, far below the post-1957 minimum guideline of 35 square feet per capita, let alone the 47 square feet per capita at the rural Tarui Home a decade earlier.[94] Worse still, at the 110-place Gifu Home, 121 people shared one packed dining hall and a basic bathroom, with three married couples accommodated in a single bedroom and twenty sick people packed into one medical ward.[95] The forty or so able residents worked in their bedrooms, as there was no workshop or communal space.

In contrast, the twenty-four residents in the 1952-built thirty-place Tarui Home had older but separate dining and living rooms and shared a bathroom of similar size to that in Gifu.[96] Yet older homes had inadequate and outmoded facilities and amenities. Minor improvements were urged by officials following their annual inspections; they demanded that older homes be upgraded to meet official minimum standards, including separate lavatory provision for men and women and laundry accommodation or storage space for every resident.[97]

Another feature of the post-1960 homes was their location. Faced with public financial constraints, municipal authorities looked for less expensive but larger out-of-town sites to offset the higher cost of enhanced facilities. With all homes in suburban or isolated rural areas, residents were remote from local communities, relatives, shops and essential amenities. Such moves also expressed a physical distancing from the earlier old people's almshouses or Poor Law institutions and their associated social stigma. New sites were often described in glowing terms, emphasizing their 'healthy and quiet environment full of nature and greenery'.[98] One newspaper article in 1975 depicted residential life in a home in the mountain town of Furukawa, eight miles north of Takayama City: 'the residents are by no means home-bound, busy growing vegetables in nearby fields, some even leaving the home as early as at four o'clock in the morning ... [they] enjoy talking with local people and exchange vegetables with each other'.[99]

The 1966 official guidelines were revised in 1973 to address residents' privacy needs by specifying an 'all double-bedroom' standard for future homes. The first to meet this was completed that year at Motosu Town, at a cost of 96 million yen, nearly three times more than the replacement facility built in 1972 at Tarui Town.[100] The new Motosu Town Home was equipped with radio and television sets, board games, newspapers and magazines, supplemented by organized activities, including an annual sports day.[101] Yet 'comfort' trips and visits from local monks and notables suggested a pre-war paternalistic ethos.[102] Residents were described in a local guide as 'unfortunate impoverished people lacking families ... [for whom] the home and the staff endeavour to create a bright and happy living environment with warm hearts'.[103] Whether these principles actually operated within the home is less clear, given the few source materials.

During 1974–5 even more impressive homes were built by Kagamihara and Seki City authorities, each costing over 110 million yen. The former was a long-awaited suburban home, 'fully air-conditioned and consisting of twenty-five double rooms, separate dining and recreation rooms with Buddhist altar and service space, a workshop and a modern bathroom with wave equipment'.[104] In the latter, 'all twenty-five double rooms had a wash basin and were soundproofed on the ground floor and corridors were equipped with handrails on both sides'.[105] Ministry of Health and Welfare officials regarded the home as 'the first of its kind in Japan to address the needs of the elderly residents so considerately ... the model for future Japanese old people's homes'.[106] Evidently, the 1973 revised official guidelines significantly improved minimum standards in *new* prefecture homes, yet it took another two decades before Gifu Prefecture could provide all single bedrooms in its homes, and even then, the eradication of the pre-war ethos and stigma attached to the homes seems questionable.[107]

Pre-1973 homes were exempted from the new guidelines and barely improved, resulting in widening variations in the environment and standards between the homes, a problem compounded as official standards were revised upwards again during the 1980s and 1990s. Eligible older applicants had little choice as regards accommodation in designated assessed institutions, something made worse by their uneven distribution. People admitted to homes remote from their home towns included thirty-four people from Kagamihara City, which had no facility before 1974.[108] And with no additional places after 1974, new applicants faced great restrictions and the rationing of places intensified. Only the neediest with few financial means and no family support had priority, leaving the rest dependent on inadequate self-help or informal arrangements. In 1971 an estimated 8,000 bedridden or frail older people across the prefecture were wholly looked after by their families at home.[109]

Nursing Homes: Restriction, 1963–99

The introduction of nursing homes under the 1963 Act addressed the problem of frail or bedridden older people with or without family support, with admissions based on need, regardless of financial or family circumstances. These, like old people's homes, were nevertheless assessed institutions and so involved compulsory means-testing and needs assessment of applicants and their families. Japan's nursing home provision developed steadily after 1963, but Gifu Prefecture initially lagged behind. The prefecture-funded social welfare corporation (quango) opened its first nursing home, Jurakuen, in 1968. It provided fifty places, which increased to seventy with extensions the following year (see Map 4.3 and Table 4.2).[110] Major national expansion followed under the government's 1970 Emergency Five Year Plan for Residential Facilities, but just three new nursing homes offering 290 more places were envisaged for Gifu Prefecture over the decade to 1980.[111] This was determined using 1971 local estimates that 'the number of frail elderly unable to obtain informal nursing assistance is 350'.[112] This echoed the prefecture's position of only '75 bedridden elderly living alone' and some 275 more frail cases lacking family as eligible for nursing homes, while ignoring at least 4,900 bedridden and thousands more frail or sick older people who were being looked after by their families at home.[113] Indeed, at the 1975 annual meeting of the Gifu Retired People's Association, the prefecture chief welfare officer affirmed that 'the family should remain a primary institution to care for their frail elderly relatives'.[114] Moreover, the prefecture seemed oblivious to 'some 10 per cent bedridden residents (120) who required nursing care, yet were accommodated in old people's homes' precisely because there were not enough nursing home places.[115] Any future accelerated demand for nursing home places as its frail older population grew was also ignored, even though the prefecture's Consultative Social Welfare Committee identified 'an urgent need for a further 900 to 1,000 nursing home places' in 1971.[116]

Community care provision to supplement informal care remained embryonic, with just fifteen home helps in 1968 and no day care or short-stay facilities at all before 1981.[117] Public hospital provision was similarly underdeveloped: in 1964 there were 12,600 hospital beds, the equivalent of 7.3 per 1,000 prefecture population, below the national average of 8.4 per 1,000 and ostensibly 3,600 beds short.[118] There were just 2,000 psychiatric beds for an estimated 20,200 mentally ill people, including dementia cases, half of them requiring urgent hospitalization.[119] The Gifu City Hospital opened its first geriatric wards for forty chronic sick older patients in 1975, but had no psycho-geriatric beds.[120] With younger and more acute cases given priority, less than 10 per cent of the beds were allocated to older patients even in the late 1980s.[121] Despite the introduction of free health care for most over-70s from 1973, community-based health care also remained underdeveloped: over 40 per cent of 110 bedridden older people living at home in Kagamihara City received no prescription medicines or home visits from doctors or nurses in 1977.[122]

In 1973 the prefecture-funded social welfare corporation completed its second nursing home, Hida-Jurakuen, for eighty-five people near Takayama. Despite urgent demand, two proposed authority nursing homes had not been realized in 1972, nor had plans been drawn up for any future homes. Yet in 1975 it was asserted that 'as local residential facilities for the elderly are adequate, there are no plans for further prefecture or prefecture-funded nursing homes ... for the time being'.[123] The two planned nursing homes were shelved. To ease the situation, prefecture officials sought to offload some of their responsibilities onto 'private' or independent social welfare corporations (non-profit quangos receiving public funding). This reflected the shift towards 'private' social welfare corporation involvement in residential care provision for older people. It started in Gifu Prefecture with old people's homes in Miwa and Sakahogi towns during 1974–5. In 1973 a branch of the National Council of Elderly Homes was established to promote the prefecture's social welfare corporation residential provision, particularly its nursing homes.[124] Yet such arrangements had a shaky beginning, despite substantial, if not full, central government subsidies for construction costs. A private social welfare corporation opened a nursing home in Miwa Town in 1974, next to its old people's home built two years earlier. But both homes went bankrupt, and their 100 residents had to be transferred to neighbouring facilities.[125] However, a more affluent corporation built the 100-place Shinseien nursing home in Ibigawa Town in 1976, followed in the next three years by five more, offering 410 places in total.[126] Thanks to these private facilities, Gifu Prefecture had 665 places in eight social welfare corporation nursing homes (two prefecture-funded and six private) by 1979, well exceeding its '360 places by 1980' target. Yet this still represented just 3.5 places per 1,000 prefecture older population, less than half the national average. Meanwhile, existing nursing homes became increasingly overcrowded. As one nursing home manager put it, 'We receive phone calls requesting admission day after day ... but our home is already overcrowded with long waiting lists ... we cannot turn down their applications as they are so desperate ... but of course we cannot take them either'.[127]

Only in 1977 did Gifu's third ten-year comprehensive local plan propose 'an urgent development of the prefecture nursing home provision up to national average levels', with a doubling of nursing home places to 1,740 being achieved by 1992.[128] Enhanced national expansion under the government's Gold Plan set the standard for Gifu Prefecture's own efforts, with a further doubling to 4,000 places (10.9 beds per 1,000 prefecture older population), again achieved by 2000.[129] Thus successive decades after 1979 saw real progress in the prefecture's nursing home provision, both numerically and as a percentage of its older population. This catching-up process was in response to growing demand and a gradual change in perception of family care. Again, as in the earlier period, this was attributable to social welfare corporation efforts and initiatives offsetting limited direct local authority provision under the prefecture's ever-restrictive policy. Nonetheless, Gifu remained substantially below the national average; it was the lowest of Japan's forty-seven prefectures in 1995, and the second lowest four years later.[130] Moreover, Gifu had no for-profit private nursing homes until 2002, whereas there were 300 elsewhere in Japan offering over 30,000 places by 1999.[131] Only in 2004 did Gifu's nursing home provision reach national average levels, with the non-profit (social welfare corporation) sector supplying almost 90 per cent of the places.[132]

The prefecture had at least 5,600 bedridden, 12,300 demented and 18,000 frail older people living at home and mostly reliant on family care in 1993, when just 1,740 nursing home places were available.[133] Its community care provision remained underdeveloped. The number of home helps rose from a paltry 174 in 1981 to over 1,000 by 1992, for 6,400 frail older people, but this represented a one-hour-a-week service, far below the Ministry recommendation of 3–6 hours.[134] Moreover, an estimated 25,600 frail older people were eligible for some form of community care services, suggesting a rationing of services to the very neediest.[135] Although some short-stay beds were available, less than a fifth of eligible frail older persons benefited, on average only once a year, compared to the official guideline of six times.[136] A further 10,600 older people were hospitalized, including 2,900 for over six months, with nearly 5,000 more in intermediate health care facilities by 1999.[137] Even so, this level of medical-led accommodation was below the national average. Thus shortages of nursing home places were offset by informal family care, supplemented by longer-term beds in medical facilities and limited community care provision.

All this echoed the prefecture's policy of family care as the primary asset for the care of older people, encouraged further under 'the prefecture's distinctive preference for the stable family function'.[138] The latter reflected its above-average cohabitation rates; larger household size with more space per capita; home-ownership ratios; household income; and consequent high ratios of family care. It is tempting to suggest that family care was inevitable because of the limited number of nursing home places, but many families genuinely preferred this.

According to the 1984 prefecture survey, over 90 per cent of the 1,050 elderly interviewees wanted to be cared for by their children within the extended family if they required assistance. This was unchanged even in 1996.[139] Similarly, over three-quarters of families already caring for older relatives at home interviewed in 1992 preferred this arrangement.[140]

Nevertheless, there were considerable social pressures concerning family obligations, particularly in rural prefectures like Gifu, where research suggested 'a strong perception that wives or daughters-in-law must take full responsibilities for the care of older members ... it is not untypical that some result in "family suicides" ... we must abandon the idea that asking for help is shameful conduct'.[141] In addition, the population rejected public welfare services because of the social stigma attached to them, particularly institutional provision. All but one of the older people living alone in Kamioka, near Takayama, expressed a determination never to enter an old people's home or nursing home in 1977, as did all but four in Kagamihara City in 1975.[142] This was true of older people living with their children within the extended family: just twenty-three of the 1,650 elderly interviewed in 1984 had ever considered admission to any type of residential accommodation, as had only sixteen of their corresponding family members.[143]

A welfare officer in rural Yaozu Town, which had no nursing home, commented in 1992 that 'the slow progress in our residential provision for older people is because firstly, there is a strong perception among the locals that care of the frail elderly should be done within families, and secondly this is a very closed community where people distance themselves from any welfare provision outside the Council'.[144] In fact, hardly any of the local elderly had applied for their own authority's community care services, let alone for neighbouring nursing homes. This was true in Gifu's other rural authorities, representing the long-standing 'gap and difficulties surrounding the prefecture welfare provision'.[145] However, other rural prefectures did develop nursing home provision: by 1989 Gifu's six neighbouring rural prefectures had achieved national-level nursing home provision, as did sparsely populated larger northern rural prefectures like Hokkaido and Iwate.[146] Gifu's lack of nursing homes was not simply a question of tradition or geography, but reflected the prefecture's restrictionist policy, which encouraged and even exploited informal family care.

In contrast, Gifu's welfare facilities for active older people at home expanded in line with the national average. Some sixty community welfare centres, offering advice, recreation, adult education and rehabilitation, had opened by 1989, from the pioneer in Gifu City in 1971.[147] Similarly, thirty-one smaller recreation centres, designed for dispersed older populations in more rural areas, were established during 1970–82.[148] The first holiday home, offering twenty affordable short-stay places, was built near a hot spring in a Gifu City suburb in 1967, followed by three more over the next decade.[149] For those who had retired but were still eager to work, the first workshop, making boxes and wrappings, opened within a community welfare centre in Gifu City in 1972.[150] It proved very popular with sixty people registered, including an 82-year-old, so three more were added by 1986.[151] Furthermore, as some moderately well-off older people lacked adequate housing, the first low-fee home for seventy such people was built in Mizunami City near a hot spring in 1965.[152] A second, in a suburb of Gifu City in 1974, provided fifty places in en-suite single or double rooms with kitchen facilities.[153] All these were provided by the municipal authorities, unlike the nursing homes which were dominated by social welfare corporations. These developments modified local opinion of public welfare facilities for older people, with 40 per cent (2,700) of elderly interviewees in 1977 expressing 'favourable' impressions of means-tested old people's homes, almost double the 22 per cent with 'unfavourable' views.[154] However, it was acknowledged, 'given that the interviewees are able-bodied far from desperate for old people's home provision, they may have responded relatively optimistically'.[155]

Day care and short-stay facilities for frail or bedridden older people developed from the 1980s. These were often built alongside nursing homes, reflecting national trends towards the 'socialization of the homes' and integration of institutional and community care. Multifunctional welfare facilities came later. One Gifu City complex, which opened in 1991, featured residential and community-based facilities, with the former consisting of nineteen means-tested small flats for twenty-seven functionally independent older persons and the latter day care and community welfare centres.[156]

Nursing Homes: Improving Standards, 1968–80s

Most early nursing homes were located on spacious out-of-town sites, similar to the post-1960 old people's homes. The first prefecture-funded social welfare corporation nursing home, Jurakuen (1968), was in 'a quiet environment with little traffic, facing a mountain full of trees and birds'.[157] The corporation's second, Hida-Jurakuen (1973) near Takayama City, was in 'a peaceful and quiet natural environment among the mountain chains', but was often cut off in winter.[158] 'Private' social welfare corporation nursing homes from the late 1970s also built 100-place facilities on spacious but isolated sites in rural districts and smaller urban buildings on the outskirts of cities.

Generally, the physical environments improved in line with revisions to official guidelines and to meet the needs of frail or disabled residents. Jurakuen consisted of twelve six-bedded rooms, seven of them on the first floor, with rather limited lavatory accommodation on each floor. There was a large dining hall, three bathrooms and facilities for the sick or disabled, two small sick wards and examination and rehabilitation rooms. Initially, there were no lifts or ramps.[159]

Although its proximity to the adjacent Gifu Prefecture Hospital implied seamless care according to the needs of residents, this was rarely achieved: there were over 200 deaths in the home but just fifteen hospital transfers during 1968–85.[160] Hida-Jurakuen had almost twice the floor space and a site five times larger, with separate dining and recreation rooms, a barber's, a Buddhist service room and a roof terrace, along with a lift, indoor ramps and wide corridors for wheelchairs. However, mostly six-bedded rooms were utilized. Separate staff accommodation improved staff recruitment and retention and provided a clearer demarcation between duty and off-duty hours, practices also adopted at Jurakuen in 1974.[161]

The 1976-built first private social welfare corporation nursing home, Shinseien in Ibigawa Town, was a two-storey concrete building and featured several extra features. It was well lit and centrally heated, and all bedrooms faced south and were equipped with patios. From the large windows, residents could enjoy the view of cherry blossoms in the spring. On each floor 'roomy and luxurious foyers analogous with a hotel lobby' were decorated with pictures, a present from Dr Imamura, its founder and chairman.[162] It cost 377 million yen to build and so considerably exceeded the 66 million yen for Jurakuen and the 177 million yen for Hida-Jurakuen.[163] This partly reflected the resources of the corporation and the founder's concerns:

> [A]fter touring hospitals and welfare facilities for the elderly in Europe and United States, I made a decision to build a nursing home next to my private hospital … I want to provide a 'home' where the elderly residents feel fulfilled with their life … future plans include a new garden and pond in front of the nursing home.[164]

Again, coexistence of the hospital and nursing home suggested 'integrated medical and social care' for patients and residents, although there is no evidence to support this.[165] In Tarui Town, Dr Asano, founder and chairman of the Ibukien nursing home in 1981, was another medical practitioner and prefecture councillor with entrepreneurial and social interests in welfare for older citizens.[166] With at least 760 bedridden older people living at home in the area, he offered a 100-place single-storey facility for frail residents. This 'spacious nursing home for resident-led life' cost 407 million yen to build and featured more living space per capita, wide corridors and central heating.[167]

Urban corporation nursing homes were different. Kikujuen, on the western edge of Gifu City, was a three-storey 25 million yen building for just fifty people.[168] There was a homely atmosphere and privacy for occupants, with a clearer demarcation between residential accommodation on the first and second floors and communal and administrative facilities on the ground floor.[169] Moreover, the bedrooms were grouped around a central garden area on the first floor and a second-floor stair well space, each floor with shared lavatories and bathrooms. Bedrooms varied from single to four-bedded to meet the residents' different requirements. Similarly, the 1980 Gifu-daisan nursing home was a compact three-storey 24 million yen building, attached to the replacement Gifu old people's home (formerly Gifu Almshouse).[170] Since they were run by the same corporation, some facilities and amenities were shared for greater economy.

Thus prefecture-funded corporation nursing homes, based on early official minimum guidelines and simple plans, were followed by private social welfare corporation homes, differing in size, plan and accommodation arrangements. Typically, the latter had higher standards and extras, reflecting uprated official minimum standards, their private origins and greater budgetary discretion, along with the founders' strong charitable and consumer-led principles. Yet both types were subcontracted quangos, providing statutory residential provision strictly in line with official guidelines and receiving public subsidies. Both were also assessed institutions, and residents had little choice as to where they would be accommodated. As the proportion of welfare corporation places increased to 70 per cent by 1989, the uneven distribution of the prefecture nursing homes worsened, because the corporations built profitably in and near urban centres where demand was higher and staff could be recruited more easily.[171] Consequently, elderly people in the sparsely populated rural areas were at a disadvantage, as their chances of access were strictly limited. At Jurakuen 40 per cent of the 335 admissions in 1968–86 were applicants from Gifu City itself, but others included some from rural districts over 100 miles away.[172]

Dementia: Responses since 1984

From the 1980s there was growing concern about dementia sufferers, who were officially excluded from both old people's homes and nursing homes as they were 'likely to cause considerable trouble to other residents or staff'.[173] However, without alternatives, both types of home accepted dementia cases. Thus in 1963 the thirty-place Furukawa and Hashima homes accommodated a handful of such cases, and twenty years later roughly 400 (20 per cent) of residents altogether in prefecture old people's homes were classified as 'confused'.[174] Nursing homes had still more, with some 42 per cent of residents at Jurakuen and 33 per cent at Hida-Jurakuen by the mid-1970s.[175] Nevertheless, 'facing long waiting lists for nursing home places, the bedridden were given priority, putting off dementia cases'.[176] Consequently, some 7,200 dementia sufferers (3.5 per cent of the prefecture older population) were looked after informally at home in 1984.[177]

That year the prefecture began to set aside funds for social welfare corporation providing residential provision designated for dementia cases, increased later by central government subsidies.[178] The first short-stay facility for ten dementia sufferers, adjoining the Toseien nursing home in Toki City, opened in 1985.[179] Two years later, permanent accommodation for this clientele was provided by building twenty-place extensions within the Hida-Jurakuen, Shinseien and Kei-waen nursing homes during 1985–8.[180] A dozen or so extensions were added at other nursing homes, and a purpose-built comprehensive facility was included in the Sawayaka nursing home in Minokamo City in 1988. Here sixty bedridden or frail cases and twenty confused residents were separately accommodated, mainly in four-bedded rooms, along with four short-stay beds and a day care facility.[181] The 1989 extension at the Hikarinosono nursing home in Gifu City included 'well-thought-out facilities'.[182] There were twenty single and five double rooms, unlike the four-bedded rooms in the main block. Such arrangements soon became standard, followed by the new Toseien nursing home in Mizunami City and extensions at Kusunokien in Ogaki City, both completed in 1990.[183] By then Gifu Prefecture had 210 designated places for dementia cases in sixteen nursing homes.[184] Their places were mostly in single or double bedrooms to minimize any disruption they might cause and to prevent them wandering.[185] The rooms were typically tiny and basic, and were sometimes locked.

With additional wards or extensions for dementia cases, the average prefecture nursing home increased by about 10 per cent to seventy-seven places during 1970–87, compared to a static fifty-seven in prefecture old people's homes and suggesting a more 'institutional' environment.[186] Nursing home residents without dementia remain in four-bedded rooms under the official minimum standards even today, and with little privacy or personal space, it is questionable whether their environment, let alone quality of care, has improved. Meanwhile, for those suffering mild to moderate dementia, new small 'group homes' were authorized and provision in Gifu Prefecture expanded rapidly, as elsewhere, with almost 2,000 places in 177 group homes by 2005.[187]

Quality of Care: Staffing

To meet increasing care requirements for frail nursing home residents, the monthly subsidy for personnel costs per nursing home resident increased to 47,000 yen by 1974, compared to 29,000 yen in old people's homes.[188] Locally, the staff establishments at Jurakuen and Hida-Jurakuen were within official minimum guidelines, and all nursing staff were full-time employees.[189] Yet austere buildings and limited equipment lagged behind the increasing needs of a larger proportion of frail residents – more than half the Jurakuen residents were doubly incontinent, and fixed 'five-a-day' pad changing was the rule well into the 1980s.[190] Care standards were problematic, and with usually just one domestic in each home, attendants and even nurses did domestic chores. This was not untypical for Japanese residential facilities then or indeed now.

From 1970 working conditions and welfare came under the scrutiny of the prefecture's Labour Standards Bureau after attendants complained about unpaid overtime, staff shortages, low wages and a seniority-based wage structure.[191] In 1973 it was noted that 'staff members are unable to take their statutory holiday entitlement because of staff shortages, as with lunch breaks; statutory pay is not given for overtime work; and resident staff undertake unpaid night duties'.[192] With no programme to remedy the situation, these issues were reiterated at the 1976 residential staff trade union meeting with the governor, Mr Hirano.[193] However, the standard working week for residential staff was not reduced to 48 hours until 1981, and unpaid or under-paid overtime continued well into the 1990s.[194]

Qualitative improvements were enhanced by local staff training, when the prefecture began to fund annual two-day training courses for managers, nurses, attendants and kitchen staff from the late 1960s. Held by rota in a local home, these consisted of general and specialized themes, followed by a tour of the home and an 'opinion-exchange reception'.[195] In 1973 the new local Gifu Council of Elderly Homes took over and organized tours to pioneering homes outside the prefecture for selected staff, the costs covered by membership fees and subsidies.[196] The participants, used to official minimum standards homes, were impressed, with one reporting: 'When I entered the nursing home, I was astonished to see piles of beer bottles … even more amazed entering the dining hall, where a buffet lunch was offered containing over forty dishes … it was like a hotel, or even more'.[197] Noting the home's underlying policy that good quality food was essential to maintaining quality of life for residents, she concluded: 'I feel sad to have nothing to be proud of in our nursing home'.[198] Meanwhile, regular meetings involving prefecture welfare officers and home managers discussed national policy issues and regulations affecting local management and practice.[199]

Other local developments included funded ten-day intensive training courses relating to dementia sufferers, launched in 1985 and based on the national course started the previous year.[200] With family carers, home helps and nursing staff in the homes all participating, there were 170 applications for sixty places, soon increased to seventy-six, as this became a regular event.[201] Similarly, the prefecture provided funding for in-home experimental research 'to motivate staff and improve the welfare of residents'. Themes covered care quality, resident-centred services, rehabilitation and activity programmes, bathing and meal arrangements and schemes to promote the 'socialization of the homes'.[202] Annual research reports were sent to all the prefecture homes to improve practice.[203] Some nursing homes ran their own induction and regular training courses for staff, with lectures and seminars for a wider audience, including family carers, home helps and students.[204]

To some extent public accountability and monitoring protected homes from exploitation or poor conditions. Social welfare corporation homes also received annual inspections by prefecture officials, although these visits were routine and reports consisted of fixed-format checklists and perfunctory notes. Essentially, compliance with state minimum standards and entitlement to full state subsidies predominated, rather than encouragement of innovative or distinct services or additional provisions, which did not attract state aid. This inevitably tended to standardize the homes.

Generally the homes could afford only minimum standards provision using public subsidies, and there were no internal or regular Ministry-level inspections. One, conducted in 1995 after a seventeen-year gap, criticized the provision. It was especially concerned about under-staffing, 'sloppy' management of residents' personal money and 'inadequate' disaster prevention measures.[205] A particular problem was the lack of residents' dignity, with the changing of incontinence pads in public and 'residents wrapped only in a bath towel were queuing in wheelchairs in the corridor outside the communal bathroom for their turn to be bathed by staff'.[206] Prefecture inspection and guidance systems were also 'inadequate' – there were no follow-up visits, and late or non-standardized reports were accepted. As 'there have been few improvements in the prefecture homes and their inspection over the last decades', the Ministry demanded radical reform.[207] By then the importance of quality issues was recognized nationally in the 1994 revisions to the 1989 new comprehensive Code of Practice for statutory residential facilities of all kinds.[208]

In summary, Gifu Prefecture's statutory residential care provision for older people lagged behind the rest of Japan, reflecting specific regional features, significantly the prefecture's conservative outlook. It regarded informal family care as a primary asset overriding public welfare provision and thereby limited nursing home places to the frailest cases lacking family support, against central legislation and directives. Yet this was largely accepted by the population, who still preferred family care for older people and associated public welfare provision with stigmatized pre-war almshouses, Poor Law institutions or *obasuteyama*. Nonetheless, as the very frail or disabled local older population grew, these perceptions changed, reflected in the expansion of prefecture nursing home provision during the 1980s and 1990s, though this was still below national averages. This catching-up process did not indicate the end of official restrictionism, but reflected more demanding central government targets and efforts by non-profit social welfare corporations underpinned by central government subsidies. Indeed, almost 90 per cent of prefecture nursing home places (3,300), created during 1976–99, reflected social welfare corporation sector initiatives.[209]

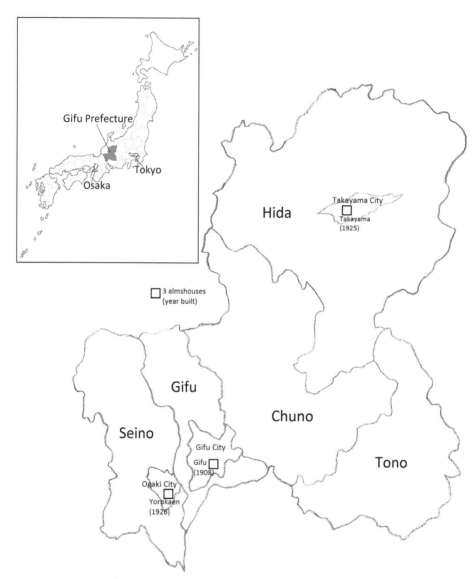

Map 4.1: Japan's forty-seven prefectures (inset) and municipal authority areas and location of almshouses in Gifu.

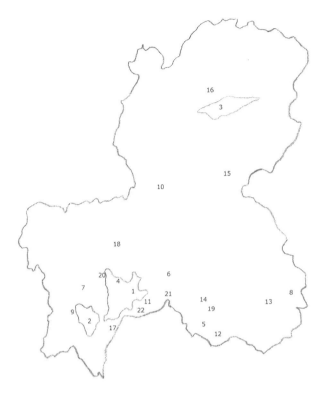

Map 4.2: Location of old people's homes in Gifu, 1974.

Table 4.1: List of old people's homes in Gifu, 1974.

ID	Homes	Location	Opened	Beds	ID	Homes	Location	Opened	Beds
1	Gifu	Gifu	1934	110	12	Keifuso	Toki	1955	50
2	Yorokaen	Ogaki	1947	100	13	Keikoen	Ena	1956	50
3	Hiyoen	Takayama	1952	50	14	Sosuien	Kamo	1956	50
4	Jumatsuen	Hino	1948	100	15	Asagiriso	Hagiwara	1958	50
5	Tayoso	Tajimi	1950	50	16	Wakoen	Furukawa	1960	50
6	Matsufuen	Seki	1951	50	17	Rowaen	Hashima	1961	50
7	Showaen	Ibigawa	1951	50	18	Miyamaso	Yamagata	1967	50
8	Seiwaryo	Nakatsugawa	1952	50	19	Chorakuso	Mitaka	1968	50
9	Seifuen	Tarui	1952	50	20	Miwa	Gifu	1972	50
10	Kairakuen	Gujo	1952	50	21	Jikoen	Kagamigahara	1974	50
11	Yamatoen	Motosu	1954	60	22	Nihonline	Shakahogi	1974	50

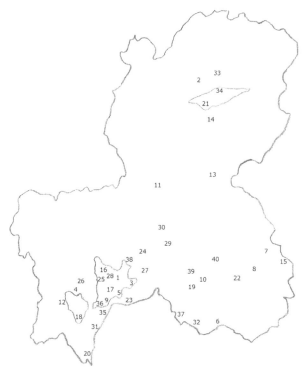

Map 4.3: Location of nursing homes in Gifu, 1996.

Table 4.2: List of nursing homes in Gifu, 1996.

ID	Homes	Location	Opened	Beds	ID	Homes	Location	Opened	Beds
1	Jurakuen	Gifu	1968	70	21	Horakuen	Takayama	1989	50
2	Hida-Jurakuen	Takayama	1973	105	22	Towaen	Mizunami	1990	50
3	Miwa	Gifu	1974	50	23	Tsutsujien	Kagamigahara	1991	60
4	Shinseien	Ibigawa	1976	130	24	Miwanosato	Mino	1991	50
5	Gifu-daisan	Gifu	1978	60	25	Daini-Zuikoen	Gifu	1992	80
6	Toseien	Toki	1978	120	26	Showaen	Ibigawa	1992	50
7	Koseiryo	Nakatsugawa	1978	50	27	Ha-tofuru	Seki	1992	70
8	Omotoen	Ena	1979	100	28	Gikyoen	Gifu	1993	80
9	Kikujuen	Gifu	1979	60	29	Juwaen	Mugi	1993	80
10	Keiwaen	Kamo	1980	70	30	Fukujuen	Kamiyahagi	1993	30
11	Kairakuen	Gujo	1980	50	31	Yasuragien	Hashima	1994	50
12	Ibukien	Tarui	1981	100	32	Toseien	Tajimi	1994	50
13	Asagiriso	Hagiwara	1982	50	33	Tampopoen	Kamioka	1994	50
14	Hakkoen	Hibino	1984	60	34	Shinguen	Takayama	1994	100
15	Seto-no-sato	Nakatsugawa	1984	80	35	Kawashimaen	Hashima	1995	50
16	Zuikoen	Gifu	1985	80	36	Asuwaen	Anpachi	1995	50
17	Hikarinosono	Gifu	1985	50	37	Harusatoen	Kani	1995	80
18	Kusunokien	Ogaki	1987	100	38	Tsubakinoen	Yamagata	1996	50
19	Sawayaka	Minokamo	1988	80	39	Sawayaka	Kawabe	1996	60
20	Matsufuen	Kaizu	1988	50	40	Minoshirakawa	Yaozu	1996	50

5 RESIDENTIAL LIFE IN NORFOLK

This chapter and Chapter 6 present institutional case studies from England and Japan respectively. The effects of their national legislation and policy goals on grassroots practices and residents' lives within each region since 1948 are examined, focusing on qualitative aspects from the residents' and carers' perspectives. Each chapter has two sections. The first covers the period 1948–73 and investigates a former workhouse or almshouse and its replacement. The history of the selected institutions is reviewed, drawing on archival and local records. The first section therefore examines the extent to which a 'homely' home and improvements in residential life and practice have been achieved. This reveals the extent to which the Poor Law legacy, stigma, and pre-war measures and mentalities have survived. These are considered by examining the environment, amenities and services, as well as staffing and care standards. Acknowledging the greater diversity in residential care for subsequent decades, the second section provides a more dynamic and complex institutional history since 1980, by exploring various long-term institutional care locations in each region, drawing on in-depth interviews with residents or patients, their relatives and staff.

The Tenacity of the Workhouse Regime

Eastgate House County Home, 1948–63

Workhouse Origins

Eastgate House started life in 1836 as Freebridge Lynn Union workhouse, near Gayton (see Map 3.1).[1] Designed by William John Donthorn, it had a cruciform and a 'rationalist, linear style of neo-classicism', the main facade featuring some ornamentation to differentiate it from earlier, prison-like workhouses, although other aspects were 'strictly utilitarian'.[2] 'A plain building' for up to 130 inmates, the two-storey structure featured a central block flanked by two short cross-wings.[3] Smaller than other workhouses in Norfolk, it cost £5,146 or £34 per capita, considerably above the £10 per capita recommended in the 1834 Poor Law Report.[4] The result was a 'pleasantly non-institutional' appearance, which 'hinted at charitable benevolence ... [and] an atmosphere of security and domesticity', albeit with strict sexual segregation and classification of the inmates.[5]

'Seldom more than 100' occupants ensured there was little overcrowding, and with the exception of a chapel added in 1907, the building was essentially unchanged during the period examined. However, its official classification changed from 'workhouse' under the 1834 Poor Law to 'Public Assistance Institution' (PAI) following the 1929 Local Government Act. It finally became a county home for frail older people, and was renamed Eastgate House on 5 July 1948, the appointed day for the 1948 National Assistance Act.[6] How far changes in nomenclature marked the transition from the Poor Law to welfare state is debatable, and improvements in the quality of institutional life and practices cannot be taken for granted.

Residents' Characteristics

As Gayton Public Assistance Institution, there was on average fifty residents between 1930 and 1948, of whom about twenty were classified as sick, with a temporary influx after the 1942 bombing of Norwich PAI and the transfer of thirty male residents there.[7] Up to thirty, mainly male, 'casuals' were sometimes housed in designated wards, but the number fell to a dozen or so by 1942. Under the 1948 Act, Gayton PAI and six other PAIs in Norfolk became county homes for non-sick, frail, mainly older people, classified as Part III residents. However, all homes were under interim joint-user arrangements and had hospital beds for sick patients under the 1946 National Health Service (NHS) Act. As a result, in addition to twenty-two non-sick and mainly older and frail Part III residents, some had lived there for over thirty years.[8] Eastgate House county home had twenty NHS patients in the sick wards, which precluded the need for transfers to NHS hospitals.[9] At first Eastgate House took mainly NHS cases from the nearby hospital, formerly King's Lynn PAI, but in 1951 Eastgate House became the first of Norfolk's seven county homes with no NHS quota.[10] However, the 1948 Act also stipulated that local authority residential/Part III provision should include temporary accommodation for those in urgent need, although it was 'not intended for persons without a settled way of living, for whom reception centres were to be provided by the National Assistance Board'.[11] People 'of no fixed abode' nevertheless comprised almost 30 per cent of Eastgate House admissions in 1950.[12] Although the Eastgate House Management Sub-Committee had already asked the Norfolk Welfare Committee to stop sending such admissions, a lack of alternatives meant that discretionary temporary accommodation was offered to people evicted by their families, single mothers with infants or young children, and the homeless, with some later discharged 'at [their] own request' or 'abscond[ing]'.[13]

Consequently there was a high turnover, with eighty admissions and fifty-nine discharges in 1954 compared to twenty-five and six respectively in 1945. The majority were under 65 years of age.[14] This was potentially disruptive for elderly residents who regarded Eastgate House as their permanent *home*, for in extreme cases some admissions were of 'undesirable characters' who had been charged with manslaughter or theft, which meant there had to be a police presence.[15] Over time abusive and inebriated residents were transferred to nearby Beech House (ex-Gressenhall PAI), which was earmarked for 'nuisances', but emergency admissions and unlawful incidents were still occurring in the early 1960s.[16] Eastgate House's complement thus reflected the legacy of the 'mixed' workhouse, with casuals, tramps and long-stay chronic sick or frail older people all housed together.

In contrast, Norfolk's new hostels were intended for 'the more ambulant and active old people' and were selective 'to ensure that only really suitable persons are admitted'.[17] Thus when Burnham Westgate Hall opened at Burnham Market in 1951, its twenty-six admissions were all aged 60 or more, and none was of 'no fixed abode'.[18] Accordingly, one poor 73-year-old resident was soon 'taken back to St James's Hospital [ex-PAI] as he did not prove suitable', an indication of Norfolk Welfare Committee's two-tier policy on its residential care development for older people.[19]

By 1955 Eastgate House was full with eighty residents, doubling from 1948, but their composition now reflected a more balanced sex ratio (earlier it had been predominantly men), with the few temporary cases and the over-80s almost equalling the under-80s by 1960.[20] Inevitably, the growing incidence of physical and mental disability resulted in briefer residency. By 1963 only three had been there for more than five years, including a 63-year-old man admitted in 1939.[21] Nonetheless, 'all the residents were able to be present in the Dining Hall' for the Christmas dinner in 1962, suggesting that few were wholly bedridden.[22]

Although the new hostels had frequent transfers to fulfil residents' location preferences, people in former PAI county homes rarely moved. When a new thirty-six-place hostel opened in King's Lynn in 1957, only three Eastgate House residents were transferred there, partly because the hostel was 'intended for the more ambulant and active'.[23] Transfers usually reflected special circumstances involving other county homes, so although Eastgate House residents were 'all Norfolk', several were from the Norwich area, over thirty miles away.[24]

Information on residents' socio-economic backgrounds is limited, but glimpses of their financial situation can be gleaned from records of their contributions to maintenance costs and the 1964–7 pensions register.[25] Most of those entitled to an old age pension received only the minimum non-contributory basic pension, and none had sufficient pensions or other income to trigger the full weekly charge of £2 18s. 4d. All but three pensionable residents in 1948–51 had the minimum weekly rate of 21 shillings deducted from their basic pensions, which left them with just 5 shillings pocket money.[26] Even in 1964 fifty of the sixty-one former Eastgate House residents (now living in Woodlands) paid minimum charges and none met the full cost.[27] Valuables or possessions were few: a 74-year-old man, resident for nine months, left in his former rented cottage 'just 3 chairs, two tables, sideboard and chest of drawers ... nothing of any real value ... only suitable for burning'.[28] Hostel clienteles were slightly better off, some paying the full cost, which was higher than at county homes.

Some residents had no nearby relatives and many had no family at their funeral: Norfolk County Council itself undertook sixteen of the thirty-four Eastgate House funeral services in 1951, including that of a 70-year-old former alderman.[29] Almost all the 1960–1 admissions were widowed (64 per cent) or single/divorced (32 per cent) and no couples were admitted between 1948 and 1963, although some couples entered hostels from the early 1950s.[30] Not surprisingly, the home received few gifts from residents or their families, and thank-you letters or small donations from distant relations came infrequently, usually after a resident's death.[31] Hardly any relatives visited even at Christmas, and very few residents spent the occasion with their relations, although more took a short leave at other times to stay with friends.

In short, Eastgate House was filled to capacity by 1955, remaining so until 1961, when thirty residents were transferred to Westfields (Swaffham), the rest moving to Woodlands (King's Lynn) in 1963. Its clientele changed from mixed age groups to predominantly older people of increasing frailty. With more transfers to and from hospitals, the average length of residency fell, even though there were fewer temporary admissions. A rough gender balance was maintained, but there was little change in residents' socio-economic background, suggesting very limited financial means and few relatives.

Physical Environment

No major structural improvements were undertaken at Eastgate House until its closure in 1963. As Gayton PAI, it had been earmarked for closure in 1931, but continued in use as a rescue service depot during the war.[32] Though it escaped bombing, the building and interior decor deteriorated under wartime restrictions. By 1944 it was noted that 'a quantity of rats were frequenting the premises ... action should be taken to destroy them'.[33] Before April 1948 the lack of electricity caused 'a great deal of inconvenience', with some parts of the buildings completely without lighting because of inadequate supplies of paraffin for oil lamps.[34] Essential equipment was missing or in poor condition: there were 'no lockers' for residents until March 1948, and 'old lath type bedsteads' 'cause[d] bed-sores', according to one resident.[35] In comparison, the neighbouring Gressenhall PAI boasted a hot water system installed in the early 1900s, with a full electrical supply from 1932 and the use of a wireless from 1945.[36]

A local clergyman voiced concern over conditions at Gayton PAI after visiting an 83-year-old resident there in 1946:

> [T]he surroundings are unnecessarily drab; the wards appear to be completely cheerless. The provision of clocks in each ward and wireless sets would relieve the unbelievable monotony of being condemned to pass the day without either of those things.[37]

Responding to local press criticism, Norfolk Public Assistance Sub-Committee Chair Sydney Dye MP visited the PAI and concluded:

> It is a great relief to me to find a pleasant and homely place for the 50 inmates and to realize that every comfort and convenience of the people is provided for. To them it must be a real home. The attention and care bestowed by the staff seems all that can be expected ... Nobody raised any complaint[38]

Such contrasting views formed the backcloth to attempts to transform an obsolete PAI into a 'homely' place. In 1948 the Eastgate House Sub-Committee envisaged this transition through structural alternations, redecoration and refurbishment. 'Most urgent' since 1943 was the construction of a dayroom attached to the fourteen-bedded male sick ward, 'at present used not only as a dormitory, but for meals and as a day room', a 'most undesirable' arrangement.[39] However, approval by the Norfolk Welfare Committee in November 1948 was overturned a month later, pending 'the closing of Eastgate House ... as soon as alternative Hostel accommodation becomes available', under the Norfolk five-year local plan submitted to the Ministry early in 1949.[40] Proposals for a covered walkway between the dining hall and sick wards and first-floor lavatories for men and women were also shelved.[41] Only after the Eastgate House Sub-Committee concluded in March 1951 that 'there is every indication that Eastgate House will continue to be used for some years' did the work begin. It was completed by 1955.[42]

The amended plan of 1955, annotated with room use and numbers of residents, shows Eastgate House's layout.[43] Male and female accommodation wings offered nine bedrooms for the eighty residents, the ground-floor male sick ward and its new dayroom adjoining the female block. First-floor sick wards accommodated fourteen male and nine female patients respectively, with the remaining forty-three more able residents in one eight-bedded dormitory and two three-bedded rooms on the ground floor and three 6–12-bedded dormitories on the second floor. A large hall with a stage doubled for meals and entertainments, along with three small dayrooms on the ground floor.

With restrictions on alternatives or structural work, additional equipment, furnishings and personal items were encouraged. By 1953 residents' rooms had 'much equipment – lockers, curtains, bedside rugs and coconut matting', instigated by Ministry of Health inspectors, although 'a shortage of bright counterpanes still exists'.[44] Hard benches were replaced with fireside or easy chairs, and long dining room tables made way for 'ten small wood dining tables each to seat four persons' in 1953, with better quality ones 'covered with Formica' in 1960.[45] Beds and bedding were considered inadequate, as some people were sleeping on 'reserve bedsteads ... the old slatted type, which were condemned many years ago'.[46] The provision in 1952 of a dozen new wooden bedsteads, each with a flock mattress and a feather pillow, was 'greatly appreciated by all'.[47]

Most rooms had linoleum flooring and hearthrugs, with 'rubber covering' on staircases.[48] 'Very shabby or inadequate' furniture in some staff quarters was replaced, while the 'worn out and unsatisfactory' kitchen range gave way to a new Aga; washing and drying equipment was updated.[49] Five electric convector wall heaters were installed in two dormitories in 1950, with a dining hall stove added in 1952.[50] Outside there were garden benches and easy chairs, with flowering shrubs planted and high stone walls lowered, but iron railings at the front were retained, despite repeated requests for their removal.[51] Officially, this transformed the home into 'a well-run establishment with a homely atmosphere', although concerns remained over 'its very isolated situation and the condition of the fabric generally'.[52] The Norfolk Welfare Committee acknowledged that a replacement facility was needed, but maintained the home 'without undertaking work ... which is likely to involve substantial expenditure'.[53] Expedient measures did not always suffice, and the impending yet uncertain closure of Eastgate House frustrated its management, staff and residents for more than a decade.

Installation of first-floor lavatories for twenty-four women was repeatedly recommended by visitors and medical officers, as 'the provision of additional night commodes' in 1956 was an inadequate substitute.[54] Without wardrobes, residents' clothing was kept in a 'wooden cupboard fitment ... [with] no partitions to provide individual compartments', or in five 'curtained off' enclosures in the corners of the rooms'.[55] Two such 'enclosures' for forty women were 'definitely insufficient'.[56] Large dormitories were divided by 'bedside screens' rather than converted into smaller rooms affording a little privacy, and with the conversion of two three-bedded rooms into dayrooms, the six beds that were removed were squeezed into the existing dormitories, making overcrowding even worse.[57] Minor renovation and redecoration in the kitchen, staff quarters and men's dayroom during 1955–7 were undertaken only after visitors repeatedly referred to 'unsafe and beyond repair', 'very poor' or 'overcrowded' conditions.[58] Some dormitories still relied on 'very old and defective' fireplaces until 1958.[59] Since the water supply came from a well, baths were severely restricted during droughts.[60] More disturbingly, 'there was no hot water during evening after the boiler was damped down and none during the night or early morning'.[61]

Substitute, piecemeal measures often involved recycling materials from the ageing building or from other institutions earmarked for closure. Compounded by overcrowding and staff shortages, the home deteriorated, and by 1957 'the provision of new premises was becoming extremely urgent'.[62] Long-awaited replacement homes – Westfields (Swaffham) and Woodlands (King's Lynn) – were completed only in 1961 and 1963 respectively. Significantly, it was specified that 'the new home [Westfields] should be furnished entirely with new equipment and ... no equipment should be transferred from Eastgate House'.[63] Yet with new expenditure on Eastgate House now ruled out, conditions for its remaining residents became unacceptable. In 1960 the superintendent complained that 'water penetrates the building during periods of heavy rain ... it is sometimes necessary to move beds', and the county architect was warned to keep the building 'habitable'.[64]

After thirty residents were transferred to Westfields in 1961, the remaining fifty shared four large dormitories on the female side. One official visitor reckoned that the rearrangement of accommodation, furniture and equipment produced 'a general improvement in the appearance of the residences'.[65] Even so, essential comforts and equipment were lacking or 'in very poor condition and ought to be replaced': there were not 'sufficient fireside chairs', and the absence of bedside lights was apparently excused on the grounds that since 'there are so many old people sharing the one room. With the switching on of a light, invariably someone would be disturbed'.[66] As for general interior conditions, 'the corridors ... are decorated in dull cream and brown. Tiled and flagged floors, worn smooth with many years of use, and large, poorly lit rooms typify the bleak atmosphere within the flint walls of the building'.[67] A public complaint in 1962 'about the condition of the room, including the furnishings, in which [a] resident was accommodated' produced a lame official acknowledgement:

> accommodation at Eastgate House is not up to the standard the Welfare Committee would normally expect to provide, but ... steps are being taken to remedy the situation by the provision of a new home [Woodlands] and that the expenditure of public money on Eastgate House is not justified at this juncture.[68]

With the opening of Woodlands in 1963, Eastgate House finally closed after 127 years. Most equipment at the home had 'no useful recoverable value', and only a few items were allocated to former PAI county homes.[69] A local newspaper described it as a 'rambling old establishment ... "workhouse" is written all over the structure ... which people still call "the Institution"'.[70] It was sold to a Cromer man for use as a smallholding and for pig keeping, confirming the unsuitability of the main buildings for residential purposes. By contrast, other Norfolk former workhouses/PAIs were converted into flats, a museum and, in one case, a hotel.[71] Such episodes pose questions about earlier, guarded comments on quality of life issues at the home, for example: 'I am very impressed at the order and all that has been done to improve a very difficult old building. The residents seemed happy';[72] and similarly, 'many expressions of appreciation of the great kindness and patience found here – they do not seem to want to be anywhere else. Some of them told me that the food had been very nice lately and that everyone is offered a second helping'.[73] Whether the substandard environment could have been offset or camouflaged by enhanced amenities, provisions and services warrants further investigation.

Amenities, Provisions and Services

Everyday life at Gayton PAI (1930–48) continued Poor Law measures, routines and an institutional regime: its residents were allowed to wear their own clothes from 1945, but most could not afford any new items.[74] Visiting remained subject to the superintendent's permission and residents' physical state and financial means. Its new beginning as Eastgate House in 1948 coincided with the installation of electricity, along with radio in dormitories and monthly film shows, which were 'greatly enjoyed'.[75] As in several of Norfolk's other former PAI county homes, a television was temporarily installed in the dining hall so that residents could watch the coronation of Elizabeth II in 1953. A set was later purchased from funds set up by the superintendent and boosted by over 150 voluntary subscriptions, although the more comfortable women's and men's dayrooms were not furnished with a TV until 1960.[76] The annual highlight was Christmas: 'From patients' point of view ... the Christmas Day celebrations ... were most enjoyable'.[77] For years Norfolk County Council provided festive extras, including a pig (later turkeys) from the on-site farm.[78] Residents also received a present of 'sponge bags, combs, hairbrushes, sweets, pipes, tobacco and so on', and many attended Holy Communion in the home's chapel.[79] After the queen's speech was relayed to all dormitories, games, solos, dances and community singing continued until late into night, with refreshments on hand.

Other measures to improve the life and well-being of the residents also featured. Medical care included appointments at nearby hospitals, dentists and opticians, with some residents hospitalized for short periods. A chiropodist attended once a fortnight from 1950, and from 1953 an occupational therapist ran weekly handicraft sessions, these 'proving very satisfactory and the number attending increases every week'.[80] In contrast, most of Norfolk's smaller hostels lacked such arrangements.[81] Eastgate House residents received regular visits from local school children and choirs, while voluntary organizations and companies in the locality and groups from the US Air Force base at Sculthorpe (Fakenham) provided entertainments and tea parties and were 'greatly enjoyed by all'.[82] The chapel held an annual harvest festival service, again 'much appreciated', as was the fiftieth anniversary of the chapel in 1957.[83] Again, such traditions and visits were infrequent or absent altogether in Norfolk's hostels, although conditions there gradually improved.[84] None of this, however, could compensate for the institutional atmosphere, so measures outside the home were introduced: Norfolk County Council funded summer days out for Part III residents, and at least half the residents of Eastgate House experienced coach trips to the Wroxham Broads, Cromer, Great Yarmouth or Skegness.[85] Voluntary organizations also arranged outings, the King's Lynn Business and Professional Women's Club's weekly summertime 'motor trips' being 'greatly enjoyed and looked forward to'.[86] The residents' 'comforts fund' covered concerts and pantomimes at King's Lynn and coach hire expenses.[87]

More personal arrangements included 'three changes of underclothing', with seasonal clothing and plain articles added later.[88] Residents could leave the home more freely and frequently, some visiting public houses within walking distance.[89] Arrangements for 'a special bus to run past Eastgate House ... to enable the residents to get into King's Lynn and back and to facilitate visiting' were made with the Eastern Counties Omnibus Company in 1954, although this was restricted to just one Monday afternoon service.[90] Otherwise, those unable to walk or take the bus, or who had no relatives or friends to take them out, were largely confined within this isolated home.

Leave of up to one week was allowed, but restrictions on 'matron's grant' initially meant that only two or three better-off residents or those with families or friends to stay with them benefited.[91] This partly explains the high rate of absconding during the early years. However, the withdrawal of the matron's discretionary powers and waiving of maintenance payments for up to two weeks a year in 1953 enabled at least ten leaves a year, mainly from 'regulars' during the late 1950s. In 1962 the voluntary Norfolk Old People's Welfare Association initiated week-long holidays at Caister Holiday Camp near Great Yarmouth, attracting mainly the better-off, less frail, regular leave-takers.[92] With most Eastgate House residents retaining just 11s. 6d. from their basic pension, self-funded holidays were an option for just four residents in 1962, compared to fifteen at a nearby hostel.[93] As 'very few ... spend any time at all reading even during the day', and residents 'did not appear to take much interest in the performances [film shows]', everyday life for the home-bound was limited indeed.[94] However, fourteen residents had earned 'extra allowances' in kind for work done in the home in 1959.[95] One male resident allegedly worked 'as a gamekeeper on a neighbouring estate'.[96] By comparison, none at a hostel in King's Lynn was involved in this kind of work, suggesting their better financial standing.[97]

Gifts from the Eastgate House Sub-Committee members, local people and voluntary organizations to residents were gradually replaced by cash donations, which were added to the residents' 'comforts fund', enabling a degree of planning.[98] However, the free tobacco or sweets allowance issued by Norfolk County Council was withdrawn in 1963 on the grounds that 'the present level of pocket money should be adequate to meet any personal needs of residents'.[99] With rising expectations, 'luxuries' such as a television, piano, organ, electric fire, hair dryer, garden furniture, pictures and carpets were purchased with the comforts fund cash, rather than from the council or home's budgets.[100] Additional income derived from a residents' tuck shop, opened in 1957 to supplement the renamed 'canteen and comforts fund', a 'very credible' bazaar, tombolas, whist drives, bingo sessions and jumble sales.[101] These modest developments enriched everyday life and, in a small way, shifted the balance from provider-driven, passive services towards more resident-centred living.

Another development was the 'residents' complaint book' (later renamed the 'suggestion book'), which was kept in the dining hall.[102] Their comments, along with those of staff and visiting relatives, were discussed at the Eastgate House Sub-Committee monthly meetings and sometimes officially investigated. Yet complaints about food were typically met with the response: 'any complaint of this nature is without foundation', 'generally the meal was satisfactory' or even 'the food had been very nice'.[103] Similarly, 'alleged complaints concerning the general welfare of the residents in Eastgate House ... were completely without foundation' and 'unwarranted'.[104] A female resident was ignored as she 'herself is a very difficult woman ... always making complaints'.[105] This reveals the gap between residents' expectations and official attitudes, the latter partly determined by financial constraints and a continuing Poor Law mentality. Those who would not comply with 'reasonable rules as to hours and behaviour' were transferred, 'preferably [to] Beech House, Gressenhall'.[106]

To a degree, public accountability and monitoring helped to maintain standards. From 1948 the twelve-strong Eastgate House Sub-Committee met monthly, with two members paying official visits before presenting their report.[107] Yet little discussion featured in the minutes, and the perfunctory comment that 'satisfactory reports were received' throughout the period suggested routine and self-serving visits.[108] The same was true of information compiled by an unofficial panel of fourteen voluntary visitors, who initially came together to 'take a personal interest in those residents who are not in regular contact with their own relatives and friends'.[109] The panel disbanded in the late 1950s, with the rota of official visits reduced to one member per month. Annual or quarterly visits were paid by inspectors and dieticians from the Ministry of Health and the Assistant County Medical Officer, who undertook general medical supervision of the home. Their reports included some direct and outspoken comments and suggestions, and occasionally led to improvements in the buildings, equipment and furnishings.

Standards of Care and Staff

For any meaningful improvements to residents' lives, good care standards were essential, but staff shortages remained a problem. It was reported in 1942 that the matron's general assistant 'was occupied practically whole time on nursing duties with the result that the matron was without assistance'.[110] In 1947 a Ministry of Health inspector visited Gayton PAI and its forty-five residents, and 'referred to the fact that one nurse only was on duty at night time and that it was advisable that not less than two nurses should be'.[111] Yet 'the isolated situation of the institution and the very indifferent transport facilities' meant that difficulties in the recruitment and retention of staff were unresolved.[112]

In 1948 Mr and Mrs O. were appointed as superintendent and matron for Eastgate House. Staff shortages certainly compounded their problems: in June 1949, for example, 'owing to the Porter being off duty [for eight months] and ... without one handyman ... all the work at present falls on the Master – Shaving; Hair Cutting; Land work; and any odd job'.[113] Early in 1950 a Ministry of Health inspector urgently requested a replacement for the retired resident nurse assistant to 'relieve the Matron of much overwork'. This was essential as Mrs O. became 'seriously ill' and died that November.[114] Mr O. stayed on, with a relief state enrolled nurse (SEN) designated as non-resident acting matron, until both retired in 1955.[115] Mr O. by then was 69 years old, and his 'efficient and loyal service' included efforts to promote the residents' quality of life.[116] He had initiated fundraising for the first television set, placed his own piano in the dining hall, rarely took annual leave and was clearly popular and devoted to the home.[117] Mr and Mrs B. took over as superintendent and matron until 1962, when Mrs C., formerly a sister at ex-PAI Beech House, was appointed matron, with her husband in a subsidiary post.[118] In 1963 she transferred to Woodlands, with her husband as the male attendant, and they worked there until 1967, when they returned to Beech House as superintendent and matron.[119]

It is difficult to form, let alone convey, any accurate impression of residents' lives from bare facts about the chief personnel. Officially, the Eastgate House Sub-Committee viewed their appointments in optimistic and generally sympathetic terms, and each retirement was recorded with warm comments.[120] Thus Mr O. was congratulated for his 'excellent and untiring work in the interests of the old folks ... of Eastgate House during the past 31 years'.[121] However, neither the superintendent's reports nor Sub-Committee minutes contain any subjective or direct accounts by residents or other staff. Other resident couples with workhouse or PAI experience included Mr and Mrs G. from Gayton PAI (1947–52), Mr G. serving for twenty-two years in total and marrying Mrs G. in 1947; Mr and Mrs H. from Beech House (1952–4); and Mr and Mrs M. from Hill House (1955–7).[122] It is debatable whether the retention of familiar or experienced former workhouse staff was better for residents than the recruitment of personnel free from association with the Poor Law legacy. Less experienced or less established key personnel could jeopardize stability in the home, whereas relatively elderly and longer-serving senior personnel offered some continuity, stability and security to residents.

Yet joint resident posts – 'porter and matron's assistant'; 'handyman and ward orderly/nurse' – proved problematic, with the former replaced six times and the latter five times between 1948 and 1952.[123] The isolated location and alternative employment opportunities made it difficult to retain kitchen staff: when the resident cook and the kitchen maid both resigned in 1955, it took six months to replace them, owing to 'the extreme difficulty of securing and retaining staff at Eastgate House'.[124] New appointees, each staying for less than two years, may explain the complaints about meals at both Eastgate House and Woodlands. It was a vicious circle: staff shortages undermined morale and time for training, which affected the recruitment and retention of new personnel, while a perceived deteriorating work environment was likely to result in resignations and a high turnover, further compounding the shortages. Occasionally, the home had no resident nurse simply because of recruitment difficulties, leading to disastrous outcomes. During the 1951 influenza epidemic, for example, five staff were absent, and six residents died in just eleven days.[125] Similarly in February 1961, 'at one time fifty residents [70 per cent of the total] were in bed as well as [nine] staff away'.[126]

There was no early improvement in attendant to resident ratios or staff training, with a nursing establishment of three female attendants/ward orderlies (including one SEN), even though the resident population almost doubled to seventy-eight by 1951.[127] An attendant notionally had less than two hours a week for each resident and was in charge of twenty-six people every day.[128] Three additional attendants appointed by 1957 improved the attendant to resident ratio to 1:13, but this was only marginally better than the 1:14 in 1948. In contrast, hostels for thirty or so mainly more active residents had three attendants by 1957.[129]

Night nursing arrangements remained unsatisfactory, with just one night orderly as in the 1940s, despite the extra residents and their 'increasing infirmity ... and ... greater attention required from the staff'.[130] The superintendent noted in November 1958 'only one young Female Night Attendant on duty to deal with eighty-two residents ... [she] looks after the sick cases at the south end of the building, washes certain of the residents in the morning and patrols the building at night'.[131] In December that year two men were wandering, and one suffered a heart attack.[132] Yet the Sub-Committee merely looked to 'the provision of a bell system to permit the summoning of assistance at night to the male wards', trusting to 'an arrangement whereby an active man in the male ward can summon assistance if necessary'.[133] This coincided with the four-hour net reduction of the night nurse's working week, and the Norfolk Welfare Committee ruled that 'no additional time is used to make up the hours lost'.[134] Lost daytime staff hours were covered mainly by 'allowing existing part-time staff to work more', which at best merely maintained attendant to resident ratios.[135]

An important shift was the emphasis on nursing rather than domestic staff. Thus two vacancies for domestics in 1960 were left unfilled 'as the work was being satisfactorily carried out by the rest of the domestic staff'; instead, an additional part-time ward orderly was appointed to meet 'the need ... for further assistance with the residents'.[136] In later discussions, the matron argued that given 'the need for continuous night duty, it would be better ... [to have] Female Ward Orderlies, bearing in mind also that it had in recent months been possible to run the premises with less than the authorized establishment of Domestics'.[137] Subsequently, the nursing staff were maintained despite decreasing resident numbers, improving the attendant to resident ratio to 1:9.3, allowing for the shorter working week mainly by readjusting the duty roster. This raises the question of whether standards of care were maintained and whether fewer domestic staff merely affected domestic tasks or undermined nursing too. Given severe staff shortages and little formal training, job demarcation between attendants and domestics was blurred, as the 1961 transfer of the part-time assistant cook to part-time female ward orderly confirmed.[138] Although such flexibility could be an advantage, more resort to part-time staff might imply less intensive or continuous engagement with residents when compared with full-time staff.

Although administrative and financial records cast some light on quantitative aspects of care, the lack of staff and resident narratives makes it difficult to convey the qualitative features. At the risk of oversimplification, nursing conditions seemingly improved in terms of numbers; yet given the increasing care needs of more disabled and frail residents, it remains questionable whether standards improved for everyone. Moreover, nursing was increasingly provided by unqualified part-time staff, rearranged shifts by domestics and the use of temporary relief staff, with no guarantees of care standards.

Woodlands Replacement Home, 1963–74

In 1963 the replacement Woodlands home opened. This was a purpose-built two-storey facility, with sixty beds in single or double bedrooms. In 1968 the Woodlands Sub-Committee was subsumed within the 'Area 7' group, which was responsible for three neighbouring homes. In 1970 Area 7 was further aggregated into a larger Area group under an expanded managerial structure following the 1970 Local Authority Social Services Act. Consequently, information on each home became limited to shorter and uninformative Area Sub-Committee bi-monthly minutes and irregular visitors' and superintendents' reports.[139] All this limits an attempt to illustrate aspects of life in Woodlands, although visitors' reports described the home as 'very clean ... almost spotless' and emphasized that its 'high standard and furnishings seem to keep a new fresh look'.[140] 'Many small luxuries' purchased from transferred residents' comfort funds included an organ, several carpets and two 'Ambulifts' (equipment to move a resident from their bed or bath), which provided 'considerable assistance to the staff and much more comfort to the residents'.[141] This helped to offset limited Norfolk County Council expenditure, as did expedients such as 'the transfer of some suitable mattresses from a [former PAI] home which had closed'.[142]

Soon after opening, Woodlands' resident population increased from the initial forty-eight Eastgate House transferees to a full complement of sixty. The oldest was 96 years old.[143] By 1972 it was reported that 'about half ... can be classed as mentally confused', among them a 95-year-old lady 'discovered in her bedroom smoking' who started a fire, and a suicidal 88-year-old man who 'cut his wrist with a razor blade'.[144] On the other hand, a few male residents still did gardening for small cash payments. Residents were nursed by twenty-three staff at the equivalent of one full-time post per six residents. Staff came from Eastgate House, including the matron, resident staff and eight attendants working 70 per cent of attendant hours, with twelve other part-time workers.[145] Whether this affected aspirations to 'homely' care and a new start and the implications of reliance on part-time carers for very elderly and frail residents seem valid questions.

Nonetheless, visitors' reports were favourable, describing the 'care and wellbeing of the residents' as 'good', 'very good' or 'excellent, and the staff 'good', 'contented' or 'all ... doing a fine job most cheerfully'.[146] Moreover, 'the relationship between residents and staff is sufficient evidence of the cordial atmosphere of this home'.[147] Evidently, Woodlands was 'altogether a happy home ... giving the right type of service to all who are fortunate enough to enjoy the evening of their lives within its shelter'.[148] Successive annual medical and hygiene inspection reports by the Deputy County Medical Officer were similarly reassuring, with 'no matters arising to which the Sub-committee's attention should be drawn'.[149] In 1972 a couple at the home were married, and their wedding reception there suggested a happy environment for at least some.[150]

Contrary evidence was fragmentary. In 1965 an official visitor drew attention to 'some deficiencies in the standard of cooking of meals ... [and] complaints from the residents', after which a cook, regarded as 'unsatisfactory ... not mentally capable of carrying out the duties', resigned.[151] A year later some visitors still 'felt very dissatisfied with the tea provided for the residents' and yet another cook was appointed, while the Sub-Committee also reviewed menus.[152] In 1968 a 'satisfactory' food inspector's report and successive visitors' notes, such as 'food was rapidly disappearing from the plates' or 'a first class meal, worthy of all praise', indicated improvements had been achieved.[153]

The opening of Woodlands coincided with greater ministerial emphasis on community care, and in 1966 the Norfolk Welfare Committee instigated day care services within its homes. A few beds at Woodlands were set aside for this in 1967 and the number of attendants increased, these arrangements being considered 'a tremendous asset in the care of the elderly'.[154] By 1973 up to six beds were also designated for short-term care, with older clients from the community spending up to a fortnight there.[155] A building adjoining Woodlands was converted into a thirty-place day centre, the first such facility in Norfolk; 'the whole atmosphere is extremely pleasant'.[156] It served meals, ran handicraft sessions, and offered communal games, television, newspapers, books and periodicals. There were three care assistants, with the superintendent and matron of Woodlands responsible for centre administration, for a weekly average of ninety-three attendees.[157] According to visitors' reports, 'all [were] very pleased to come in for a meal and pleasant surroundings', and 'everyone [was] … most grateful for all that is done for them'.[158] It was noted that 'more would come if transport was available', so a minibus fitted with a hoist was procured.[159]

Nonetheless, there was a shortage of daily attendants, bathing, washing and kitchen facilities. Nor did this address growing demand for permanent Part III accommodation in the locality: 'not a single bed [was] vacant' and at least 100 people were awaiting admission, including ten 'considered to be first degree priority cases' in 1972.[160] In these circumstances, an administrative reorganization to facilitate transfers between the Area's homes was unlikely to produce real gains, with at least ten people also hoping to transfer outside the Area in 1973.[161] Such difficulties were compounded by 'an acute shortage of geriatric beds in hospitals', reflected in a doubling of monthly referrals within two years to sixty by 1974.[162]

Community care also implied better links with other older people in the locality, with Woodlands' kitchen facilities doubling for a meals-on-wheels service from 1967 and for day care provision from 1972. An over-60s club held monthly meetings in the home, attended by twenty or so non-residents; the Red Cross weekly 'trolley service' from 1969 also proved 'very successful'.[163] Sharing amenities with local older people boosted residents' interests and led others to engage with them more. Volunteers continued to provide entertainments and gifts, but others visited for training purposes or to offer help. In 1966 twenty local technical college students were shown around, while several district nurses attended for a training course and 'were interested in all sections concerning the running of the home and the channels through which residents are admitted to the home'.[164] These visits led to more 'voluntary helpers', 'taking some of the cripples out in wheelchairs etc.' and, noticeably, 'all these youngsters are a great help and enjoyed by the old folk'.[165] Other helpers included police cadets, scouts, guides and a 77-year-old man 'who comes in almost daily … a wonderful voluntary worker', all adding interest and complementing the care provided by established staff.[166]

Despite the limited source materials on Woodlands, it can be inferred that with the expansion of community care, the role of the home expanded considerably. Day and short-term care benefited a wider local older population and could obviate the need for a permanent admission for some. Residents were evidently buoyed by visitors and volunteers, and began taking a more positive role in social activities or helping around the home. Yet the demand for permanent accommodation remained high, as confirmed by long waiting lists and overcrowding.

Official records do not provide sufficient insight into the lives of Eastgate House or Woodlands residents, but this may be partly offset by the more direct, if subjective, accounts of personnel, residents and relatives closely involved in the life and practices in long-term institutional care provision for older people from the 1970s.

Diversity in Residential Care Locations since 1970

In Norfolk there were roughly 1,500 Part III older residents in local authority homes in 1962, with some 2,000 more in geriatric, psycho-geriatric or psychiatric NHS hospitals.[167] Many of the latter failed to satisfy strict Norfolk Social Services' 'Part III fit' criteria for its homes but were arguably unnecessarily institutionalized.[168] With the policy focus on de-institutionalization following the 1959 Mental Health Act, a few hospital patients were discharged to 'group homes' under limited supervision, with a few others requiring constant care being moved to (private) nursing homes. Yet hospitalized older patients awaiting transfers to 'residential' places still featured in the 1990s, and given their numbers and linkage with local authority Part III accommodation, they are considered in this section. Similarly included here are private home residents, who became dominant by the late 1980s under the post-1979 accelerated privatization within the increasing mixed economy in residential care delivery in Norfolk, as elsewhere. Comparisons between private and local authority homes and their residents are also provided, as private homes, to some extent, are dependent on public subsidies by taking publicly funded residents and are subject to central regulations and inspections.

Consequently, this section includes the recollections or experiences of residents, their relatives and care staff in various long-term institutional care settings, with the weight on the latter two groups. It begins with the St Andrew's and Hellesdon psychiatric hospitals (Norwich) and the Vale psycho-geriatric hospital (former Swainsthorpe workhouse near Norwich) during 1970–88, along with group homes and an NHS nursing home ancillary to St Andrew's, to which some patients were transferred. It then examines two local authority care homes – Heartsease Hostel and Foulgers House (Norwich) – during 1976–85, and finally several post-1980 private care and nursing homes in the East Anglia region. Attempts to recognize greater diversity in long-term institutional care provision must acknowledge that each older resident/patient had a unique story, and overall assessments of institutional life can never be genuinely representative or wholly accurate. Nor can reliance on the indirect experiences of staff and relatives wholly compensate for the absence of direct evidence, though residents' deaths, confidentiality issues, difficulties in accessing individuals and the need to respect their privacy limit the value of such testimony. Nonetheless, it is useful to examine whether the common features of ageing and declining energy or abilities produced recognizably similar or shared experiences. Oral testimonies too can partly offset the dearth or unavailability of other primary material.

Psychiatric and Psycho-Geriatric Hospitals, 1970–85

St Andrew's psychiatric hospital (originally Norfolk Lunatic Asylum) was generally overcrowded – 'dangerously' so in 1960 – with some 1,200, nearly 500 of whom were elderly inpatients.[169] Typically, they were accommodated in fifty-bedded wards with 'three, even four rows of beds'.[170] Work to improve or maintain standards was long overdue, leaving many wards 'very cold and uncomfortable', 'dingy and drab' or 'very shabby'.[171] Officially, de-institutionalization policies were signalled after the Ministry of Health Hospital Plan (1962), with a near-50 per cent reduction in regional psychiatric hospital beds by 1975 and closure of St Andrew's envisaged.[172] Yet without alternative accommodation, St Andrew's retained over 1,000, increasingly elderly, inpatients, their higher care requirements compounded by staff shortages and limited resources. Nevertheless, inspectors and visiting officers 'almost invariably praised the attitude of the St Andrew's staff and the quality of care provided'.[173] Staff during the 1950s and 1960s remembered it as a 'kindly' place, with 'caring' relationships and 'genuine friendship' between nurses and patients.[174]

A sharp reduction of beds in use from 925 to 560 during 1971–4 and a corresponding increase in discharges of younger, short-stay patients left a core of elderly long-stay and very dependent patients. Yet there was very little affordable or suitable alternative accommodation, and it was only in the 1980s and 1990s that designated units and purpose-built nursing homes for the elderly mentally ill opened.[175] Most of St Andrew's patients remained there for the rest of their lives, though some of the more able were discharged to group homes.[176]

Mrs S., who started at St Andrew's as a nursing assistant in 1970, recalled her first visit for a job interview:

> It was intimidating ... smelly and vast and the ceiling was so high. I've never been into a place with so many old people in ... they [the staff] took me into one of the wards to meet some of the people ... they all came towards me, talking to me and touching me. I was horrified ... I was apprehensive about everything.[177]

In contrast, 42-year-old Ms N., who began psychiatric nurse training in 1972, was more relaxed:

> I was surprised at the size of the hospital; it was massive and rather overpowering ... But as soon as I entered inside, I liked the friendly atmosphere. Staff were all very welcoming, and so were patients.[178]

She recalled the forty-bedded Ward 7, which had two rows of beds on each side with some small side rooms, although bed numbers were gradually reduced to twenty or so and some wards were subdivided. Between the beds there were small, individual lockers, but no partitions to afford any privacy. There were corner hanging spaces and shared wardrobes, and staff placed the patients' clothing on their bed at bedtime. Patients had very few personal belongings, but a weekly allowance from 1971 represented 'a big change because elderly long-stay patients could buy and wear their own outfits rather than hospital clothes for the first time'.[179] Ward 7's forty elderly female patients were

> mostly long-stay, 'burnt-out schizophrenics', having been in the hospital since [the] 1920s and 1930s. Although they had calmed down ... they weren't sufficiently able to live out in the community ... because they sometimes became aggressive or violent and still needed constant medical supervision. A few ... had to come to the hospital fairly recently because they became too demented or frail to cope with living in a community either by themselves or with their families.[180]

In other wards patients were even 'older and more frail, needing full nursing care, with many doubly incontinent and several bedridden'.[181]

In the early 1970s nursing was by pairs of sisters or charge nurses during either the morning or afternoon shift. Elderly long-stay wards had a charge nurse and two or three untrained part-time nursing assistants, working from 8 am to 4 pm and on some evenings. At night there was usually just one qualified nurse and an assistant on each ward. Staff shortages were a problem, although the nursing establishment had a higher proportion of qualified or trained full-time staff than in many private nursing homes in the 1990s or even now.

Hospital life remained heavily institutionalized. Typically, day staff woke the patients at 7 am and helped them to wash and dress before breakfast at 8:30, by which time the care assistants had arrived. Most patients spent the morning in the lounge area. Their weekly bath also took place in the morning. In the afternoon, able patients joined in sing-songs or games or watched films; some had occupational therapy. The sick attended hospital appointments, with a few receiving electro-convulsive therapy sessions. After tea most returned to their wards, while 'staff tried to get patients, especially the more dependent, put into bed before night staff came on duty at 20:45'.[182] Some patients attended Sunday services in the on-site chapel or joined the hospital choir. Occasional days out were organized and much appreciated, since most had no family or relatives.

This institutional routine was generally justified by the nursing staff:

> Patients ... [were] used to the routine and loved it; that was their safety net and one of the things they most appreciated. They didn't like any change at all. When you introduced something new, it would be a shock to them ... invariably they would want to go back to the original ideas.[183]

Patients often regarded 'nursing staff as part of their family and, for many, they were all the family they had'.[184] Nurses were generally on first-name terms with patients, although 'some old institutionalized sisters and untrained care assistants tended to play a motherly role or treat patients as "naughty stupid children"'.[185] One strength of psychiatric nurse training was that 'you learnt to communicate with the patients; to treat the whole person not just their complaint'.[186] These principles featured at St Andrew's, where all care staff were encouraged to talk with patients as much as possible and we often spent our break, sitting and talking with them. In those days, all of the patients smoked and we used to have a cigarette with them and chatted with them ... They liked nothing better than to talk especially about their old days and families.[187]

Patients rarely communicated with each other, a common feature in other geriatric or psychiatric hospitals and old people's homes, though 'a lot of them were "drugged up" and "zombie-like" and might have been unable to communicate with each other or had been institutionalized for so many years that they lacked social skills'.[188] This helped to maintain an orderly atmosphere, with relatively few conflicts between patients. All wards were unlocked by the time of the deinstitutionalization, but greater freedom of movement was seemingly achieved at the cost of tighter control of 'aggressive' patients by increasing their medication, indicative of continuing institutionalization for a minority.

Other measures improved informal and patient-oriented hospital life at least for the more able, by recognizing their abilities and preferences. By the early 1970s most wards had side-rooms, and one was fully converted into twelve single rooms. 'Self-governing' accommodation was converted from a former nursing home for a group of twenty long-stay male patients and from a former isolation block for six female patients.[189] Residents ate in the dining hall and received medical treatment and occupational therapy, but otherwise lived independently. They included 80-year-old Doris. She shared the hospital routine, but

freely went back to her room and listened to a radio or took a nap. She washed all her clothes by hand in the washbasin and hung them up in her room. She also went to the Griffin Pub, opposite to St Andrew's ... before lunch.[190]

'There were lots of old long-stay male patients, who used to walk into the pub by themselves or with male staff. They mixed with local people, who knew them very well'.[191]

Many patients were restricted to places within walking distance, since most could not use public transport unaided and had very few relatives who could accompany them on visits or trips. Long-serving nursing staff often volunteered their off-duty time, males arranging outings to Norwich City football matches and females taking patients into the city for meals or shopping. Several older sisters and nurses even invited patients, usually in pairs, to their own homes at weekends, although this covered 'only a few most able patients' and left the very dependent elderly hospital-bound.[192]

For able patients, weekday occupational therapy 'played a large part in their lives',[193] and 'Those who attended associated together more as they had something in common to talk about'.[194] A few patients were rehabilitated to the point of discharge and 'went out into the city ... and learned to get used to the buses and new money'.[195] Five former female patients, aged between 58 and 75 years, moved into the first group home, opened in 1966 by the voluntary National

Mental Health Association.[196] A local domiciliary (community) nurse recalled her visits to a similar group home a decade later:

> Six elderly women, all ex-psychiatric patients, lived together in a group home ... They were attended by a domiciliary nurse twice a day for the administration of medication but otherwise they lived independently. One old lady was the most reliable and responsible for the rest – literally looked after them – ordering all the shopping, doing the cooking and helping to bath, etc.[197]

However, there were cost intimations in the reliance on patients' support, minimum nurse supervision and lack of social provision, of contact with care staff and of activities associated with the hospital. Accordingly, 'most of them did not want to go and live out in a community'.[198] One elderly patient, discharged to live in unstaffed accommodation,

> didn't like the new home and kept coming back to the hospital but was repeatedly sent back out into the community. On the seventh time, she drowned herself ... Perhaps, it was too lonely for her with no family of her own and missing the nursing staff ... but that was a *policy* you see ... people like her, who were able, had to be sent out into the community [my emphasis].[199]

Ms N., a former student nurse, concluded that 'long-stay patients had been institutionalized for thirty or forty years and suddenly had to do things they'd never done before ... some never adapted'.[200] Even 'changes of ward upset the elderly long-stay residents. Within days a patient died'.[201]

In contrast, six older women discharged from hospital went to live with their former ward sister when she resigned and opened a nursing home to look after them. They 'were much happier than others in unstaffed group homes or private accommodation because they could continue to be looked after by her, whom they had known for many years'.[202] Evidently, some continuity and companionship with nursing staff were critical for elderly patients, who 'regarded the hospital as their home and nursing staff as part of their family'.[203] Such voluntary arrangements were rare, and it is unclear whether residents received public subsidies or the nurse met the entire cost. Given nurses' modest pay, it seems unlikely that many could have subsidized ventures like this.

Other patient-centred arrangements included an auxiliary NHS nursing home for the elderly mentally ill, which offered thirty places in single and double rooms in a more homely, if remote, location. Mainly former St Andrew's older long-stay patients settled into a rather ordered existence and 'appreciated the "hospital" atmosphere, the routine and nursing staff. They liked leading their own lives in an enclosed, safe environment, as they had done for many years in hospital'.[204] Again, the staff's understanding of patients was reflected in relaxed and patient-centred arrangements:

While we were having a break in a staff room, quite a few residents used to come and sit and talk with us over a cup of tea. Others liked walking into the garden and around [the] neighbourhood, whilst more 'responsible' ones were allowed out on their own ... Mr E., tripped out by bus as far as Great Yarmouth ... [while] some ... did fruit-picking for pocket money.[205]

Yet with alternative accommodation in short supply, most older long-stay patients remained at St Andrew's:

There were very few discharges and bed turnover only occurred when patients died, and these were filled by other elderly long-stays ... Most patients needed long-term total nursing care which could only be provided at psychiatric hospitals ... Hospital was thus the end of their road: indeed, none of the elderly patients in the 40-bedded Wards D and 12 was discharged into the community during my time [1972–5].[206]

Another nurse, working during the 1970s, stated: 'I don't think there were any discharges of elderly long-stay patients into the community ... it was unrealistic ... [for] those who had been there almost all their life'.[207] Thus St Andrew's remained 'the provider of comprehensive care for an ageing group of long-term residents ... more like a nursing home'.[208] Some staff later left the hospital as 'it was getting very run-down. You couldn't go much further. You got only old long-stay patients'.[209]

Other patients were transferred in the 1970s to the Vale psycho-geriatric hospital, Swainsthorpe, a former workhouse with some 180 patients in thirty-bedded wards. Again, a somewhat rigid daily routine was combined with an understanding nursing staff and a tolerant local community:

An ex-farmer senile patient used to slip himself out to a private farm next to the hospital at six o'clock every morning and was taken back by the farmer in time for breakfast ... the farmer didn't mind him at all and we understood his motives and allowed him a space familiar with his past.[210]

The hospital had its own coach for outings and held occupational therapy classes, but 'many were too senile and frail to participate in any activities at all'.[211] Accordingly, 'there was nothing for them in the community, although a local vicar used to come'.[212] In short, the Vale hospital was very similar to St Andrew's but much quieter, since 'most of them just sat or slept all day'.[213]

In contrast, Hellesdon psychiatric hospital had more acute new and admission patients. A staff nurse on forty-bedded mixed Ward 6 recalled the very different atmosphere:

There were some elderly long-stays; a few very recent admissions; and many middle-aged or elderly admission patients, the latter coming to the hospital only for short, usually six-week, treatment ... some didn't like the other patients and often had fights and quarrels.[214]

The able ones went to occupational therapy, and a few were successfully discharged. One 80-year-old woman, admitted with depression,

> was really good at cooking and used to bring back cakes and things she had made at the occupational class ... She got better and was later transferred to an old people's home where she helped to cook for the residents.[215]

Other patients were less compliant:

> They didn't like the hospital routine at all, because they hadn't been used to it ... they didn't want to get up so early or be told what to do ... They wanted to look after themselves and have breakfast later or in bed. They hated restrictions.[216]

Tension between a rigid hospital routine and more flexible domestic, private lives was evident, and partly explains why institutionalized older patients found it very hard to adjust to a new setting after discharge from hospital.

Generally, the established but closed lifestyle marked by a timetable and routine in the three psychiatric/psycho-geriatric hospitals was repeated in the new auxiliary NHS nursing home and was, arguably, appreciated by older long-stay patients. Patients were grateful for their care, which included personal as well as physical nursing, along with kindness and understanding. Genuine friendships between patients and staff, and community toleration sufficient to offer extra-institutional opportunities, might feature, although freedom of movement was very restricted for those with severe disabilities or dementia and some 'drugged-up' patients.

Nevertheless, these arrangements sat less comfortably alongside Hellesdon's increasingly short-term treatment for new patients, who expected more freedom, flexibility and privacy. Where the smooth running of the hospital took priority, their expectations might be ignored or considered selfish, especially 'when you had a big ward and a small staff and those demanding having meals in bed were able and capable'.[217] With insufficient staff at St Andrew's, 'welfare of the whole rather than individuals had to come first'.[218] This became more pressing from the mid-1970s, when some patients fell victim to over-medication and further institutionalization to secure life for the rest. Both St Andrew's and Hellesdon found it difficult to improve living conditions for a more diversified patient population without enough staff. Emerging concerns over freedom, privacy and flexibility, appreciated by able short-term patients, at Hellesdon sometimes represented a threat and disruption for the older 'long-stays'.

Older people discharged from hospital to 'group home' community care missed hospital life and nursing staff. The official community focus often involved manipulation of concepts of independence or privacy, which did not necessarily matter to long-term institutionalized older patients, although lack of alternative arrangements kept many in hospital well into the 1980s. Yet they possibly fared better than elderly mentally ill residents in the post-1990 era, because the manageable ones were often simply 'warehoused' or 'suffering tedium and apathy' in private care or nursing homes, while severe cases 'were moved around between hospital assessment wards and [private] nursing homes'.[219]

Local Authority Residential Homes, 1976–80s

In 1976 Ms I. became deputy matron at Heartsease Hostel, a local authority residential home in Norwich. Built in 1972, the two-storey facility provided double and single rooms for thirty female and six male residents:

> [Q]uite a few were infirm, who needed some degree of physical nursing but could manage to get around. There were also three ex-psychiatric patients and one or two dementias from the community, but again they were all quiet and harmless and none got aggressive, violent or wandering off.[220]

Though not confined, 'a lot of them didn't go out at all because they didn't have any relatives'.[221] Many were effectively home-bound. However,

> There were no everyday organized activities ... life there was generally boring ... they used to sit mute in a long row in arm chairs, snooze and vegetate ... Social Services and people all say that this is a very bad thing and they need to be motivated ... I used to try to get them [to] knit but they didn't want to know ... it was just too difficult to stimulate them.[222]

Residents' views were unrecorded, but 'everything was organized for them, whereas, in their own homes, they had to do things themselves ... some women might have liked being looked after ... but quite a few did miss independence and responsibilities for their own lives'.[223] Their relationship with staff was 'generally cordial' and staff care was 'generally good', but there was little time for chatting.[224] 'Care over physical things' took priority, and care assistants were unqualified and had little training, although some were 'experienced'.[225]

By 1980 Norfolk local authority residential homes had changed: 'all looked very similar with a certain design ... [and] inside, big white corridors ... it was clean and always smelt antiseptic', yet they were 'more homely than hospitals, with thirty or forty residents and a bit of more privacy ... and smaller lounges'.[226] The resident populations included more very frail and disabled people who, at the admission stage, had once met the 'rather narrow and strictly-set' Part III criteria, which excluded 'anybody who would have needed nursing procedure'.[227] Despite growing demand for Part III residential provision, no increase of Part III places and limited (public) community alternatives, this restrictionist approach continued.

Norfolk Social Services field/community social worker Ms C., who assessed frail older people and arranged local authority Part III accommodation, recalled 'placement meetings' in the early 1980s:

> [W]hen we [community workers] presented elderly people who required long-term residential care, the people in charge of the council homes were able just to say whether they could take them or not. They always said that they ... needed a balance of people ... but invariably they refused to take less able people and we were always left with the problem of where to place them.[228]

Over time many who met Part III criteria on admission became frail or disabled. In practice, staff 'did try to keep them there ... until they could not be physically managed ... and, indeed, very few people were moved', according to a Norfolk Social Services relief care assistant.[229] Mobility was a critical factor: 'once somebody is immobile, that had huge implications for transferring them'.[230] Thus Part III criteria might be loosely interpreted for existing residents. Indeed, Foulgers House was equipped with hoists in 1983 to help to move 'many incontinent and quite a few severely demented or confused residents'.[231]

As workloads increased, it became increasingly difficult to meet the needs of a diverse group of residents, some of whom could not lead anything resembling a communal life. At Foulgers House most remained in basic double rooms: 'Staff tried to put together residents who might get on and, as long as both roommates were active and mentally alert, a lot of them didn't mind sharing that much. They ... kept an eye on each other, and told staff if there was a problem'.[232] Indeed, 'many women were local people, who had grown up in big families; lived in crowded houses; always shared rooms; and never had privacy in their lives'.[233] Yet problems arose

> if they shared with somebody who was or became very difficult ... This was very disturbing, frightening, stressful, or upsetting for the other occupant of the room, who really felt very deprived because they lost their privacy and dignity.[234]

Moreover, resident-centred arrangements involving independence, choice and personalized rooms or routines were ignored by some staff, who

> felt that they knew best. They felt that, because the residents needed to come into a home to be looked after, they should just put up with it and be grateful ... There wasn't a lot of sympathy from many of the staff who didn't seem to feel that residents should be allowed to have much independence or choices.[235]

Thus 'we used to wake them up quite early and take them to the lounge because we had to clean the bedrooms ... We also had to take them to bed quite early'.[236] Many were left 'just to sit in a chair all day, do nothing, watch TV or sleep. It's just a waiting room to die ... Some of the more independent and better-off residents had their own rooms and TVs and would spend more time in their rooms'.[237] In 1983 Norfolk Social Services introduced a choice of meals in their care homes, but some longer-serving staff in Foulgers House resisted this. They 'felt they were given more work and argued "if somebody was confused or had

Alzheimer's and would or could not remember the next day what they had chosen, why give them a choice?"[238]

This compared well with many private homes in the 1990s, where 'residents weren't given menus or choice at all ... meals were prepared and if somebody didn't like pork or something, they didn't get it'.[239] Foulgers House residents were allowed to stay in bed later or spend more time in their rooms rather than in the lounge, but 'a lot of staff didn't think they should be allowed'.[240] Staff training was encouraged, with a 'first aid course at least' for everyone and other courses for permanent staff dealing with frail older residents, although 'a lot of them didn't bother and just did what they did'.[241] Work conditions featured 'proper pay' and additional payments for extra hours or 'dealing with the most incontinent residents'.[242] Such measures were again absent in many private homes.

In-home or attached day centres were new, offering 'at least some daily activities ... for residents and people from their own homes'.[243] They offered hairdressing, music and games, including bingo ('the one they liked best') for the more active and mentally alert, although the confused and very dependent simply sat in the lounge. This reflected the underlying principle that 'everyone, even those confused, should at least be tried because by doing so they might benefit from a degree of stimulation and interaction with others and lively atmosphere'.[244] Once again, many private homes lacked day care provision. Short religious services were held at weekends for home-bound frail residents, while the more able were taken to local churches by volunteers. Quite a few families and friends visited or took out residents; 'some confused people did recognize their relatives and behaved normally for a short time or felt better' after a visit.[245]

Overall, from the 1980s various measures to improve, or at least maintain, the quality of residential life began to feature in Norfolk local authority residential homes. Yet residential life remained largely communal, and some care workers ignored or dismissed the wishes or needs of those with severe disabilities or dementia who were unable to express themselves, even though generally staff followed good management practice and guidelines. Without residents' own accounts, the main perception of residential life was still that 'some valued having company or a safe place to live, and for those disabled, having care'.[246] Foulgers House needed

more activities and a lot more time to spend with residents ... but it's all about money. The manager could only work within the budget ... but, in general, the management was good, and staff were caring and had basic training. It was far better than many private homes I worked in or knew.[247]

Private Sector Homes since the 1980s

With direct local authority home provision limited by the mid-1970s, private sector provision expanded rapidly. Yet there was no liaison between the sectors. Private home applicants could bypass Norfolk Social Services needs and financial assessments in relation to the Part III criteria. All older people, except the minority better-off, could apply directly for Department of Health and Social Security supplementary benefit, and might receive the benefit to pay for their home costs in part or in full. In the 1980s Norfolk Social Services social workers 'weren't supposed, in any way, to be involved in the private sector and ... we weren't allowed to express our opinion ... Precisely because of this, we didn't know anything about private resources'.[248] With no needs assessment, the profile of private sector home residents was more diverse: an able spouse might live with a frail partner, whereas local authority provision under Part III criteria would separate them.[249] Some independent individuals entered private homes for better accommodation, security or company. One single lady moved into a private care home in 1988 because 'I missed company and thought a care home was an ideal place where I could keep privacy but at the same time easily meet other residents in common spaces if I wished'.[250]

Meanwhile applicants for local authority homes were increasingly more disabled or confused and thus did not meet the Part III criteria, particularly as long-stay NHS hospital beds were closed and patients were discharged. One attendant in a private care home felt that:

> The people going into [private] care homes in the early 1990s were in far worse health than a decade earlier. More ... should have really been in nursing homes, but care homes were cheaper ... However, they often ended up in a nursing home, which was very disruptive and upsetting for them and probably they would die quicker than those who remained in hospitals or went straight into a nursing home.[251]

Most were fully or partly state-funded through the supplementary benefit. Many small business private homes faced financial difficulties because they relied on very frail residents who needed extra care but had minimal state funding. Accordingly, most of these homes pared provision to official minimum guidelines and sought to offset extra nursing costs by providing additional fee-paying services for better-off self-funders. Inevitably, this meant that variations in standards of provision widened. A self-funded resident might enjoy a single room, with privacy, independence and a personalized lifestyle. One better-off 85-year-old woman moved into a private care home in 1983. Her daughter recalled:

> She had a very nice big single room with a big window ... overlooking the well-maintained, beautiful garden. She was surrounded by her own furniture and belongings and had her own TV, which she never did before ... she seldom left the room and even had meals there. She really valued the maintenance of her privacy and freedom.[252]

In contrast, the publicly funded had to share double and sometimes multi-bedded rooms, and could only afford the bare essentials. Disturbing cases of 'residents, who had enough money to pay for single rooms at first, but were moved very quickly to the shared rooms once their money ran out' suggested a clear distinction in living arrangements according to residents' financial means and a two-tier system in residential care provision.[253]

Generally, private homes had fewer physical aids despite their higher proportion of residents with severe disabilities than in local authority homes, so that 'once residents became very disabled or infirm, private homes could and did move them to nursing homes a lot quicker than the council [local authority] homes'.[254] In many private homes organized activities and amenities beyond hairdressing were limited even for the better-off, but they could purchase services within or outside the home to enrich residential life.[255] Thus 'some had their own telephones and quite a few had newspapers delivered', and 'a female resident used to go to the city by taxi on her own to have lunch with her daughter'.[256]

Private home residents also moved between homes, often with the help of relatives. Thus in 1985 an 83-year-old woman chose a small private home, which was run by a resident couple with small children and catered for just four older women, each in her own bedroom. This seemed ideal, yet 'she didn't like it because the children ... used to come into her room', so her daughter found a nearby private home where she was 'much happier because she could maintain her privacy in a bigger single room'.[257] Transfers of state-funded residents were less frequent and more restricted because of their financial status. Ms M., aged 78, shared a double room in a private care home with a lady who became a good friend. When this lady died, her next roommate was very noisy and selfish so Ms M. asked to be moved, but 'they simply said they couldn't, so her family eventually moved her ... she had to share with another resident ... [but] she was told that she could always move to another room if there were any problems'.[258] The second home 'had a bit more understanding'.[259] Yet given limited Social Services involvement, those lacking financial resources or relatives were in a much weaker position as they had to make arrangements for themselves. Moreover, although general care was theoretically available to all residents, 'the self-funded tended to receive more attention from staff, and more was done for them ... with some reminding the staff of their status'.[260]

Care standards varied not only within but also between homes, the latter affecting the whole resident population. One care assistant, employed in a local authority home in the mid-1980s and a private home in the early 1990s, candidly stated that 'the private home was far, far worse than the council [local authority] one. No training, worse pay, long hours, a lot fewer staff, worse quality of staff ... absolutely bad'.[261] She was particularly concerned about the lack of staff training: 'one resident was having a fit and a care assistant was sitting her up ... I could not believe that staff didn't even know the basic principles'.[262] Staff shortages meant that 'you often ended up doing things on your own, like lifting a resident, which you really shouldn't have done legally'.[263] Similarly, although it was prohibited 'to tie residents into their chairs to stop them wandering or falling down', staff in one private care home in the early 1990s 'used to put hospital trays in front of somebody so that they couldn't get out of the chair very easily'.[264]

Insufficient supervision of staff could lead to abuse: 'a young care assistant used to bring her boyfriend in while she was on night duty … They had food and drink meant for the residents and he even took some of it back home'.[265] In another home, 'one care assistant was sacked after stealing money and posses-sions from residents' rooms'.[266] With just one qualified staff member on call but not necessarily on duty, under- or untrained care assistants often did not take residents' privacy, independence or dignity into consideration. Some staff in one private care home

> showed a sense of power over vulnerable residents. They treated residents like children, not as responsible adults with respect, ordering them to do this and that and some inter-vened into residents' privacy, demanding they tidy things up or buy a new set of pyjamas … on which occasion the resident was most upset and felt very disrespected.[267]

Even worse were cases involving very confused or disabled residents, who were more vulnerable or unable to express their feelings or exercise their rights. Pri-vate homes notionally endorsed choice and dignity, but generally provided few free or low-cost activities and programmes for their clientele. Some relatives of residents with dementia criticized their parsimony or mean-spiritedness, calling it 'abuse in the form of neglect'.[268] Staff might feel that 'there was no point for the confused in attending outings because they would only spoil the enjoyment of other able residents'.[269] In one extreme case, a staff member slapped a confused resident because he was aggressive and did not listen to her.[270] Quite a few staff informants confirmed that 'there was definitely abuse' in some homes, and one traced problems in the latter to poor management:

> A lot more decisions were made by staff on behalf of residents. This did happen in council [local authority] homes but not as much because they had much better man-agement systems, under which staff had to or at least try to follow the principles, which were clearly set out and emphasized resident-centred provision … at private homes the principles or decisions were very much down to who was on duty.[271]

Better management could raise private home care standards, and one former staff member witnessed positive effects: 'the new manager arranged more trips and said that everybody who was able to go should go … but if some staff didn't like her ideas, they just ignored them or only followed when she was there'.[272] With limited staff training or unrealistic workloads, effective management was hard to achieve, leading one informant to question widespread preconceptions that 'private homes are better than council [local authority] ones, because people generally pay more, so they get better quality of care'.[273] She concluded:

> Money matters terribly but if people are vulnerable or have dementia, they still don't always get what they should ... Even with the same fees, one would find excellent homes with very positive attitude, a lot of activities and encouragement to be independent and others concerned only with money or a persistent old attitude that residents should not make a fuss or demand things.[274]

A self-funded private care home resident agreed, recounting a conversation with the home owner soon after he entered it in 1993:

> The owner said that good management was to treat residents as a group, in his words 'animal husbandry' ... during the last fifteen years the manager changed several times and the old building was replaced by the modern one. But the owner remains the same and so does the home ethos ... monthly calendars show quite a few activities and events but they are just show-off lists for inspectors ... He puts money and healthy finance of the home first.[275]

Overall, resident profiles, whether in local authority or private homes, became more diverse in terms of their socio-economic and physical conditions, while more very dependent or disabled, notably dementia sufferers, required more intensive nursing care and personalized arrangements beyond basic and universal services. In an uncertain and straitened financial climate, with public expenditure constraints and continued ageing populations, both local authority and private homes face an uphill struggle if these needs are to be met.

6 RESIDENTIAL LIFE IN GIFU

Like Chapter 5, this chapter is divided into two sections. The first covers the period 1947–73, examining the Yorokaen institution and its replacement home in Ogaki City, Gifu Prefecture (successors of Ogaki Old People's Almshouse), and drawing on records held on site and at Gifu Record Office. The second section provides institutional histories of Yorokaen (both the 1963 replacement and its 1994 reconstruction) after 1970, and the city's first nursing home, Kusunokien, opened in 1987, mainly using interview material.

The Tenacity of the Almshouse Regime

Yorokaen Old People's Institution, 1947–63

Yorokaen originated in 1926 as Ogaki Old People's Almshouse and retained its official assessed institution status and title (literally, 'flower garden for the elderly') throughout the period examined.[1] However, its location and physical appearance altered in 1963 when the modest 1947-built building on the former almshouse site was replaced by a purpose-built larger facility on the outskirts of the city. Similarly, Yorokaen's management changed in 1959, from the non-profit Ogaki City Relief Foundation, officially recognized as a social welfare corporation (technically, a quango acting as a subcontractor of public residential care), to Ogaki City Council. Equally, Yorokaen's official definitions and aims changed, along with its institutional ethos, regulations and practices, ostensibly to match these. Thus Yorokaen operated as a 'publicly sanctioned general public assistance institution' under the 1946 (Old) National Assistance Act, then as an old people's institution under the 1950 (New) National Assistance Act and finally as an old people's home under the 1963 Elderly Welfare Act. All this has affected the lives of the residents and staff. Whether it has resulted in a 'homely' environment is questionable.

Residents' Characteristics

Following the bombing of the original Ogaki Almshouse in July 1945, twenty mainly older survivors were evacuated to adjoining accommodation for vagrants

and casuals and then to makeshift accommodation for up to forty people, utilized as a publicly sanctioned general assistance institution under the 1946
National Assistance Act, in which older people were the majority.[2] The forty
places served the surrounding western Seino region, which had nearly 4,000
public assistance recipients living at home, including 570 in need of institutional
care, along with hundreds more sick or disabled.[3] Overcrowding at Yorokaen
was eased in 1949 when its bed capacity doubled to eighty after extension work
was undertaken. Under the New National Assistance Act, Yorokaen was reclas-
sified as an old people's institution exclusively for needy people aged 60 or more.
Designated as an assessed institution, its admissions were subject to compulsory
means-testing and needs assessment of applicants and their family. Throughout
the 1950s Yorokaen operated at 70–80 per cent capacity, even though the eligible older population in Ogaki City and surrounding towns increased steadily.[4]
Up to 20 per cent of places were available for self-funded residents with above-
threshold income and/or with family support, but none applied and the publicly
supported eligible residents 'did not reach the planned number'.[5] This can be
explained not by stringent criteria but from lack of older applicants in a rural
community where the tradition of family care and the stigma associated with
public welfare provision remained strong.

During the 1950s the gender imbalance at Yorokaen switched from being
overwhelmingly male to 60 per cent female.[6] At a time when average life expectancy in Japan was 65 years, forty-three of the sixty-seven Yorokaen's residents
were aged 65–79, and thirteen were aged 80 or more.[7] A few under-60s were
admitted, but Yorokaen's regulations excluded 'elderly with contagious diseases,
severe disability or disruptive characters'.[8] The first group was referred to the few
public hospitals across Gifu Prefecture or to its only public institution for disabled adults in Gifu City, although Yorokaen did accept a couple of blind people
as there was no special accommodation for them in the prefecture until 1992.[9]
Most required little assistance: in 1952 just six residents were 'sick, confined to
bed', although thirteen saw a doctor once a month and thirty-three took some
form of medication.[10] All but a couple with short-term illnesses did unpaid or
underpaid work, and five, including a 75-year-old woman, became employees
of Yorokaen during 1950–2, when they no longer satisfied the criteria of public
assistance.[11] However, by 1958 fully 80 per cent of residents were diagnosed with
some form of physical or mental disability.[12]

Turnover was high: almost a third had spent less than one year there in 1958
and another third less than three years.[13] Mortality too was high, with twenty-
two deaths in that year alone, including fifteen from 'decrepitude'.[14] Very few
were transferred to hospitals – just four to general or psychiatric hospitals during
1953–9, for example.[15] People supposedly 'active' on admission might die after
three years or so. Inadequate treatment or nursing and limited access to hospital

needs to be examined in the context of life in post-war Japan. A comprehensive health care system did not exist until 1961, and even then the majority had to pay for half their medical costs, which placed hospital care beyond the reach of most older people. No residents died from malnutrition, something that occurred in the 1940s almshouse period. Altogether, Yorokaen residents fared better with basic treatment and nursing care, and rudimentary, brief doctor's visits. Their average age of death – 76 years in 1955 – exceeded the national average by ten years.[16]

Only glimpses of residents' education and religion can be found in Yorokaen's annual reports for 1952–8. No one had more than six years' primary schooling, and twenty-four women and four men had no education whatsoever.[17] Although below the national average, this was not untypical among those born in rural areas before 1900.[18] Most had been agricultural or manual labourers, and all were Buddhists, mainly *Jodo-shinshu* (literally, 'pure land' Buddhism), the most widely practised form of Buddhism in Japan.[19] All residents received public assistance, with most drawn from the very poorest, with their funeral costs covered by public subsidies and institution expenses.[20] Yorokaen provided funeral services for thirty-six of the forty-three deceased residents in 1955–7, and the remains of thirty of them were sent to nearby hospitals for dissection as no relatives or friends claimed them.[21] Similarly, just one of the seven people discharged from Yorokaen in 1955–62 was taken by a distant relative.[22] It is unclear whether relatives or friends ever visited Yorokaen, but regulations were hardly conducive to this and excluded visitors entering residents' rooms.[23]

To summarize: Yorokaen's restrictive assessed institution status ensured that only the neediest elderly, without financial means or family support, received residential care. The numbers of very old and frail residents increased marginally, but declined as a percentage of the growing eligible older population, suggesting the strong stigmatization of the institution through association with the pre-war old people's almshouse, public welfare or *obasuteyama*. Considering it as a last resort, local older people and their families limited Yorokaen's resident population, reflected in 70–80 per cent occupancy rates and no ineligible self-paying residents, even though up to 20 per cent of the home's beds could be allocated to such cases.

The Physical Environment

The 1947-built makeshift building consisted of three parallel, single-storey, terraced wooden houses, with a central connecting corridor.[24] Initially, there were four dormitories, each for about ten people, with shared lavatories, a communal bath and a dining hall. In 1949 extensions, costing over 1.2 million yen in public subsidies, converted the dormitories into twelve smaller bedrooms, with two sick wards and additional lavatory accommodation.[25] The kitchen and bathroom were expanded, with medical facilities; offices and staff accommodation were renovated; and extensions, using recycled materials from a nearby house, added ten small bedrooms. All bedrooms had floors covered by *tatami* (straw mats), and most were partitioned with *shoji* (sliding doors made of paper). Residents slept on futons, which allowed flexibility of resident numbers per room and compensated for the lack of communal dayrooms.

Officially defined as an old people's institution under the 1950 Act, Yorokaen's dormitory occupancy at that time was better than the 1957 official minimum 'four people per room' standard, and it was one of thirty-six among 146 such institutions to provide medical facilities.[26] Conditions there were far better than those that thousands of people in the vicinity experienced. Further expansion during the 1950s was made possible by money from the Community Chest Fund, which replaced emergency public subsidies and provided a quarter of Yorokaen's annual income.[27] In 1951 the adjoining institution for vagrants and casuals was taken over to provide an assembly hall, with a new workshop added in 1953 and accommodation for five married couples completed in 1956.[28] Marking the thirtieth anniversary of Yorokaen, a memorial tower for ancestors was erected within enclosed gardens planted with trees and shrubs.[29] Redecoration and additional equipment and furnishings meant that bedrooms now had a shared closet, wooden cupboard and low table, and were heated by charcoal burners in winter and equipped with mosquito nets and later window screens in summer. Items such as shoeboxes, mirrors, hair-clippers and a sewing machine were shared, as were improved washing and drying equipment, while communal rooms and spaces were decorated with curtains, vases and pictures, and a new Buddhist altar was placed in the assembly hall in 1953.[30] New dining tables and chairs were purchased, as well as a wireless set (1950), a television was donated in (1954) and a *shamisen* (three-stringed musical instrument) acquired (1957).[31]

Whereas the 1957 Ministry Code of Practice recommended the provision of workshop facilities, a memorial building for the deceased or nurses' room only when considered necessary, Yorokaen already had these and other amenities, and its spare capacity allowed a little private space.[32] Nonetheless, problems were acknowledged by the end of the 1950s. The timber construction was a potential fire hazard, and the expansion of Ogaki City increasingly encroached on the site, producing noise and air pollution and adding to the fire risk.[33] Flooding, notably during the 1959 Vera typhoon, caused considerable damage.[34]

Amenities, Provisions and Services

Yorokaen's association with the pre-1945 Ogaki Almshouse implied a continuing almshouse legacy and underlying mentality. Its 1958 brochure claimed it offered a 'bright and happy life for the pitiful and least fortunate elderly who have lacked financial and moral support ... by no means *obasuteyama* but a rest place to provide a quiet and relaxing life',[35] yet its regulations required that 'residents must follow the daily routine'.[36] Typically, the residents rose at 6 am to clean their bedrooms and lavatories, followed by a twenty-minute Buddhist service and ten minutes spent listening to a newspaper résumé by staff before breakfast at 7:30.[37] Two hours of 'communal work' before and after lunch covered basic chores, such as cleaning, washing and 'mutual nursing', along with 'communal side-jobs' according to residents' ability. These varied from preparing meals or working in the kitchen garden to sewing, making artificial flowers or packing goods.[38] A few men helped local farmers during the rice harvest. Following dinner at 5 pm and another twenty-minute Buddhist service, residents were free until they went to bed at 9 pm, but usually resumed the communal side-jobs.

Both communal work and side-jobs were considered 'voluntary' and so usually were unpaid, but sometimes residents were paid a token sum, even though the regulations required that 'all residents, health permitting, must participate in communal work'.[39] This emphasized the institution's financial situation rather than the residents' independent means. In 1955 critical Ministry of Health and Welfare inspectors noted that 'the residents are paid for only a part of their assigned work in the institution, which is not only unlawful but may lead to exploitation'.[40] Accordingly, their work was redefined as 'voluntary according to each individual will and health ... rewards ... are to accrue to the residents concerned, with ten per cent to be reserved and redistributed to everyone equally at the end of the year'.[41] Whether residents were paid is doubtful: official reports described work as fulfilling, since 'by working, residents dispel their idle fears and instead discover pleasure in life'.[42] Given their disadvantaged socio-economic status, residents may have taken the work-dominated institutional life for granted and did not expect an easy lifestyle or free leisure time; in this they had little choice.

Residents' work helped to ensure basic standards were observed, with accommodation kept clean and disinfected twice a month 'to prevent spreading infections among the residents'.[43] With fire safety paramount, duty staff conducted daily checks and able male residents undertook night patrols in rota, with monthly fire drills for all residents and staff.[44] Medical care included check-ups on admission and regular doctor's visits to those in the two sick wards, who were nursed by attendants from the adjoining duty room.[45] An on-site clinic was approved by the Ministry in 1954, and the temporary examination room built that year was replaced in 1960 by a new clinic, equipped with an examination couch.[46] A doctor arranged hospital referrals for any seriously ill patients. Otherwise, a qualified nursing assistant dealt with emergencies. Free medical care was a bonus, as most older people living at home did not receive any professional health care because of its prohibitive cost until the introduction of free health care for most over-70s in 1973.

Under Japan's post-war food rationing, Yorokaen's menus were simple and monotonous, averaging just 1,700 calories per person a day in 1952 and 1,800 by 1958.[47] Barley substituted for rice, with meat or fish served only twice a week, as were puddings. Yet this was better than those living independently and struggling to make ends meet could expect. Moreover, residents received regular donations of staples and 'extras', including bread, milk, cheese, butter, sugar, fruit and sweets. However, variety and taste were only acknowledged in 1959 in efforts to 'plan the monthly menus'.[48] Special diets for the sick were taken into consideration, as were the needs of those requiring different meals from others, but there was little choice throughout the period examined.[49] For most Japanese people, taking a daily bath was a highlight of the day. As many people lacked bathroom facilities and had to pay to attend a public bath, Yorokaen residents greatly appreciated the free use of their own spacious communal bathtub, which could be used between 1 pm and 5 pm three times a week.[50] (In comparison, half the sixty or so male older residents in one Norwich Home had only one bath a fortnight even in 1960.[51]) Thanks to volunteers from the Barber Association, Yorokaen residents also enjoyed free haircuts every three weeks, something that was beyond the means of many Japanese people at that time.[52]

Religion was a crucial support, and various Buddhist services, rituals and events featured prominently. Twice a day people sat in front of the assembly hall altar to meditate on their conduct and pray, with monthly communal sermons delivered by Ogaki Relief Foundation members and invited Buddhist monks.[53] Yorokaen still arranged funerals for residents with no family, placing unclaimed ashes in the new memorial tower rather than in public graves, a measure greatly appreciated by terminally ill residents as it offered them reassurance about their likely status in the next world. Residents typically performed daily Buddhist rituals to relieve anxiety about their own deaths and make peace with the deceased. Whenever a resident died, a Buddhist farewell ritual was followed by monthly and annual communal memorial services, the latter including at the spring and autumn equinoxes, *Obon* (a Japanese Buddhist custom to honour the deceased spirits of one's ancestors) on 15 August, and on the anniversary of the death of a benefactor, Ms Yoshioka.[54] Discrimination on the grounds of religion, race, sex, belief or social status was strictly forbidden, as was obligatory participation in religious activities: given the predominance of Buddhism in Yorokaen, it is unknown who organized the Christian missions that visited every first and third Friday of the month in the early 1950s.[55]

Recreational activities included free access to newspapers, magazines, books and board games, with a radio installed in communal and residents' rooms in 1950.[56] A television set, donated by a local benefactor, was set up in the dining hall in 1954 and was appreciated as a tremendous luxury, as only a tiny percentage of people owned one in Japan.[57] Various 'comfort events' included twice-monthly film shows, comic operas, sing-alongs and talks, highlights being New Year festivities, the Ogaki Festival (15 May) and Old People's Day (15 September), to which were added residents' birthday parties.[58] Annual resident/staff 'joint theatricals'

aimed 'to enhance the intimacy in the institution', while days out offered a welcome change for many institution-bound residents.[59] 'Comfort visits' provided
rare opportunities for residents to mix with people in the community.[60]

Acknowledged as vital in enhancing institutional life, annual 'comfort expenditure' was 26,000 yen in 1950 and almost quadrupled to 100,000 yen by 1958.[61]
Yet even the latter figure represented just 3 per cent of Yorokaen's annual outgo-
ings, and as almost all 'comfort' services were confined to Yorokaen, they did not
necessarily diminish the institutional atmosphere. Arrangements sensitive to each
resident's preferences were barely considered, and there are seemingly no extant
records about individual life or activities. Indeed, regulations were deliberately
restrictionist: 'residents must report all their belongings and moneys and follow
the superintendent's instructions ... they must obtain the superintendent's permission whenever they bring in or take out their belongings and receive personal
gifts'.[62] Typically, people could not have any personal furniture, household goods
or family Buddhist or Shinto altars in their rooms, and bedding and clothing were
'to be kept in shared closets and cupboards and ... not taken without permission'.[63]
Essential articles for daily living were limited to a set of underclothing and a pair of
geta (wooden clogs) yearly, tobacco twice a year and a bar of soap and toilet tissue
monthly.[64] Clothing and bedding were 'loaned to those lacking their own' by the
institution, supplemented by second-hand items sent from the Licensed Agencies
for Relief in Asia (LARA) and later donated by local people.[65]

From 1952 every resident received an annual 'compassion allowance' of 300
yen, gradually rising to 1,000 yen by 1958, while some received token payments
for communal side-jobs.[66] This was significant, given the lack of a comprehensive
pension scheme before 1961, but sat uncomfortably with the annual 12,000 yen
means-tested, non-contributory minimum old age pension ('welfare pension'),
introduced in 1961. Such meagre provision had to be supplemented by gifts or
donations from city officials, the Ogaki Relief Foundation, voluntary groups or
individuals and relatives. Thus in 1958 cash donations from twelve benefactors
totalled 45,000 yen, and gifts, worth over 300,000 yen, included towels, clothing, magazines, eye-glasses, cooking equipment, food stuffs, festival gifts and
decorations.[67] Cash donations supplemented 'comfort' provision rather than
offering 'extras', but allowed a degree of planning for residents' needs.

Officially recognized as a 'good' institution, Yorokaen still received gifts and
discretionary subsidies from Gifu Prefecture on Japanese Constitution Memorial Day, reflecting shared principles between the Constitution and the 1950
National Assistance Act, as did testimonials and 'blessing moneys' from the
emperor on his birthday, culminating in an imperial visit in 1957.[68] When the
emperor showed compassion for the residents, exhorting them to 'take care of
your health', they 'cried for joy'.[69] This was the experience of a lifetime for people
instilled with pre-war familistic nationalism based on worship of the emperor

as a living deity. The event enhanced Yorokaen's reputation. Meanwhile public accountability and monitoring contributed to maintaining official minimum standards. Ministry visiting inspectors' reports covered various issues and occasionally featured direct comments and recommendations, which led to improved care or rewards for residents' work. Yet these were rare, and barring perfunctory annual inspections by prefecture officers, there were no systematic or regular inspections by internal officials or external visitors. Quarterly committee meetings of the Ogaki Relief Foundation, the management body until 1959, mainly dealt with financial and personnel matters, but there were no official committees as such after Yorokaen's management transferred to Ogaki City Council, since its assessed institution status and state regulation required only statutory annual inspections by prefecture officials.

If Japan's post-war welfare society increasingly conceptualized welfare as a right, Yorokaen still regarded welfare as a favour or act of compassion bestowed by the state or the emperor. Japan's new welfare ideology maintained the pre-war regime and ethos. An age hierarchy, fortitude, harmony and cooperation were also reflected in near-obligatory 'communal' work, services and strict, managerial-centred regulations and rules. Collectivism, consideration, mutual give-and-take and humility were thus features of communal living, but basic individual rights, privacy or choice were not.

Paradoxically, this tended to suit the older residents, born in the Meiji period (1868–1912) and familiar with such norms. Among the poorest, expectations of institutional life were relatively low, as were concepts of individualism, civic rights, political participation or welfare policies. Imbued with familistic nationalism and traditional values, people had a strong sense of filial obligation and believed that elderly parents should be cared for by their children. Institutionalization conferred loss of social prestige, causing trouble to society or the emperor and negative feelings of being abandoned. A sense of shame made residents submissive. In short, life in 1947–63 Yorokaen exposed the survival of the pre-war regime and ethos through its emphasis on tradition and cultural values.

Staffing and Care Standards

Driven by the need for cost-effective labour, in the early 1950s Yorokaen depended on mutual help, which meant that residents undertook near-obligatory communal work. For example, the Ogaki Relief Foundation Committee responded to the superintendent's request for temporary domestic assistance in 1954 by suggesting 'further utilization of residents' labour', even while noting its appreciation of near-obligatory voluntary night patrols by able male residents.[70] There were then just seven full-time personnel for nearly sixty people.[71] Demarcation between attendant nursing work and domestic tasks was blurred, as posts such as 'general helpers including cooking' confirmed.[72]

Moreover, the Foundation acknowledged that 'staff members have been working for very low salaries', particularly the former resident employees.[73] In 1950, 63-year-old Mr H. was employed as a welfare supervisor after he became ineligible for public assistance. He was followed by others, including a 75-year-old woman in similar circumstances.[74] The 65-year-old Ms T. had a nursing qualification and could work in the clinic in 1954, but was paid only 5,000 yen a month, 20 per cent less than younger, qualified nurses received.[75] Each simply accepted a new role and remuneration, serving for relatively long periods and evidently grateful to have free accommodation and a regular income, with a lump sum gratuity on retirement.[76] Thus Ms T., after five years' nursing, received a further 18,700 yen and stayed on in Yorokaen as a resident until her death sixteen years later.[77] Arguably, these full-timers fared better than some of the casual workers who received a daily wage only when work was available, and able residents performing voluntary or under-paid work.

Staff in the early 1950s were often members of the superintendent's family. In Yorokaen Mr I. (superintendent in 1947–54) shared modest quarters with his wife and five children, who were employed as a clerk, two attendants and two general helpers.[78] This was considered efficient rather than nepotistic, since running costs for in-home staff accommodation were much lower than housing and travel allowances for outside staff; recruitment expenses were negligible and a family-based resident staff could better adjust to 24-hour working.

At the same time, the Foundation applied the pre-war familistic ideology to its workforce, viewing employees as dependent, obedient children. When Mr I. died, it arranged his funeral on behalf of the family and provided his wife, an attendant, with moneys additional to the lump sum gratuity.[79] It also produced a testimonial honouring his 'dedicated, long-term service' and presented gifts on Mrs I.'s retirement a year later.[80] For their part, employees were fiercely loyal to the institution and their employer. Traditional family values were a prerequisite, and staff members undertook a considerable amount of voluntary work. Reinforcing this, Foundation members were themselves involved: a local private GP, Dr J., regularly attended the sick and arranged weekly nurse visits out of his practice's expenses from 1954, and others visited the residents and provided gifts on Old People's Day.[81] Cultural norms such as harmony and fortitude, team work, and observation of an age and gender hierarchy were also encouraged.

All this became increasingly important as more non-related employees were recruited. Acknowledging that family-centred arrangements, heavily dependent on unpaid overtime and low wages, were no longer sustainable, Yorokaen's staff regulations, which were mainly based on the 'president's discretionary powers', were revised in 1956.[82] The new regulations were more pragmatic and generous though strictly budgeted, with the working week set between forty and forty-eight hours and overtime pay of 25–50 per cent introduced, alongside travel and clothing expenses and dependent family benefits.[83]

Even so, Dr J., now Foundation Deputy Chair, claimed that 'it was unrealistic to afford overtime pay for all actual hours worked within the restricted budgets and I am not convinced of such a piecework approach, as the institution's work represents social work'.[84] Others felt that 'formal regulations like those employed by the City Council should be avoided, although minimal regulations are necessary', or reiterated perceptions of an ideal workforce associated with charity or dedication.[85] Accordingly, a clause which noted that 'the aforementioned regulations can be amended within annual net budgets for the time being' was added in 1956.[86] In 1958 modest overtime payments were given to every employee from surplus funds at the end of the year, rather than paid to individuals for the actual hours they worked.[87]

Transitional arrangements thus echoed the familistic workforce, a charitable spirit and traditional values. Although the staff increased to eleven, the growing resident population meant that the attending/nursing staff to resident ratio of roughly 1:14 barely improved.[88] However, no near relatives were now employed; job demarcation between attendants and non-attendants were clearer; and more specialist appointments included a part-time qualified doctor and dietician. Overall, Yorokaen's average wages increased from just 15 per cent of total annual expenses in 1945–50 to 30 per cent in 1950–5, and exceeded 40 per cent after 1956.[89]

While personnel records indicate quantitative aspects of care, the absence of staff and resident narratives precludes close examination of care standards or staff roles and relationships with residents. With some oversimplification, it can be inferred that care provision began with basic nursing undertaken largely by residents. This was gradually taken over by under-staffed and low-paid nursing labour. This functioned tolerably when the staff was mainly made up of family members, supplemented by residents' mutual help and voluntary work, but it could not last. Staff and residents alike simply accepted minimal nursing and limited services and amenities, perhaps because resident-oriented care was not the overriding ethos. With dependent residents assigned to the institution by a superintendent administration, the resident–staff relationship, sustained by the pre-war familistic ideology and a charity-based outlook, was seemingly that of subordinate–superior, rather than close or friendly. As Foundation President Mr Yamamoto remarked in 1957, 'We devote ourselves to protect pitiful, solitary and poor elderly residents with a deep spirit of compassion'.[90]

With local authorities encouraged to take a more active part in welfare provision, Ogaki City Council terminated Yorokaen's contract with the Ogaki Relief Foundation and assumed direct management in 1959. To develop the institution in a more suitable location, it earmarked a 1.5-acre site in residential Makino, where it built a larger facility in 1963.[91] This coincided with its official approval and regulation as an 'old people's home' under the 1963 Elderly Welfare Act.[92]

Whether relocation, transfer of management and revised nomenclature marked a genuine new beginning, particularly from the residents' point of view, should be investigated rather than simply taken at face value.

Yorokaen Replacement Old People's Home, 1963–73

The 'extremely modern and bright', single-storey concrete complex consisted of three long parallel residential blocks, containing twenty-seven Japanese-style *tatami* (straw-matted) bedrooms for 100 people in total.[93] These were fronted by a building comprising staff offices and quarters, dining hall, kitchen, laundry, communal bath, barber and medical facilities, with a clinic, large sick ward and nurses' accommodation. Dormitory facilities were austere, with a 'four people per room' standard, but carefully delineated to provide more homely living space, greater privacy and security. Dormitories had between eight and eleven rooms with lavatory accommodation and an attendant's room, offering basic group living arrangements for thirty-two or so people. Adjoining the Home was the reconstructed public institution for seventy disabled adults completed in 1964 and managed by Ogaki City Council but within public assistance measures under the 1950 Public Assistance Act.

The relocation and new management interrupted records on Yorokaen. The Annual Home Inspection Reports are incomplete, and there are no indications of residents' or staff views in Gifu Record Office.[94] This limits what can be reconstructed concerning life at the new Home. Under the 1963 Act, its residents were meant to be at least 65 years old, eligible for public assistance and dependent for physical, mental or environmental reasons. Those requiring constant nursing care because of serious physical or mental impairment were supposed to be assigned to newly regulated 'nursing homes' under the 1963 Act, but since Ogaki City did not have any until 1987, they numbered among Yorokaen's residential complement.

By 1967 the new Yorokaen was running at full capacity, and within six years the over-70s comprised 85 per cent of its residents.[95] All were able-bodied when they arrived, as their principal reason for admission was financial, and most could undertake communal work and physical exercises, a third even doing communal side-jobs too.[96] The doctor saw an average of sixteen people twice a week, and a dozen might be in a sick ward, but in 1973 just eight of the eighty-eight residents were classified as 'chronic infirm'.[97] Mortality rates almost halved to 17 per cent during 1958–72 and longevity increased, the decennial average age at death rising from 75.9 to 77.5 in 1953–73.[98] This can partly be accounted for by the increased transfer of sick residents to hospitals, with five cases in 1972 compared to just four for the whole of 1954–60.[99] With hardly any other discharges, roughly 45 per cent of the residents had lived in Yorokaen for at least five years, compared to 30 per cent in the late 1950s.[100]

With eligibility criteria now including an unsuitable environment, older people living with their families had a greater chance of admission to a Home. Yet no one at Yorokaen was admitted for this reason, and 85 per cent of residents in 1971 simply had no families or relatives while the rest had relations themselves too poor to look after them.[101] All residents qualified for public assistance, which exempted them from making maintenance contributions. Thus, despite the 1963 Act's relaxed eligibility criteria, the continuation of the 1950 Act's assessed institution measures left Yorokaen's clientele essentially restricted to the neediest. The situation was broadly similar in other prefecture rural Homes, although 20 per cent of the Gujo Home admissions were due to 'tensions within the family' in 1973, compared to just 4 per cent a decade earlier.[102]

At the new Yorokaen, older staff typically worked well into old age and the few younger ones for a decade or more, with the new superintendent, Mr W., who served for seven years until his retirement at 65, succeeded by other relatively long-serving men.[103] This reflected the City Council's lifetime employment policy. Thus in 1964 personnel expenses exceeded state subsidies by 35 per cent, even though they were three attendants short, the deficit covered by the City Council.[104] Whether this policy could be sustained was doubtful, as was the likely focus on quality of care issues, with only one qualified nurse and official qualifications in care and social work not introduced until 1987.[105]

Staff shortages could be acute, with just four attendants for seventy-seven people in 1964, the ratio of 1:19 worse than in the late 1950s when it stood at 1:14.[106] Under pressure from inspectors, the nursing staff increased to nine in 1973, a ratio of 1:11.[107] Moreover, as younger personnel were recruited, the average age of the nursing staff fell to 41 years in 1973, compared to 58 years in 1963, with three aged under 30 and five in post for less than one year.[108] Arguably, the last two former institution staff offered some continuity and stability, even if their experience was anchored in the old regime. However, owing to the wage structure their combined salaries exceeded 30 per cent of the total nursing costs.[109]

Revised regulations in 1968 emphasized greater personalized care for residents, within a 'communal' order:

> The superintendent and welfare officer must endeavour to offer individual meetings to listen to residents' concerns as much as possible ... [and] provide communal sessions and guidance to help residents live out an orderly, cooperative and homely life under a bright environment.[110]

Yet daily life still followed a rigid timetable, and 'communal' services and daily chores had to be performed, although 'physical exercises ... to maintain residents' independence and to help them be motivated for living' had replaced a four-hour period of 'communal work'.[111] Thirty or so people undertook 'communal side-jobs' which earned them a monthly wage of 1,000–1,200 yen in 1967, but this ceased in 1970, and no alternative or supplementary activities were put in their place.[112] These residents may have regretted having to adapt to an income based on monthly pocket money of 1,200 yen.[113]

To offset staff shortages and heavy workloads, meal times were brought forward and the communal bathroom was open for shorter periods. For economy and efficiency reasons, older residents were offered the same menus as younger disabled residents who lived in the adjacent public institution, despite their different nutritional requirements. Inspectors' demands that 'separate menus should be introduced' in 1970 were ignored until 1973, when twenty 'special meals' were served each day for those requiring different diets, and the monthly menus were changed 'to reflect residents' tastes'.[114] But with just three kitchen staff and no domestics, Yorokaen continued to rely on its residents for cleaning and washing up duties.

Only minor improvements in treatment, provisions and services were required to fulfil the revised official minimum standards, with twice-weekly doctor's visits for the sick by 1967 and twice-yearly health check-ups for all residents by 1971.[115] Two more televisions and an electric massage chair were obtained, and trips out now ventured beyond prefecture boundaries, but articles for daily living remained basic, although items of clothing were supplied three times a year.[116] The cycle of 'comfort' events hinted at continuity with the pre-war era. From the late 1960s monthly staff meetings were held to discuss individuals as well as managerial matters. This acknowledged the need for personalized care, yet heavy workloads jeopardized this and inspectors repeatedly urged staff 'to record [their discussions] more frequently'.[117] Even then, the prime requirement was not resident-centred, for 'case records are the only official proof of whether an institution is providing required services to residents and whether its staff are doing their job satisfactorily'.[118]

Resident-centred measures might be seen in holidays and outings, with two sets of travel tickets a year, paid for from public subsidies, given to any resident wishing to use public transport.[119] Nonetheless, Yorokaen's regulations required written permission from the superintendent in advance, and everyone 'must carry identification … at all times while away from the Home'.[120] In practice 'the Home keeps a slack rein on outings', but hardly anyone applied for free tickets because the Home was well away from public transport and most simply could not afford to go on outings anyway.[121]

Thus, although the new Home's resident population increased, grew old and lived there longer, their socio-economic situation stayed the same. More nursing staff were employed, but their numbers barely exceeded official minimum standards, and less experienced, unqualified and younger staff raised doubts about the quality of care, even though all were on permanent and full-time contracts, unlike the majority of part-time staff in Norfolk's care homes.[122] Increasing administrative demands, with compulsory recording and documentation to comply with state guidelines, probably meant that staff had less time to engage with residents, let alone provide resident-centred care, suggesting few grounds for optimism or the end of an institutional regime. With so few official insights into the actual experiences and lives of residents before 1970, more impression-istic sources are now considered, using oral testimony from current and former residents and personnel at the present-day Yorokaen (rebuilt in 1994) and the first Ogaki City Council Kusunokien nursing home (purpose-built in 1987).

Latecomers in Development: Ogaki City, Gifu

Although Ogaki City Council had considered expanding Yorokaen and estab-lishing its own nursing home since 1970, only two social welfare corporation nursing homes – Shinseien in neighbouring Ibigawa (1976) and Ibukien in Tarui (1981) – had opened, each with 100 places.[123] By 1980 at least 750 bed-ridden older people were being cared for by their families at home in the western Seino region, including 140 in Ogaki City.[124] In 1984 the mayor, Mr Iwata, again announced plans for a city council nursing home, but meanwhile the council was subsidizing thirty places for residents at Ibukien at a cost of 50 million yen.[125] Finally, in 1987 the Kusunokien (literally, 'camphor tree lodge') nursing home opened. It provided fifty places for frail or bedridden older people along with a day centre for a similar clientele living at home.[126] In 1990 an extension block was built. This offered fifty more places, including twelve for dementia cases and twenty for night- or short-stay purposes.[127] A year later a 'home care support sta-tion' was added to provide home-based services and counselling for older people and their families in the community, so that Kusunokien became central to a more comprehensive and integrated service, a belated response to government policy which called for normalization and 'socialization of the homes'.[128]

Yorokaen also built a day centre in 1991, rebuilt three years later as a mod-ern four-storey structure, providing seventy places in single rooms, along with twelve short-stay beds in single or double rooms.[129] A matching multi-purpose welfare facility, Okachiyama, connected to the new Yorokaen Home, was com-pleted in 1998. Okachiyama had a day centre, a new home care support station, a 'community welfare centre' and a 'care house' for thirty physically independent, moderately well-off older people, while also integrating the new Yorokaen.[130] The city-funded social welfare corporation, established in 1990, took over management of Okachiyama (including Yorokaen), along with the Kusunok-ien complex, reflecting the mixed economy in welfare.[131] In 2000 Kusunokien and other nursing homes and all community care services were integrated into the new national Long-Term Care Insurance (LTCI) scheme, but Yorokaen remained outside. Retaining an assessed institution status under the 1963 Act, its admissions are still determined by the city's welfare office, using compulsory means-testing and needs assessments and leaving applicants with no choice about which institution they would be admitted to.

In contrast, and at least in theory, LTCI recognized a client's right to choose any LTCI residential and home-based services, which took the form of a contract between the client and service provider(s). It also acknowledged the part LTCI residential facilities could play in addressing the care needs of very frail or bedridden older people whatever their financial means or family situation. This suggests that specialized, person-centred care was emerging. This contrasts with the Yorokaen old people's home, which was still being run in line with public assistance measures within the 1963 Act.

Oral testimony from former and current residents and staff at Yorokaen and/ or Kusunokien are included, some staff having been involved also with older people in the community as day care staff or home helps or in other institutions. Others are or were informal carers for older relatives, some with experience of Kusunokien short-stay and residential care. Each older resident's life story is unique, so attitudes and perceptions cannot be taken as wholly representative or objective; the same is true of the staff accounts. Nonetheless, it is worth considering whether the almshouse mentality and reach, seen in the 1947–73 Yorokaen, could be detected in the contemporary homes.

Life in Yorokaen Old People's Home, 1980–94

The 1963 Yorokaen was demolished in 1994. The 22-year-old Ms K. recalled the last days of Yorokaen:

> When I looked at the rundown, bare concrete exterior of the Home, I was utterly shocked ... inside ... my first impression was of a very chilly and grim atmosphere. The windows and doors were too old and hard to open or close and the floors were made of plain, thin veneers ... I imagined that life and residents here would be grim and dull too.[132]

In contrast, the attendant Mrs F., transferred from the adjoining 1963-built public institution for disabled adults in 1992, found that:

> Yorokaen was very old and made of plain concrete, but it was a single-storey, cosy home with a pleasant garden ... I associated it with a somewhat heart-warming, homely community like a big family, where elderly residents helped each other, did cleaning and washing together, chatted with staff members, and shared multi-bedded rooms, meals and bathroom.[133]

This may have reflected her previous experience at the adjoining public institution, 'similar to Yorokaen but homely and very friendly inside'.[134]

With rising living standards, more hospitals and less visible destitution, fewer people needed assessed institutions, something reflected in Yorokaen's shrinking resident population, which almost halved from eighty-four in the mid-1980s to forty-eight by 1993.[135] In the mid-1980s the majority of the residents were female and had lived there for at least five years; their average age was 76 years.[136] Nearly all were physically independent, and 'quite a few were even ... participated in dash and relay races ... at annual sports'.[137] Although almost everyone had a relative or friend they could get in touch with, a third received no visitors at all and a mere handful had more than four visits a year.[138] In the early 1990s they all qualified for public assistance and, as before, were 'functionally independent but poor and solitary'.[139] They were seen by some staff as 'pathetic' or 'unfortunate', but unlike many nursing home residents with severe disabilities or dementia, they were 'communicative' and 'capable of putting their affairs in order by themselves'.[140]

Despite claims in the Yorokaen brochure, its daily life in the 1980s and early 1990s was almost unchanged since 1970, although an extra television set was set up in the dining hall and two-hour club activities had been introduced by 1980, which finally filled the gap left when residents' communal side-jobs came to an end.[141] Each activity attracted an average of eighteen members, and all signed up for the singing club.[142] Those not attending were assigned tasks rather than being allowed free time, reflecting the continued emphasis on the collective norm and identical routines.[143]

Ms K. found that 'the residents were lively, very lively indeed' in the early 1990s and that there was little interference from long-serving older staff: 'as long as residents could follow the set daily routines and adhere to the basic rules, we leave it in residents' own hands to regulate their lives'.[144] Officially given little scope for a private life, residents utilized 'very strict power-driven interrelationships' based on an age hierarchy and traditional values.[145] Thus:

> if some lazy or frail people were late coming to the dining hall for meals or other communal services, domineering residents told them off ... Cleaning and communal tasks were undertaken through teamwork.[146]

In practice private life was more relaxed than the Home's rules stipulated, since 'residents went out when they wished ... although they usually just went for a walk in the neighbourhood, as there were no shops or public transport nearby'.[147] Most residents washed their clothes by hand and starched their sheets. One young attendant, Ms C., 'had seen neither washboards nor rice water starch before, and wondered if the astonishingly crisp sheets could be folded'.[148] Such arrangements respected personal preferences and traditions. Some residents collected and burned rubbish, delivered meals and did the washing up or gardening.

Whether assigned or voluntary, these tasks offered residents a measure of continuity and reassurance that they could still undertake and maintain their previous routines and rituals, which made them feel independent, contented and useful. Some even instructed the personnel: when Ms K. tried to help clean the Buddhist altar, a resident told her, 'You must not wipe the Buddha with a wet cloth ... cooked rice for Buddha should be placed here not there'.[149] Younger attendants trying to introduce 'new' forms of care found that residents resisted change and kept 'the newcomers' at arm's length, as did experienced older staff who favoured a less interventionist approach. In these circumstances, Ms K. 'was bewildered as to what on earth my work meant and involved ... I wasn't helping or supervising residents ... but had to follow and learn the ongoing old regime from them'.[150]

During construction of the new Home (July–December 1994), residents and staff moved to a nearby small, overcrowded, prefabricated facility:

> When you stood in the central corridor, you could see all the bedrooms and residents at a glance on both sides. Yet it ... made us [young attendants] and residents close at last. We slept in rooms next to each other, ate together and shared the communal bathtub and lavatories. We went to residents' rooms or they called in ours ... They talked about their memories of childhood, families and home town, showing us pictures and keepsakes. They gradually ... accepted us into their community.[151]

As closer relationships developed, the younger staff organized activities and recreations, although older staff complained that 'our workloads increased considerably'.[152] Ms K. felt that 'we finally developed close-knit ties with residents like a big, extended family', exemplified during a trip to a hot spring resort: 'I was helping a disabled resident with a wheelchair in a souvenir shop. She turned to me and said, "Take whatever you want, dear K. I will get it for you" ... I was very touched by her generosity'.[153] She concluded that 'the six-month period at the prefab was the happiest time in my administration at Yorokaen'.[154] A significant difference between her current role as a nursing home care manager and as Yorokaen junior attendant was

> the psychological feeling toward the Homes and their residents ... now when I finish work ... I shut out all matters surrounding the Home. At Yorokaen, the Home and residents stayed in my heart all the time ... In this way, I had two families.[155]

Life at Yorokaen in 1994 thus was characterized by a rigid regime and routines, offering residents continuity and stability yet allowing a degree of autonomy, facilitating a sense of independence and satisfaction. Significantly, the power-driven relationships among the residents were essential to its smooth running. However, it was never organized on democratic or modern lines, but manipulated cultural norms. This spoiled the quality of life for some, yet this same structure created a sense of solidarity and belonging, particularly before 1994 when the institutional ethos was communal and public and residents came from broadly similar backgrounds.

A Fresh Start? Yorokaen Reconstructed, 1994–2008

Opening the reconstructed Yorokaen in December 1994, Mayor Ogura anticipated that the 'modern Home will deliver satisfactory welfare provision to its
elderly service users'.[156] The new building offered spacious accommodation for seventy people, although the staff generally found it 'too large without garden space'
and 'somewhat like a large hospital or medical institution rather than a homely
place'.[157] Many residents disliked the multi-storey structure and a few 'were con-
stantly lost ... and took a good while to learn where their bedroom was'.[158] Others
felt that 'it was too big to do the daily activities smoothly and to maintain a group
life'.[159] It also reduced interaction, particularly with staff, since communal or
administrative and residential sections were more strictly delineated.

Nonetheless, the single bedrooms exceeded the post-1973 official minimum
of 'all double bedrooms' standards, and unlike recent Westernized versions, the
Japanese-style bedrooms suggested a degree of continuity and domesticity to
older residents, unused to sleeping in beds. Each had a *tatami* (straw-matted)
sleeping space, with sliding door, entrance hall and built-in storage on one side
and a French window opening onto a balcony on the other. Rooms were small:
they put attendant Ms C. in mind of a 'prison cell'.[160] Staff generally 'preferred
the older multi-bedded but larger rooms'.[161]

Single rooms ensured residents' privacy and autonomy, and avoided quarrels
or psychological stress caused by other roommates – something that could occur
under the old arrangement. Each room had basic amenities, including a TV, a
folding low table, a small cabinet and two large floor cushions. While the Home
discouraged residents bringing in personal possessions as there was so little space,
88-year-old Mrs H. had a bedroom cluttered with personal possessions.[162] These
hardly represented a lifetime's accumulation, but she acknowledged that 'I keep
too many things here and my room is a bit chaotic, but I need everything'.[163]
Among her possessions were the ashes of her late husband, and she chanted Buddhist sutras before his ashes to console herself and make peace with him, as she
was not allowed 'a proper Buddhist altar'.[164] Overall, she led a monotonous and
lonely life, 'just lying, dozing, reading, listening to the radio or watching TV'.[165]

Other residents' lives were similar, not least because women especially disliked
any intrusions even by staff. Mrs F. 'felt a sense of alienation' after offering to help
one very old lady clean her room, only to be told, 'No thanks. I can do it myself!'[166]
Similarly, she 'found that the small glass panes set in the entrance door of some of
the bedrooms were completely covered by clothing or calendars to prevent us from
even glancing in'.[167] Greater privacy and autonomy, with so little social interaction,
came at the expense of support, especially from staff, and was hardly ideal.

Yet those wanting interaction with staff found only one attendant's room
on the first floor, where sick or frail patients in the temporary sick ward or bed-

rooms resided. The able majority on the second or third floors had only a bell connection to the attendant's room, which merely identified the floor on which they were calling. 'It took ages for us [staff] to find out who had actually pressed the bell and we somehow discouraged residents from using it ... Consequently, they felt reticent about ringing the bell and its use soon ended'.[168] The 'top floors' now had even less opportunity to interact with attendants, and some looked back nostalgically to the old or temporary Home, where 'attendants were always around ... now ... I hardly see any attendants ... and whenever I want them, I have to press the bloody bell, but how can I press it just to say "hello"?'[169]

Clearly, some envied the 'first floors' who had easier access to the attendant's room, care and attention. They generally felt special and more satisfied after an attendant's visit, but this could also incur jealousy: Ms K. 'had to sneak in and out of residents' bedrooms to avoid being seen by neighbouring residents. It was very stressful and I even felt guilty as if I was doing something wrong'.[170]

Overfamiliarity was discouraged to avoid tensions like these. Younger staff were aware of this and sought to 'maintain formality, as we were not friends or families of the residents but providers of welfare services'.[171] Older kitchen staff tried to retain close relationships, one being reprimanded after she chatted with some of the residents about her private matters. Then, in 2007, meals were contracted out to a private company and the kitchen staff were made redundant. One felt that:

> although the new arrangement may be more cost-effective, I don't think it is any better from the residents' point of view, especially because they have lost the chance to talk with us about their personal preferences ... which, to a certain degree ... we could take into consideration through special arrangements such as swapping fish with Tofu ... or boiling Japanese noodles for a few more minutes.[172]

Elements of communal life did continue in shared bathing, the dining hall and daily cleaning or help routines. Yet a greater degree of freedom, choice and flexibility was also apparent, which was important particularly as the resident population became more diversified, including very frail and moderately well-off people still within public assistance measures. With property development in neighbouring areas, able residents could take a bus into the city centre, and their access to personal and everyday articles was facilitated when several shops opened within walking distance. Residents could now bring food, purchased in local shops, into the dining hall, while bathroom and laundry opening hours were extended to cater for residents' differing lifestyles.

There were more covert changes too. Older, power-driven but stable relationships were replaced by 'more complicated and irrational' ones based on residents' financial and physical status.[173] A sense of inequality, unfairness and envy could be detected between those with means and good health and those without: at mealtimes, for example, 'the poorer, unable to afford extras, felt miserable eating with those who had their own additional dishes bought from nearby stores or given by relatives'.[174] Able residents tended to be assigned more work and house cleaning chores to make up for the frailer or less capable residents, although 'a few able residents felt unfairly treated and could not understand or accept the fact that they had to do extra work'.[175] Worst of all, 'a few wealthier domineering residents got poorer and compliant people to do their personal tasks ... in return, allowing them to get on their side or in their circle or giving them a tiny amount of pocket money or sweets'.[176]

Staff who had worked in Yorokaen found 'highly charged personal relation-ships among the residents ... so challenging to handle that tips and advice were detailed in the Home Manual handed on from previous employees'.[177] One recalled, 'I did very little physical nursing ... My work was mainly just to deal with discord among the residents, but emotionally I felt utterly shattered, much worse than physically exhausted'.[178] Another attendant noted:

> I was ... often annoyed to have to intercede on behalf of residents about trivial inci-dents day after day, such as quarrels over who should eat first, do the laundry first and get into the bathtub first, and complaints about who didn't flush the toilet or used too much toilet tissue.[179]

In these circumstances, most residents stayed in their bedrooms and 'quite a few felt lonely and cut off, but were too intimidated to get involved in a quarrel with the dominant ones'.[180] Some longer-term residents regretted that 'a well-ordered, united group life in the old Home had disappeared ... A few dominate the rest with their money. There is no mutual help or warmth among the residents any more'.[181]

In order to overcome this, the Home changed its focus from being resident-centred to imposing more communal activities, which meant that interaction among the residents was unavoidable, and making impartial or standardized provision. Thus people were not allowed to watch TV in their bedrooms before 4 pm, and a 'no extras' rule was introduced in the dining hall, which, it was hoped, would reduce the variety of dishes seen and consumed.[182] Yet whether restoring communal life and cultural norms was appropriate or well received by the residents remains uncertain, as Ms K. explained:

> Residents demanded privacy and said they preferred being alone ... Yet, they were actually lonely and longed to mix with the others ... They were in fact very Japanese; they pretended that they were adopting the modern Western value of individualism and so weren't interested in others superficially, but actually they were still deeply traditionalist and felt extremely ill at ease and insecure if they didn't belong to a group ... no matter how testing they were.[183]

This, though, does not indicate whether a communal life was preferable. Atten-dant Mrs F., who had worked at Yorokaen and the adjoining contract-based 'care house', concluded:

[I]n the past, everyone at Yorokaen was absolutely poor, so their relationships were untainted by the power of money. But now, the poorest cannot fully exercise freedom and choice in their daily life, while the slightly better-off can. Accordingly, the poor tend to be jealous ... [or] sometimes subservient ... some slightly better-off people feel superior to the rest and boss them ... By contrast, those moderately well-off at the adjoining care house engage in some communal life but are very supportive of each other, because everyone there has enough to lead a comfortable life of their own, plus extras to treat others. I myself used to think that it was OK to be admitted to Yorokaen ... but now I cannot imagine living here, suffering such spiteful, money-fuelled relationships.[184]

Life in Kusunokien Nursing Home, 1987–99

Kusunokien nursing home opened in 1987. It was run by the Ogaki city council and later by the city-funded social welfare corporation. Like Yorokaen, it was an assessed institution under the 1963 Act, so that applicants and their families underwent compulsory means-testing and needs assessments, but here the focus was principally on needs and there was no upper financial limit, with residents paying a sliding scale of fees according to their means. It purported to embody a modern welfare ethos, and new staff were informed that they 'are not providers of care for residents but are honoured to care for [residents] ... with loving hearts and respect'.[185] Nonetheless, recruitment policy was specifically 'to utilize existing city officials and family connections', with all but one member of staff taken on in this way. The exception was Ms A., a graduate with a background in care and social work but without practical experience.[186] The staff were consequently 'completely inexperienced in nursing the frail elderly', their training being a three-day crash course at the neighbouring Ibukien, followed by visits to two other Gifu Prefecture nursing homes.[187] There was back-up from two qualified nurses, but it was immediately apparent that 'the heads of the nurses' and attendants' sections loathed each other'.[188] From the outset, a clear boundary between social and medical care existed, undermining the quality of care offered.

Furthermore, the chief attendant imposed a traditional work ethic, based on a rigid age hierarchy, loyalty and subordination to the institution. This 'forbidding, absolute autocrat' thus oversaw a staff-centred rather than resident-centred working environment.[189] Ms A., astonished by a ruling that residents must be served breakfast in bed, took them to the dining hall as usual and was 'severely reprimanded by the superintendent and chief attendant ... [who] said that this behaviour was utterly unacceptable'.[190] Vulnerable staff reluctantly complied with the regime. One, finding that her increased daily workload allowed little contact with the residents, voluntarily came early and stayed late to spend time with them: she was reprimanded by the chief attendant on the grounds that she was undermining the work environment. She summed the situation up in this way:

'The nail that sticks out gets hammered down'. Even though I was unpaid, I did it for the residents' sake ... in the end, those with administrative power and strong characters won and dominated other staff, residents and the whole Home. I couldn't risk losing my job ... I gave in.[191]

Another, divorced and with children, listened to residents as much as she could, but 'was told ... "Don't chat with the residents. Get back to work"'.[192] Time spent with residents was not considered work and, as the daily workload increased, was even regarded as undermining basic nursing: 'we were so busy with daily business that, whenever called or stopped by residents ... we couldn't help them straight away and used to reply "Sorry, wait a minute, as we have to do our tasks first"'.[193]

Further contradicting the official care ethos, there were just two night attendants for 100 residents, including many dementia sufferers. Restraints were common, with special clothing, belts or straps used to tie patients to beds or wheelchairs, and single rooms locked. Dementia sufferers were consequently excluded, something that was reinforced by staff 'undressing residents and covering them with just a bath towel in their bedrooms before taking them to the downstairs communal bathroom'.[194] Basic rights counted for little, with occasional

> incidents involving violence which would be a scandalous disclosure in contemporary Japanese society ... For example, a senior attendant shouted at a disabled resident to walk quickly and pulled her by the hand so harshly that she fell ... I [a young attendant] was about ... to help but just watched while she cried instead, as I was too scared.[195]

A male volunteer found that in 1989:

> Care standards were astonishingly poor ... no attendant had qualifications, professional skills or training. Female staff used childish terms to speak to residents ... believing that these expressed affection ... but male residents in particular were appalled ... A few male attendants threatened senile patients by shouting abuse at them in order to get things done ... One female attendant said accusingly to a doubly-incontinent lady: 'Oh dear, again! ... I only changed your pad a moment ago'. The poor woman was utterly humiliated ... and begged me, 'Not that attendant again, never' ... Attendants violated residents' dignity every day, but were simply too ignorant and unprofessional to realize it.[196]

One experienced attendant bluntly summarized the situation in the 1990s: 'Superior staff members gave state basic welfare services to the subordinate poor and vulnerable elderly dependent on public assistance on behalf of the government'.[197]

A New Departure? Kusunokien since 2000

How typical experiences in Kusunokien were is unknown, but the enactment of LTCI in 2000 changed things considerably. Nursing home applicants were now assessed only on their physical and mental status under standardized assessment procedures; before, 'it was common that a fairly able applicant got round the long waiting lists with a simple reference from a city councillor'.[198] Yet shortages of long-term care facilities and the growing frail older population meant that Kusunokien's waiting list exceeded 400 by 2002 and entailed rationing prioritized applicants with the most disabilities or severe dementia and lacking family support.[199] Consequently, Kusunokien became

> An absolute last resort for the most disabled, sick or demented ... their condition requiring 24-hour care was beyond psychiatric or geriatric hospitals or other long-term care institutions. Meanwhile, there were hardly any discharges ... none during 2000–8 and just two in the decade prior to 2000 ... about a dozen patients are fed by [nasogastric] tube to keep them alive, just within manageable numbers, but if they live much longer, the Home will not be able to cope[200]

Artificial feeding was by no means atypical, as suggested by an unofficial 'maximum of 10 per cent designated places for the tube-fed'.[201]

One innovatory LTCI concept was 'the socialization of care'. As the Home was no longer an assessed institution, nursing home provision became part of a social contract, involving mandatory contributions, universal entitlement and some consumer choice. Subsequently, staff attitudes acknowledged older residents as 'important clients choosing the Home on contract'.[202] Residents' needs were prioritized: 'Whenever I was called by residents asking for assistance, I would reply, "Yes, I am coming", not "Wait a minute". I then left work in hand on hold, no matter how busy I was'.[203] To improve the quality of care, more attendants were given subsidized home help training, and some qualified as social workers or care managers. The Home Manual covered everything from basic nursing and medical skills to daily workloads and advice, and emphasized more equal and professional interpersonal relationships: 'Staff members should use honorific language to elderly customers and address them by their surname ... to respect their dignity'.[204] There was to be no restraint or confinement policy, and special arrangements were to be made to meet residents' need and wishes. Thus a toothless resident was allowed to eat festive dishes without them being cut into small pieces. Although staff were worried that he might choke, he managed, remarking, 'I've been dying to eat dishes in their proper shape for years and my dream has now come true'.[205] Resident-centred arrangements like this raised questions about the boundaries between the residents' wishes and staff judgements, and about attitudes to those unable to articulate their needs and wishes.

With more qualified staff, a collegial atmosphere emerged among the workforce. One attendant, with seventeen years' experience, explained: 'The current work team is the best ... we hold daily meetings to ensure the smooth operation of our team, ending with chanting our monthly slogan: "Mission, passion, high tension, let's work hard cooperatively"'.[206] Nevertheless, some newcomers felt less able to express their views freely or kept their frustration and dissatisfaction to themselves 'in order not to upset the senior staff or be thrown out of a work circle'.[207]

Kusunokien ensured the official minimum standards of nutrition, security, shelter, care, amenities and daily necessities, a blessing to most residents who had often experienced family discord prior to admission. One attendant said: 'When I cleaned and changed a frail lady, recently admitted, she was in tears as she thanked me, saying, "I've never been cared for by my daughter-in-law with such gentleness and affection."'.[208] A former day centre assistant regarded many Kusunokien residents as 'lucky' compared to those living alone, neglected or abused: 'I went to collect an old lady, not living in the main house where her son's family lived, but put in a dilapidated barn ... it was so appalling ... I've seen similar elderly people, living in a modern *zashikiro* (prison cell within the home)'.[209] This suggests that domestic *obasuteyama* persists in contemporary Japan and is actually getting worse.

Despite advanced age and frailty, 'residents lived out fairly long lives, a dozen for over twenty years'.[210] Better care, a balanced diet, medical check-ups and good nursing all contributed to improved health and longevity. As a 94-year-old lady remarked, 'I suffered from asthma for years, but as soon as I came here, it's all gone and I became healthier and stronger. I hadn't expected to live so long ... maybe it's because I keep regular hours and finish every meal'.[211] Whether a healthy but rigid institutional life is better than an irregular but homely one is open to debate: a one-hour interview in Kusunokien was interrupted three times by loudspeaker announcements reminding residents of the daily routines.[212] Similar uncertainties surround the treatment of bedridden or severely frail people, particularly the tube-fed. Attendant Ms W. felt that: 'Wards for those fed on tubes are a living hell. Once you entered the Home, you had no choice but were forced to live bed-bound ... when I become very ill or disabled, I won't go to hospital or ask Social Services for help'.[213] Tube-fed patients now number some 400,000 or 40 per cent of long-stay elderly hospital population in Japan.[214]

Increasingly, enhanced care services resemble commodities, reflected in increasingly standardized care plans with packed timetables. These employ various recreational and rehabilitation programmes to help maximize residents' independence and minimize bed stays. Yet more programmes without additional staff due to economic restraints mean heavier workloads, compounded by preparation, recording and evaluation procedures and staff meetings. Attendant Ms T.'s workload became 'like a train timetable, scheduled to the minute ... new activities one after another and corresponding paperwork'.[215] Once again staff lacked time to interact with residents, as 'even during activities, we are keeping records of residents' case files, while keeping an eye on them'.[216] Ms N., a 64-year-old nurse, recalled:

[I]n the early 1990s, my duty consisted only of professional nursing and I spent ten minutes or more listening to each resident. Now, I deal with residents one after another, spending less than a minute, something like a conveyor belt. I have many more residents requiring daily treatment and additional domestic and caring tasks. Worse still, we [nurses] were recently told to take over the new rehabilitation programme. I do too many extras on the same salary.[217]

Despite deteriorating working conditions, nursing staff were typically dedicated, remarking, 'I miss the residents when I am off work' and 'I feel attached to residents like they're my parents'.[218] In return, residents demanded little and expressed their appreciation: a 78-year-old man said that the 'attendants take good care of me ... I keep some worries to myself as I owe a lot to the Home and its staff'; and an 86-year-old lady noted, 'I am very grateful to the staff and am trying my best not to be a burden to them'.[219] These comments imply better, if not necessarily equitable or close, staff–resident relationships, although some longer-serving staff do retain friendly, personal contact. (In contrast, some residents in English care homes confided that 'staff are discouraged from personal chats and hardly talk to us'.[220]) Kusunokien nursing staff still undertook domestic tasks, including collecting rubbish, cleaning and laundry, but generally took those chores for granted:

[W]e look after the Home as well as its residents, just the same as a housewife in an ordinary home does all the housework, plus looking after her elderly family member. Whenever we have a bit of spare time, we scrub the floors, water the plants, and so on.[221]

In English care homes, job demarcation between nursing and domestic staff is normally strict, with workloads precisely set out.[222]

There were concerns whether some residents should have an easier time. According to Nurse Ms N., 'If I were a resident, I would go mad. They are tied hand and foot by the hectic daily routine with no free time at all'.[223] Attendant Ms T. sympathized:

in the open-plan, noisy dayroom ... many are not joining in activities, but dozing in wheelchairs or simply staring at the floor ... I feel sorry for them and my inclination is to take them to their bedrooms so they can have a proper rest ... But I also think we should follow the set routine and engage them in activities to stimulate them or prevent them deteriorating.[224]

Care manager Ms K. expressed mixed feelings:

[D]uring rehabilitation programmes, a few residents complained 'I don't want to do it ... Why do I have to make an effort to keep fit in old age?' I totally agreed ... But what we actually did was the opposite. We typically encouraged them saying, 'Keep at it, and you will get better and can return home'. How cruel it was: we know their families won't take them back and so do the residents ... with the dementia sufferers, we left them for a bit and, when they calmed down, we said the same thing.[225]

This is typical of the traditional Japanese life ethic, as noted by one attendant: 'A good life means not being free [to do as you wish] or relaxing, but a *fulfilling* life and consequently, the daily routine is packed with *meaningful* activities. The more, the better' (my emphasis).[226] Work is a virtue, and the merit of days off or holidays has not gained full recognition; workaholism and *karoshi* (death from work) are common; free time is associated with futility, laziness or boredom. Thus, rather than reflecting the actual lives or preferences of elderly residents, remote policymakers encourage routines packed with purposeful programmes and enhanced activities. Japanese tradition embraces conformity to the majority, the state or institutions, whereas asserting individual rights or preferences is characterized as being self-centred or uncooperative. In this context, Kusunokien's regime was imposed whether or not residents liked or wanted it. Those unable to express their preferences had care plans drawn up by the care manager on their behalf, sometimes after consulting their families, who often asked for unrealistic recreational and rehabilitation programmes. However,

> families seldom visited residents, let alone took them back home if they got better, making demands not for the sake of residents but for themselves, feeling safe to stick to official objectives ... typically reflecting the differences between words and intentions in Japanese society.[227]

What constituted a 'good life'? Care manager Ms G. felt that the policy objective of restoring or maintaining independence through rehabilitation was critical, particularly for Kusunokien residents, who were very hesitant or reluctant to seek nursing assistance even when they needed it.[228] Chief attendant Ms A. disagreed, arguing that it should replicate their former family life: 'A resident can continue to carry out her own daily routine in her own way, pursuing maximum privacy and autonomy in a familiar environment surrounded by personal possessions and in close touch with the local community and family'.[229] Attendant Ms T. recalled how able Yorokaen residents had a less rigid regime: 'They used to go to their rooms after lunch and take a nap ... I think that is absolutely normal, the same as other older people do in their homes, resting, watching TV or dozing, as I do when I'm off work'.[230]

As for the growing majority of frailer residents, some staff felt that they required a different lifestyle, sensitive to their needs, rather than an *excess* of imposed programmes and routines. Yet the latter seek to stimulate those with severe disability or advanced dementia, creating opportunities for interaction and integration. Others pointed to arrangements and services which might enhance residents' quality of life, such as simple outings, as 94-year-old Ms Q. confirmed:

> [A] staff member took me to a city-centre Sushi restaurant with three other residents by car about four years ago. It was the happiest time in my five-year stay here and I would like another. But it won't happen again as I can't walk and have no relatives who drive to come to the Home and take me out.[231]

Family support was valued, yet very few residents received regular visits, even from family members who lived near the Home. In 2007 just two had daily visits and ten received monthly visits, leaving the majority (88) with only occasional visits or none at all.[232] No one had an annual holiday, compared to a dozen or so during the early 1990s.[233] Stigma was still attached to the institutionalization of older people. Families placing older relatives in a nursing home felt very guilty, something that was compounded by criticism from relatives, neighbours and even staff, who considered them irresponsible or callous, while sympathizing with the elderly. As a result most families avoided the Home to evade facing their 'undesirable' decision.[234] Although Kusunokien is effectively the last resort for almost all residents, LTCI emphasizes rehabilitation to enable residents to return to their homes. Yet due to limited affordable or accessible alternatives in the community, families inevitably have to assume the prime responsibility for those discharged and fear being considered an alternative care provider.[235]

Not only did Kusunokien's isolation impact on residents' quality of life, but the building was also inadequate for current standards or the perceived needs of the residents. Staff viewed its four-bedded rooms with particular concern, as they were noisy and lacked basic amenities and space, let alone privacy. Interestingly, the residents interviewed accepted these arrangements and even preferred them to single rooms, because 'I can ask roommates for help, if something happens at night', and 'I don't feel lonely as I have roommates to chat with'.[236] Relationships among the residents themselves were important, although not necessarily close: 'I get on with my roommates, although I don't talk to them much'.[237] Most staff recognized that 'conflicts among residents are insignificant, particularly compared to Yorokaen ... because many Kusunokien patients are so severely demented or disabled that they were not communicative'.[238] To satisfy residents' preferences, some Western-style bedrooms were turned into traditional *tatami* (straw-matted) rooms with futons. This was much appreciated by less frail residents, although it was unsuitable for the bedridden, who required intensive nursing or tube-feeding.[239]

Finally, changing staff attitudes to residential care provision reflect the transition from a government-assigned 'assessed institution' under public assistance measures to a 'commodity' under LTCI. Ironically, current deficiencies and limitations in the 'basic' Kusunokien – the city's oldest and only city-funded nursing home – might now be justified when based on the concept of a 'contract' between an older client and the Home. As attendant Mr L. stated, 'Once residents decide to enter Kusunokien voluntarily, they have to accept a certain loss of privacy and freedom and abide by its rules and communal lifestyle. Otherwise, they shouldn't have come here ... they should go to another nursing home and pay extra'.[240] Another attendant put it bluntly: 'Residents are here because they cannot afford other luxurious nursing homes. So it cannot be helped, they have to put up with what currently happens here'.[241] Attendant Ms P. arranged for her mother-in-law to enter Kusunokien in 2004:

> because it was the cheapest and the only home we could afford. For worse-off families like us, single rooms, nice food, high care standards, a welcoming atmosphere or convenient location didn't matter at all, but only *money* mattered. I myself loathed multi-bedded rooms with little privacy and space, but if you didn't have money, that was it [my emphasis].[242]

This suggests a tiered market of residential care under LTCI: an upper end offering exclusive care with extra 'hotel costs' for the well-off, and a minimal lower end for those with limited personal means, a feature seen also in England. With little further government intervention and exemption from the official uprated guidelines, the 'basic' early built nursing homes have lapsed into public assistance minimum levels. Indeed, these correspond to the stigmatized Yorokaen old people's home for the minority on public assistance, even though these 'basic' nursing homes were integrated into LTCI. Significantly, staff members working at Yorokaen and Kusunokien could barely see a difference between the two in terms of the care, provisions and amenities, regarding both as 'second class' and expressing a strong determination 'to avoid entering either of these at all costs'.[243]

CONCLUSION

By presenting national, regional and local institutional perspectives and using a variety of sources, this study has revealed the diversity and complexity of the way residential care for older people in England and Japan has evolved. It has identified that the root of the problem of residential care in both countries is their Poor Law legacy and cultural norms, specifically the stigma associated with the English workhouse and *obasuteyama* in Japan. This final chapter reviews the findings for each country in a cross-national and comparative context at the national, regional and grassroots institution levels. The analysis highlights commonalities and differences, continuities and change, and achievements and failings, while acknowledging the different national contexts. These are also considered in relation to current policy trends and debates, along with the implications for professionals and for further research.

National Contexts

Chapters 1 and 2 contrasted elderly care provision in England and Japan in the early twentieth century. While some needy older people in England received outdoor relief after the New Poor Law came into force in 1834, many were accommodated in mixed workhouses or special facilities; there was also a little charitable provision. Comparable state involvement in Japan began almost a century later with the implementation of the 1929 Poor Law, under which a tiny minority of the destitute, frail elderly without any family support were assisted, often in publicly sanctioned charitable old people's almshouses. Although very different in scale and history, England and Japan shared deterrent features in their respective Poor Laws, their stigmatized workhouses/almshouses often invoking fear, loathing and shame in response to degrading levels of care.

Welfare in post-war Japan was still profoundly rooted in historical and cultural norms and traditions and continued to be seen as a family responsibility; as a result there was only restrictive and supplementary state involvement. Thus the 1950 National Assistance Act and, to a lesser extent, the 1963 Elderly Welfare Act both incorporated restrictionist and supplementary measures, with entitlement to the old people's institution/home limited to the neediest without financial means or family support. In contrast, England's 1948 National Assistance Act was distinguished by state commitment and universality, with entitlement to a residential home or Part III accommodation based on need, regardless of income or family support. In short, entitlement to post-war statutory residential home provision for older people under each country's respective Acts was different, although Japan moved somewhat closer towards England's provision after the 1963 Act came into force. Nonetheless, admission to mainstream provision in both countries involved means-testing. This focused on applicants' financial status and suggested the tenacity of restrictive and degrading treatment, even as needs assessments were increasingly emphasized. Again, significant differences were found between the two countries, since Japan's admission procedure also involved assessment of the applicants' families, which underlined the supplementary nature of state aid in that country.

Post-war government policy objectives also differed, approximating to the legislation and its underlying ideology, though attempts to improve residential provision were seen in both countries. In order to bring an end to Poor Law and workhouse associations, the 1945–51 UK Labour government proposed the construction of homes accommodating 20–30 persons. These would be analogous to private hotels for those 'in need of care and attention which is otherwise not available to them'.[1] In the same period, and within Japan's 1950 Act's limited commitments, old people's institutions with 30–200 places were provided under minimum public assistance measures for the neediest clientele. Overall, policy objectives were closely linked to the respective legislation and its underlying ethos, so that these were also imbued with the Poor Law legacy and cultural norms and traditions. While England's aspirational targets derived partly from political and popular hostility to the Poor Law and workhouse, Japan's disappointingly low goals were attributable to strong family obligations and the corresponding stigma associated with the institutionalization of older people.

The same was true of outcomes, which were limited by economic restrictions. This was particularly the case in England where policy goals were very ambitious, but post-war austerity dictated that many former workhouses were designated as Part III residential homes and stayed in use for much longer than planned, while the number of 'small' homes proposed under the 1948 Act was strictly rationed. This two-tier approach partly echoed Japan's restrictionist approach, although it did not openly entail financial or family ineligibility. It also anticipated the current tiered market of residential care within a mixed economy. In contrast, Japan's modest targets were less affected by post-war austerity, and its minimum-level old people's institutions under the 1950 Act were at least guaranteed for their highly limited clientele. For these reasons the old people's institutions were relatively small, almost two-thirds of them with fifty or fewer beds, and suggested a domestic setting. Once again, stigmatized public (local authority) residential home provision in each country deterred potential applicants and embarrassed residents. This was especially significant in England because so many older people in large (former workhouse) Part III residential homes experienced directly the physical and symbolic association with the Poor Law. More than half the Part III residents in 1960 were housed in these facilities, and even in the late 1970s there were still 7,000 people living in a former workhouse.

Cross-national comparisons of residential care present problems. When Japan's legislation, policy goals and outcomes are measured against the English equivalents, its residential home provision was clearly lagging. Yet in its national and cultural context, Japan's provision was arguably closer to its policy goals. Older people cared for in this way fared relatively well compared with many needy older people living alone or receiving very limited support from their families, who were also suffering the dire poverty and upheaval of post-war Japan. In fact, the state of elderly people dependent on minimal family care suggested that *obasuteyama* was now emerging in domestic settings. Local authority and local authority-funded residential home provision in England and Wales greatly exceeded that in Japan, both in absolute numbers and proportionate to their respective over-65s populations, although the 'genuine' small home provision (some 49.8 per cent of the total places) was not very different from Japan's total statutory residential home provision in proportion to the older population by 1960.

However, England by then provided considerably more places in smaller voluntary and private homes, mainly for the better-off, than did Japan. This growing diversification of residential care beyond mainstream local authority residential home provision can be traced to the mid-1970s in both countries, although elements of the mixed economy of residential care were always present. It was a response to the problem of growing numbers of frail or disabled older people requiring constant or intensive nursing who were initially excluded from mainstream provision under each country's National Assistance Act. Both governments sought to include this clientele, in England by extending the definition of 'in need of care and attention', and in Japan under the 1963 Act by opening nursing homes for frail or bedridden older people with or without family support. Yet neither measure was wholly successful due to the persistent stigma attached to public (local authority) residential provision and squeezed local authority budgets, while free, 24-hour care alternatives, such as long-stay hospital beds and family care, continued to decline.

Later, insufficient local authority measures were partly compensated by alternatives, notably central government-funded subsidies to private sector homes in England and to hospitals in Japan. Since each could bypass local authority assessment procedures, they grew significantly, with such 'unplanned' extension of entitlement to statutory residential care provision resulting in soaring public expenditure. Both governments therefore revised their systems, restricting entitlement and public subsidies and simultaneously emphasizing care *by* the community, including informal (family) help. This seemingly confirmed that policy aspirations to greater entitlement and expanded services did not override economic factors and highlighted the question 'Who is entitled to what?' when it came to the care of older people, as the state rolled back its responsibilities to the family and to older people themselves – an issue all too familiar today.

Another theme that emerges from the national survey chapters is that any understanding of the diversity and complexity of residential care needs to extend beyond statutory provision, to encompass long-term arrangements involving the health and social care sectors, alongside supplementary institutions such as 'housing with care' or sheltered housing in England, and Japan's equivalent, the 'care house'. The latter may be further extended to include some reliance on family care. This is of particular importance in Japan where it is seen as the best and preferred option, associated as it is with commitment and compassion, nationally endorsed and seen internationally as a commendable practice. Yet the sources examined here reveal neglect and abuse of older persons by their family, which seems to have been getting worse in recent years. Similar abuse and mistreatment of older residents by care staff were also found in some 1980s English private homes, though little is known about these or voluntary homes before that date, even though they played a relatively important role. Consideration of residential care for older people also highlighted the gaps in the statistics, particularly concerning Japanese data, in which narrow definitions of residential care facilities have led to an underestimation of the size of the institutionalized older populations. This is compounded by the lack of national data, for example, on 'socially hospitalized' older patients, who are effectively resident in hospitals. The implication from other information and estimates is that Japan's overall ratio of institutionalized older people was not significantly less than in some Western European countries or the United States by 1990, while older patients had the longest hospital stays in the world. The inference is that Japan's tradition of a strong family orientation in the care of older people, and assumptions about low numbers of institutionalized older people there, are doubtful. Conversely, in England, poor quality evidence of family care and assumptions about the breakdown of the nuclear family may have led to an underestimation of how much the family actually contributes to caring for older people.

Regional Contexts

Chapters 3 and 4 focused on regional perspectives, examining Norfolk and Gifu Prefecture to illustrate how respective national legislation and policy objectives were assimilated by local authorities, the bodies responsible for their implementation, since the 1920s. These case studies mirrored national trends and highlighted the complex process of implementation. Regional interpretations, based on existing facilities and perceived needs, and shaped partly by local traditions as well as by the local economic and political climate and socio-demographic trends, determined outcomes. The studies suggest that regional variations were also, in part, attributable to poorly specified central government initiatives or guidelines.

Following the 1948 Act, Norfolk's county (Norfolk) and county borough (Norwich) councils initially developed their relevant flagship Part III residential home provision proportionate to national levels. However, the two councils experienced contrasting transitions from workhouse to 'small' homes, reflecting their different post-war starting points and corresponding local interpretation of their obligations. Norfolk clearly had a major task, given its inheritance of large, obsolete former workhouses, the county's size, and a widely dispersed and growing older population. Its initial two-tier residential care policy necessitated the continued use of former workhouses for frail or disabled older people and some so-called 'nuisance' cases, along with the strict rationing of 'small' home places to a minority of the more active and 'well-behaved' elderly. This approach was thought to be necessary to secure adequate residential care places, especially given the lack of 24-hour care alternatives. In contrast, Norwich's only workhouse was severely bomb damaged in 1942 and wholly appropriated as a NHS hospital in 1948, forcing the county borough council to seek alternative accommodation by acquiring and converting older, modest but relatively small premises, a process completed by 1954.

Post-war Gifu Prefecture also initially developed its old people's institutions in line with Japanese national averages, but these achieved low occupancy rates. As with Norfolk, this partly reflected the uneven distribution of the institutions, the sheer size of the area and the sparse population. Yet local traditions and culture were also clearly important, specifically the family orientation of care for older people and persistent stigma surrounding institutional forms of public welfare. Local people avoided local authority old people's institutions at all costs, while prefecture officials regarded family care as a primary and cost-free asset, and restricted public welfare provision to a tiny minority totally lacking financial means and family support.

By 1963 local authority residential home provisions in Norfolk, Norwich and Gifu were consistent with the respective national averages in proportion to their over-65 populations, although Norfolk and Norwich had contrasting stocks of residential facilities. However, national-level assessments did not necessarily match local need: Norfolk's former workhouse accommodation had few vacancies but its waiting list was short, and Norwich's small homes were full and had long waiting lists, whereas Gifu's institutions were underused. Continuing use of former workhouses in Norfolk and stigmatized institutions in Gifu seemingly deterred potential applicants, yet the small home arrangements in Norwich clearly appealed to new applicants. Local information on bed occupancy rates and waiting lists highlighted demand and perceptions of local authority residential provision, which were not always clear from central statistics, usually based on total bed numbers. Yet few local records deal with actual assessment procedures to determine the eligibility of applicants. Nor is there any information on potential demand, which would indicate those in need of residential care but reluctant to ask for it because of the stigma attached. Political features, such as the preponderance of Conservative voters and local councillors in Norfolk and Gifu and of Labour counterparts in Norwich, may also have been influential, but this cannot be confirmed due to the absence of evidence. Such problems cloud any speculation on the extent to which local authority residential provision matched actual demand.

By the mid-1970s residential home provision in Norfolk, Norwich and Gifu did not proportionately exceed that of other local authorities. Early efforts in Norfolk and Norwich were effectively penalized by government policy during the 1960s and early 1970s. A focus on loans for capital projects to local authorities with too few residential places disadvantaged local authorities which had plenty of places in former workhouses (as in Norfolk) or had actively opted for older, converted 'small' homes (as in Norwich). Without ministerial prioritization, and given central government financial restrictions, Norfolk's ex-workhouse closure programme and Norwich's modernization project might have been completed well before the mid-1970s and both authorities might have provided more places to meet local need. In these cases central control and funding priorities impinged on local initiatives and developments. This may have suited local political inclinations, but Norfolk had little alternative but to use local revenues to fund a few smaller residential homes and sheltered housing accommodation, supported by local housing associations. Worse still, Norwich lacked any local funding and so opened just one new home, using central subsidies, during the decade after 1963.

Acknowledging the needs of a growing frail or bedridden older population typically wholly looked after by family carers, Japan's 1963 Act introduced nursing homes for this clientele regardless of their income or family support, though applicants *and* their families continued to be means-tested and needs-assessed. Subsequently there was a steady national expansion, particularly from the 1970s, although Gifu Prefecture lagged behind the rest of the country for four decades after 1963. Yet this situation did not reflect central legislation, government policy controls or financial restraints. As with the earlier old people's homes, the demand for nursing homes was low in rural, traditionalist Gifu, where the customary family orientation in the care of older relatives remained strong. Indeed, it was reported that many families genuinely preferred family care, although considerable social pressure was exerted on families. Above all, the prefecture's own restrictionist policy limited nursing home provision to the frailest elderly lacking any family support, simultaneously encouraging or even manipulating the family care ethos concerning the others by emphasizing the prefecture's preferences. This local policy position seemingly contradicted central directives and the principles of the 1963 Act.

From the mid-1970s the enlarged unitary Norfolk council (now incorporating Norwich) saw considerable growth in private sector residential places, which doubled to almost 1,000 by 1979 to represent over a third of those available. This mixed economy of residential provision in Norfolk began under a Labour government, fully five years ahead of the Thatcher era. Similarly, Gifu's catching-up process in nursing home provision from the late 1970s was largely attributable to non-profit (social welfare corporation) initiatives with the help of central government subsidies, although the process was slower, the period extending into the 1990s. In short, although local authority provision in all three areas declined after 1963 and was limited by the mid-1970s, the causes differed: delays in Norfolk and Norwich reflected the impact of central controls and funding targets, but Gifu's stagnation was due to its own policies and objectives, along with a rural, traditionalist outlook. Subsequent shortages of local authority provision in the enlarged Norfolk and Gifu were offset by the private or non-profit sector helped by central government subsidies, indicating limited local authority spending and the stigma still attached to public (local authority) provision, and furnishing local examples of outcomes subjected to economic factors and stigma.

Region-wide variations in the environments, standards and locations of post-war local authority residential homes reflected unclear, and sometimes lack of, central directives, regulations and guidelines. Thus, without specifications regarding the location of old people's institutions, Gifu's early establishments were built in or near a temple or shrine, reflecting the prefecture's continuing association of public welfare provision with charity, based on religion (Buddhism) or the emperor (Shinto). They typically invoked the Confucian association with a 'paradise for the unfortunate elderly', this frequently used expression echoing the pre-war ethos and mentalities, while paradoxically something resembling the counter-Confucian *obasuteyama* legend emerged. Nonetheless, barring a few urban institutions, these typically modest wooden buildings for 30–50 people offered a fairly domestic environment. In contrast, the larger replacements were less homely and were located in spacious out-of-town locations. They echoed economies of scale rather than least cost.

Similarly, the lack of detailed central guidance was one reason why Norfolk's (former workhouse) Part III homes remained essentially unchanged until they were closed in the 1960s and 1970s. Converted small homes generally had higher standards, with smaller bedrooms and a homely atmosphere, but these varied considerably within and between Norfolk and Norwich. Whereas Norfolk adopted a mixed-sex policy at the outset, the early Norwich homes were all single-sex, echoing the sexual segregation of the workhouse, which continued in Norfolk's former workhouse accommodation too. However, new and replacement homes were purpose-built, providing small living units, with many single or double bedrooms, although again these varied in size and style. Norfolk built several complexes, consisting of a Part III residential home with twenty or so places and adjoining flats or bungalows for independent older people from the late 1960s, while Norwich switched to larger and separate forty-eight-place replacement homes in the early 1970s.

Given such local variations, it is difficult to make cross-national comparisons. Seemingly until the mid-1960s Norfolk's residential home provision was more diverse than the standardized Gifu institutions, with the Norwich accommodation somewhere between the two. In 1960 living arrangements in Gifu's institutions were within the official minimum 'four people per room' standard, but many Norfolk ex-workhouse residents shared bedrooms with ten or more, although some Norfolk and Norwich residents in small homes already had single en-suite rooms. The post-1960 new or replacement homes in Norfolk and Norwich addressed the residents' needs for privacy and personal space more effectively than did Gifu's equivalents. Yet it is debatable whether Gifu's residents actually fared worse than those in Norfolk given their preference for communal living. Ironically, as official minimum standards were revised upwards in both countries, variations in the physical environments and standards actually increased, since new or replacement homes followed most recent guidelines, whereas existing ones were left unchanged. The historical regional surveys thus confirm great diversity in residential care provision with certain continuities in 'bottom-end' homes, which were not necessarily apparent from any overarching narrative based on policy guidelines or ideological frameworks.

The ambiguities in central policy directives concerning residential provision for growing numbers of dementia sufferers also led to different regional policies. Again, Norfolk and Norwich had contrasting approaches: Norwich adopted a policy of integration of the confused with other residents, whereas Norfolk provided a specialized home designated for dementia cases. In a further contrast, the shortages of nursing homes in Gifu left dementia sufferers with other residents in ordinary old people's homes until 1984, when local funds were allocated to provide special accommodation for them. In effect, Gifu experienced a transition from Norwich- to Norfolk-style practice.

In summary, the regional case studies show the value of analysing the development of local authority residential provision in some depth, acknowledging their particular contexts rather than fitting them within broad or assumed national trends. In this way, they reveal region-wide variations and specific features, but it would be interesting to explore whether apparently distinctive interpretations and practices in Norfolk and Gifu were mirrored in or contradicted by other local authorities in England and Japan. For example, Norfolk's retention of former workhouses was not unusual – it occurred in Cambridgeshire, Lancashire and Essex too.[2] In contrast, Japan's national surveys revealed that other sparsely populated and larger rural prefectures, similar to Gifu, had achieved national-level nursing home provision by 1990.[3]

Institutional Studies

Chapters 5 and 6 looked at the experiences of the residents and grassroots practices at a number of long-term care facilities within each region. Each chapter offered a history of two mainstream local authority residential homes, Norfolk's Eastgate House and Gifu's Yorokaen (1947/8–63), and their replacement facilities (1963–73). Both institutional histories suggest the continuity of Poor Law measures and mentalities, despite the official emphasis on a transition to 'welfare state' arrangements. Eastgate House's earlier complement of casuals, the homeless, evicted families and a few 'nuisances', as well as frail older people, contrasted with Yorokaen's tiny minority of the neediest poor and solitary elderly. Each reflected corresponding national Poor Law characteristics, retained under the respective local authorities' own policy position: the mixed workhouse with its confined 'residuum' and the old people's almshouse (used as a publicly sanctioned Poor Law institution) for the neediest elderly destitute. In both examples, resident populations became predominantly increasingly aged and frail females, largely without financial means and family support. But potential applicants and their relatives felt the continuing stigma of the workhouse or almshouse and viewed residential homes as a last resort. This limited applicants, despite growing eligible older populations in both localities.

Creating a 'homely' atmosphere was a shared policy goal, but Eastgate House fell short even of official minimum standards and received inadequate public investment pending its closure. Consequently, its residents experienced the direct physical association with the workhouse as well as overcrowding and deteriorating conditions. Yorokaen was a temporary rebuild in 1947, but did meet (admittedly minimal) official guidelines. Their respective replacements, both coincidentally opening in 1963, offered better physical environments, but with few major improvements in amenities, provisions and services, both also bore the hallmarks of an institutional regime. Any improvement in residential life largely reflected unofficial or informal and often overlooked efforts, including work by the residents themselves, voluntary resources in kind and cash, and the homes' own initiatives, ranging from religious services and rituals to fundraising events and the accruing of residents' funds to provide 'extras'.

In principle, residential life in Eastgate House was more 'advanced' than in Yorokaen in that it operated under a modern welfare ethos, acknowledging basic rights and equity. Under Yorokaen's familistic nationalism, welfare was seen as a favour or mercy bestowed on unfortunate older people by the state or emperor, exemplified by 'comfort visits' and 'comfort allowances', the emperor's 'blessing money', and birthday testimonials. Yorokaen residents did not necessarily fare worse than their Eastgate House counterparts, however, although the absence of staff and resident narratives during the whole period reviewed (1947/8–73) precludes any definite conclusion.

The second sections of Chapters 5 and 6 provide a more dynamic and complex institutional history, illustrated by interview materials from the post-1970 era, which shows the greater diversity in residential care in both countries. Resident-centred provision and services sensitive to privacy, choice and even dignity began to replace communal and institutional arrangements. Yet changes and improvements were slow to take effect in some of the larger, obsolete psychiatric and psycho-geriatric hospitals in Norfolk and the earlier local authority basic homes in Gifu. Once again, such provision was not always perceived as undesirable or outmoded: multi-bedded rooms and communal, near-obligatory 'voluntary' work were appreciated by some Gifu residents, who preferred shared living arrangements, as they provided a feeling of belonging and, indeed, a degree of independence and sense of purpose. Similarly, the sustained institutional regime and environment were key factors providing continuity, security and stability for many older long-stay Norfolk hospital patients.

Contrasting perceptions were also identified regarding apparently improved residential life and services for less frail residents. Japanese policymakers and professionals interpreted a good residential life as 'fulfilling' rather than unrestricted or relaxed, and so imposed a timetable packed with 'meaningful' programmes, activities and rehabilitation, which were usually included in the standard fees. Yet the residential staff questioned whether a healthy but strictly regimented residential life was superior to an irregular but homely one, and suggested that instead the home life of each resident should be replicated. English homes notionally endorsed freedom and choice by emphasizing individuality and person-centred care, but offered fewer programmes and activities (other than in luxury private homes), and these were usually charged for. Some of the interviewees characterized such measures as 'cost-conscious' or even 'abuse in the form of neglect', leaving some residents 'warehoused' or 'suffering tedium and apathy'.[4]

Policy directions concerning 'model' residential life and services for severely frail or ill residents were similar, focusing on longevity rather than preference or choice, and were perceived critically in Norfolk and Gifu alike. Some interviewees thought that tube-fed or bedridden residents were experiencing 'a living hell' and stressed that they should have the choice to die.[5] Others wanted to be in control of their lives, by which they meant not having to 'linger on' and expressing a wish to 'end it all' if they became gravely ill.[6] Recently, the 'right to die' has been attracting greater public and political attention around the world. This opens up very different perspectives on long-term care, posing the question of whether choice for terminally ill patients should include the option not to receive long-term care but to end life peacefully by 'assisted suicide'. In the UK, Dignity in Dying campaigners emphasize greater personal control over the process of dying, whereas opponents, such as Care Not Killing, warn that any legislative change to allow 'assisted suicide' would bring pressure to bear on many of the vulnerable elderly. Some allege that in societies where 'assisted suicide' has been legalized, the culture and value of the lives of the disabled are diminished.[7] Yet since 2002, 160 British citizens have opted to travel to the Swiss Dignitas centre to end their lives.[8] In Japan 11,700 of the 30,700 people who committed suicide in 2009 were aged 60 or over, in a country with one of the highest suicide rates in the world.[9] A key motive is age-related illness, suggesting that vulnerable older persons in the UK and Japan are already – illegally – achieving the 'right to die'.

Broadly, the interviews reveal some positive aspects to residents' lives in the outmoded or 'bottom-end' basic homes, but also expose negative features within improved or officially promoted 'model' conditions. In other words, oral testimony has demonstrated distinctive and complex categorizations concerning *undesirable* and *ideal* residential care models between policymakers and grassroots service providers or older recipients, as well as between the two countries. The interviews also confirm the importance of personal experiences and perceptions, and background social and cultural factors, as critical in devising appropriate forms of care from the residents' perspectives. This poses questions concerning current policy direction and goals as perceived by policymakers and professionals who, in popular discourses, are often detached from practice.

Current Debates and Prospects

The provision of socially equitable and financially viable long-term care for frail older people ranks among the most urgent of the political issues facing Britain and Japan today. At the time of writing, the governments of both countries are reviewing their long-term care arrangements in the light of a fast-growing ageing population and economic uncertainties. This last section considers what the experiences of both countries suggest for current debates and future policy planning. One trend in both countries is a mixed economy approach, featuring expansion in services and providers, particularly involving the private and non-profit sectors. Japan's Long-Term Care Insurance (LTCI) scheme, introduced in 2000, has combined commercialization and wider socialization of care to replace reliance on the family. Yet as this study demonstrates, aspirations to expand statutory care provision for a wider older population in need have hardly overridden economic factors, while notions of rights or choice have been increasingly undermined by rationing and charges, a feature also seen in England's means-testing and targeting social care system, which is always constrained by spending caps. Such approaches have created a tiered market of residential care in both countries, polarized around private (or in Japan, non-profit social welfare corporation) homes for the well-off part- or full self-funded and basic local authority and private homes for those reliant on public assistance or with limited financial means. This leaves many, mainly female, poor and vulnerable older people to experience remnants of the Poor Law legacy and its associated stigma in each country. Significantly, even in 2006, 88 per cent of all residents' bedrooms in Japan's three pillar LTCI residential facilities were shared, mainly four-bedded, rooms.

Worse still, tens of thousands of poorer older people requiring long-term support receive no form of residential care whatsoever, but struggle unassisted in their own homes. They are the unwitting victims of the tension between ideology and resource allocation. Both governments have promoted de-institutionalization and have limited the number of residential places, but without establishing matching capacity within the community. Similarly, both governments have emphasized the benefits of community-based care at the expense of residential care, without making available the funding necessary to support it. Thus in England the number of older people receiving local authority-funded care fell by 11 per cent between 2010 and 2012.[10] Consequently, nearly 800,000 older people with care needs (40 per cent of all those elderly requiring care) receive no support whatsoever from public or private sector agencies and struggle on alone or with limited family support, while large numbers of older long-stay patients have been discharged from hospitals without an adequate alternative, the most severe cases being 'moved around between hospital assessment wards and [private] nursing homes'.[11] Locally, at least three Norfolk and Norwich council-run day centres face closure following the withdrawal of local funding, which will adversely affect most vulnerable elderly people in the community. Among these were an 89-year-old female and 94-year-old male who bluntly expressed their anxiety: 'It would be the end of the world if it closed'; 'I live on my own. I depend on this place'.[12] In Japan in 2009, 420,000 people were on nursing home waiting lists, the figure matching the total nursing home places then available.[13] One Gifu nursing home alone had 800 applicants on its waiting list.[14]

Meanwhile both governments have manipulated the concept of community care to emphasize care *by* the community, thereby stressing the family's role. In 2009 there were six million unpaid carers (one in six adults) in the UK, with 1.25 million providing care for more than 50 hours a week.[15] A quarter of these were themselves aged 65 or over, while half of the cared-for were aged 75 or over.[16] Many of the carers themselves were not in good health as a result.[17] In

Japan the consensus was, until recently, that families had an obligation to provide care for older relatives. Yet with changing demographic and residence patterns, gender roles and employment practices, the role and function of family care have also evolved, with a shrinking pool of carers and heavier burdens placed on them, producing the social phenomenon of the so-called *kaigo-jigoku* (care-giving hell).[18] In extreme cases, family care culminates in the murder of the whole family, with no fewer than 200 incidents reported during 1998–2003 and in excess of fifty cases a year since then.[19] Thus family care is not a feasible or desirable alternative to relatively expensive statutory community-based provision, particularly for severe cases.

Nonetheless, statutory community-based care packages do not appear to be a panacea, especially in the current financial climate, and institutional care remains the only feasible and realistic option for many of those most in need. Some suggest that residential homes will always have an institutional ambience and are therefore not ideal; others acknowledge that under-resourced community-based alternatives cannot address needs which only institutional provision can meet. There are parallels here with Scull's Dilemma, and finding solutions to the complexities of long-term care is likely to exercise researchers and policymakers for the foreseeable future.[20] In light of these problems, both governments have recognized the attraction of voluntary initiatives in the care of older people, seen in the UK government's 'Big Society' concept and the Japanese government's equivalent, *Atarashii-Kokyo* ('New Public Commons'). These call for a radical shift in relations between citizens and the state, and promote popular participation, not least by older people, a theme explored by the author in recent and current research.[21]

Increasingly, the problem of the care of frail older people is gender-related – 'a problem of women' – since 72 per cent of those in need in Japan were women and two-thirds of informal (family) carers in Britain looked after a female sick or disabled person.[22] As this study shows, institutionalized older people have been predominantly women, many of whom are vulnerable financially and physically. They are consequently placed in the 'bottom-end' homes. Institutional care is also largely dependent on low-paid female workers, who will most likely experience poverty in their own old age, while domiciliary care adds to the burden of largely female low-paid or unpaid (family) carers. In Japan in 2009 over 92 per cent of domiciliary care workers under LTCI were female, and 80 per cent of these workers had non-regular (part-time or on-call) work contracts.[23] In recent years small but increasing numbers of men have become involved in caring for older people.[24] Optimists view this as a harbinger of changes in attitudes and gender roles which are likely to produce a new social contract, ensuring that mainly older females do not suffer disproportionately.[25] However, broader trends suggest otherwise. Japan's Democratic Party proposed a 40,000 yen monthly pay rise to encourage residential care staff in its 2009 manifesto, but only a 14,000 yen monthly pay rise was finally sanctioned.[26] In Britain both the former Labour and current Coalition governments have recognized the contribution of unpaid (family) carers, embodied in the National Carers Strategy of 2008 and 2010, but it is doubtful whether planned additional funding for projects supporting carers will keep pace with the demand for informal care, expected to increase by around 45 per cent from 2003 to 2026.[27] Nevertheless, it is imperative that observers in Britain pay close attention to the Japanese experience when evaluating Japan as a model.

In conclusion, given the entrenched economic downturn, public expenditure constraints, population ageing and social and cultural transformations, the prospects for long-term care for growing frail older populations are both challenging and unpredictable. This does not invalidate attempts at planning, but suggests that they need to be based on the evidence of real experience rather than on guesswork driven by moral panic, popular discourse or assumptions set by policymakers or professionals remote from grassroots provision of older residents. Feasible solutions are not likely for problems whose origins are not fully understood. This study of historical perspectives has confirmed that certain policy issues, dilemmas and problems facing the care systems in both countries partly reflect the cumulative impact of former decisions and commitments and are profoundly rooted in the Poor Law legacy and influenced by cultural norms and the stigma attached to institutionalization. The multilayered approach adopted here, which has revealed the great diversity and complexity of provision and need, confirms the value of a holistic approach, encompassing health, social and housing provision in all sectors. Longer-term national surveys of past achievements and failures may hold lessons for policymakers today, just as close scrutiny of regional studies highlights the importance of the role played by local authorities in implementing national goals, while the life experiences of residents and grassroots practices shed light on current public discourses. Finally, cross-national coverage can address distinctive as well as common experiences, obstacles and achievements, helping to expand perspectives to deal with problems and pressures which clearly transcend national boundaries.

If this study interests not only social and welfare historians but also a broader audience concerned with long-term care for older people in Britain, Japan or elsewhere, its research findings are gladly offered to address gaps in the existing literature and for wider evaluation or reinterpretation towards more practical ends.

NOTES

Introduction

1. B. R. Mitchell, *International Historical Statistics, Europe 1750–2005*, 6th edn (Basingstoke: Palgrave Macmillan, 2007), pp. 41–3; B. R. Mitchell, *International Historical Statistics, Africa, Asia and Oceania 1750–2005*, 5th edn (Basingstoke: Palgrave Macmillan, 2007), p. 25; United Nations, *World Population Prospects: The 2010 Revision Population Database*, at http://esa.un.org/wpp/unpp/panel_indicators.htm [accessed 10 August 2012].

2. United Nations, *World Population Prospects: The 2010 Revision Population Database*.

3. Cabinet Office, *White Paper on the Ageing Society 2012/13*, p. 2, at http://www8.cao. go.jp/kourei/whitepaper/w-2012/zenbun/24pdf_index.html [accessed 10 August 2012].

4. E. Charles, *The Twilight of Parenthood: A Biological Study of the Decline of Population Growth* (London: Watts & Co., 1934), pp. 75–6; E. M. Hubback, *The Population of Britain* (London: Penguin Books, 1947), p. 99. For a discussion, see P. Thane, 'The Debate on the Declining Birth-Rate in Britain: The "Menace" of an Ageing Population, 1920s–1950s', *Continuity and Change*, 5:2 (1990), pp. 283–305, on pp. 283–99.

5. Cabinet Office, *White Paper on the Ageing Society 2012/13*, p. 6; M. Dickie, 'A Fiscal Frailty', *Financial Times*, 4 August 2009, p. 7.

6. Commission on Funding of Care and Support (Dilnot Commission), *Fairer Care Funding: The Report of the Commission on Funding of Care and Support* (July 2011), p. 5, at https://www.wp.dh.gov.uk/carecommission/files/2011/07/Fairer-Care-Funding-Report.pdf [accessed 10 August 2012].

7. HM Government, *White Paper: Caring for Our Future: Reforming Care and Support*, Cm 8378 (Norwich: Stationery Office, 2012).

8. N. Tamiya et al., 'Population Ageing and Wellbeing: Lessons from Japan's Long-Term Care Insurance Policy', *Lancet*, 378:9797 (24 September 2011), pp. 1183–92, on pp. 1184–5.

9. M. Hayashi, 'Testing the Limits of Care for Older People', *Society Guardian*, 29 September 2010, p. 3, also available at http://www.guardian.co.uk/society/2010/sep/28/japan-elderly-care-mutual-support [accessed 10 August 2012].

10. Figures from Laing & Buisson, *Care of Elderly People: UK Market Survey 2008* (London: Laing & Buisson, 2008) (hereafter *Laing Survey 2008*), pp. 16, 23.

11. Figures from Ministry of Health, Labour and Welfare (hereafter MoHLW), *Summary of the Year 2010/11 Long-Term Care Insurance Expenditure Survey* (Tokyo: MoHLW, 23 August 2011), at http://www.mhlw.go.jp/toukei/saikin/hw/kaigo/kyufu/10/ [accessed 10 August 2012]; MoHLW, *Summary of the Year 2010 Social Welfare Facili-*

ties Survey (Tokyo: MoHLW, 30 November 2011), at http://www.mhlw.go.jp/toukei/saikin/hw/fukushi/10/index.html [accessed 10 August 2012].

12. Tamiya et al., 'Population Ageing and Wellbeing', p. 1184.

13. S. Fukazawa, *Ballad of Oak Mountain* (Tokyo: Shincho-sha, 1964), pp. 33–94.

14. This perspective is developed e.g. by P. Thane, *Old Age in English History: Past Experiences, Present Issues* (Oxford and New York: Oxford University Press, 2000), *passim*.

15. M. Hayashi, 'The Care of Older People in Japan: Myths and Realities of Family "Care"', *History and Policy* (July 2011), at http://www.historyandpolicy.org/papers/policy-paper-121.html [accessed 10 August 2012].

16. S. Macintyre, 'Old Age as a Social Problem', in R. Dingwall, C. Heath, M. Reid and M. Stacey (eds), *Health Care and Health Knowledge* (Beckenham: Croom Helm, 1977), pp. 39–63; A. Walker and C. Phillipson, 'Introduction', in C. Phillipson and A. Walker (eds), *Ageing and Social Policy: A Critical Assessment* (Aldershot: Gower, c. 1986), pp. 1–12, on p. 2; P. Thane, 'Gender, Welfare and Old Age in Britain 1870s–1940s', in A. Digby and J. Stewart (eds), *Gender, Health and Welfare* (London: Routledge, 1996), pp. 189–207, on p. 194. See also C. R. Victor, *Old Age in Modern Society: A Textbook of Social Gerontology*, 2nd edn (London: Chapman & Hall, 1994), pp. 9–11; and C. R. Victor, *The Social Context of Ageing* (London: Routledge, 2005), pp. 11–17.

17. Exceptions include N. Johnson, *Voluntary Social Services* (Oxford: Basil Blackwell, 1981), Japanese translation available; H. Qureshi and A. Walker, *The Caring Relationship: Elderly People and their Families* (Basingstoke: Macmillan Education, 1989).

18. An exception is I. J. Norman and S. J. Redfern (eds), *Mental Health Care for Elderly People* (New York and Edinburgh: Churchill Livingstone, 1996).

19. R. Jack (ed.), *Residential versus Community Care: The Role of Institutions in Welfare Provision* (Basingstoke: Macmillan, 1998), Japanese translation available.

20. Y. Wu, *The Care of the Elderly in Japan* (London: RoutledgeCurzon, 2004), p. 11; K. Jones, 'The Development of Institutional Care', in E. Butterworth and R. Holman (eds), *Social Welfare in Modern Britain* (London: Fontana, 1975), pp. 286–98, on p. 290.

21. E. Goffman, *Asylums: Essays on the Social Situation of Mental Patients and Other Inmates* (New York: Doubleday, 1961). Japanese translation available; see below, p. 194 n. 24.

22. R. Barton, *Institutional Neurosis* (Bristol: John Wright & Sons, 1959).

23. B. Robb, *Sans Everything: A Case to Answer* (London: Nelson, 1967); M. Meacher, *Taken for a Ride: Special Residential Homes for Confused Old People – A Study of Separatism in Social Policy* (London: Longman, 1972).

24. D. G. Cooper, *Psychiatry and Anti-Psychiatry* (London: Tavistock, 1967); R. D. Laing and A. Esterson, *Sanity, Madness and the Family* (London: Tavistock, 1964); M. Foucault, *Madness and Civilization: A History of Insanity in the Age of Reason*, trans. R. Howard, abridged edn (London: Tavistock Publications, 1967).

25. P. Townsend, *The Last Refuge: A Survey of Residential Institutions and Homes for the Aged in England and Wales*, abridged edn (London: Routledge & Kegan Paul, 1964), p. 190; P. Willmott and M. Young, *Family and Kinship in East London*, 2nd impression (1957; London: Routledge & Kegan Paul, 1960), pp. 155–66; P. Willmott and M. Young, *Family and Class in a London Suburb* (London: Routledge & Kegan Paul, 1960), pp. 123–32.

26. D. W. Plath, 'Japan: The After Years', in D. O. Cowgill and L. D. Holmes (eds), *Aging and Modernization* (New York: Appleton-Century-Crofts, 1972), pp. 133–50, esp. pp. 133, 138–9; D. L. Bethel, 'Life on Obasuteyama, or, Inside a Japanese Institution for the Elderly', in T. S. Lebra (ed.), *Japanese Social Organization* (Honolulu, HI: University of Hawaii Press, 1992), pp. 109–34, esp. pp. 112–13. See also Chapter 2, pp. 39–40.

27. Goffman, *Asylums*, trans. T. Ishiguro (Tokyo: Seishin-shobo, 1984). Exceptions include works by Kazuo Okuma, an *Asahi* journalist, who reported on the lamentable conditions in psychiatric and geriatric hospitals and later private nursing homes: K. Okuma, *Non-fiction Report: Psychiatric Hospitals* (Tokyo: Asahi-shinbun-sha, 1973); *Non-fiction Report: Geriatric Hospitals* (Tokyo: Asahi-shinbun-sha, 1988); and *Non-fiction Report: Private Nursing Homes* (Tokyo: Asahi-shinbun-sha, 1995).

28. E. Grundy and T. Arie, 'Falling Rates of Provision of Residential Care for the Elderly', *British Medical Journal*, 284:6318 (1982), pp. 799–802.

29. K. Jones, 'We Need the Bed', in Jack (ed.), *Residential versus Community Care*, pp. 140–53; P. Higgs and C. Victor, 'Institutional Care and the Life Course', in S. Arber and M. Evandrou (eds), *Ageing, Independence and the Life Course* (London: Jessica Kingsley in association with the British Society of Gerontology, 1993), pp. 186–200.

30. I. Allen, D. Hogg and S. Peace, *Elderly People: Choice, Participation and Satisfaction* (London: Policy Studies Institute, 1992), p. 309.

31. D. Jerrome, 'Introduction', in D. Jerrome (ed.), *Ageing in Modern Society: Contemporary Approaches* (Beckenham: Croom Helm, 1983), pp. 7–10, on p. 9.

32. A. Digby, *British Welfare Policy: Workhouse to Workfare* (London: Faber, 1989), p. 1.

33. Thane, *Old Age in English History*. See also M. Pelling and R. M. Smith (eds), *Life, Death, and the Elderly* (London: Routledge, 1991); P. Johnson and P. Thane (eds), *Old Age from Antiquity to Post-Modernity* (London: Routledge, 1998); and P. Thane (ed.), *The Long History of Old Age* (London: Thames & Hudson, 2005), Japanese translation available.

34. D. Thomson, 'Workhouse to Nursing Home: Residential Care of Elderly People in England since 1840', *Ageing and Society*, 3 (1983), pp. 43–69; R. Means and R. Smith, *From Poor Law to Community Care*, 2nd edn (1985; Bristol: Policy Press, 1998); R. Means, H. Morbey and R. Smith, *From Community Care to Market Care* (Bristol: Policy Press, 2002).

35. Y. Ogasawara, '100-Year History of Homes for the Elderly', in National Council of Social Welfare (hereafter NCSW) and National Council of Elderly Homes (hereafter NCEH) (eds), *Fifty-Year History of National Council of Elderly Homes* (Tokyo: NCSW and NCEH, 1984), pp. 3–154; Y. Ogasawara, 'Homes for the Elderly in the Past Decade', in NCSW and NCEH (eds), *Sixty-Year History of National Council of Elderly Homes* (Tokyo: NCSW and NCEH, 1995), pp. 25–74.

36. Jerrome, 'Introduction', p. 10.

37. K. Wrightson, 'The Social Order of Early Modern England', in L. Bonfield, R. M. Smith and K. Wrightson (eds), *The World We Have Gained: Histories of Population and Social Structure* (Oxford: Blackwell, 1986), pp. 177–202, on p. 202.

38. A. I. Harris, *Social Welfare for the Elderly: A Study in Thirteen Local Authority Areas in England, Wales and Scotland*, 2 vols (London: HMSO, 1968).

39. M. Brown, 'The Development of Local Authority Welfare Services from 1948–1965 under Part III of the National Assistance Act 1948' (PhD dissertation, University of Manchester, 1972).

40. Wu, *The Care of the Elderly in Japan*.

41. D. L. Bethel, 'Alienation and Reconnection in a Home for the Elderly', in J. J. Tobin (ed.), *Re-made in Japan: Everyday Life and Consumer Taste in a Changing Society* (New Haven, CT and London: Yale University Press, 1992), pp. 126–42; L. L. Thang, *Generations in Touch: Linking the Old and Young in a Tokyo Neighbourhood* (Ithaca, NY: Cornell University Press, 2001).

42. J. Kayser-Jones, *Old, Alone, and Neglected: Care of the Aged in Scotland and the United States* (Berkeley, CA and London: University of California Press, 1981).

43. Y. Ichibangase, 'Meaning and Challenges of Research on Institutional History', *Journal of History of Social Work*, 2 (1974), cited in Y. Ichibangase (ed.), *Historical Sources for Social Welfare*, 5 vols (Tokyo: Rodo-shunpo-sha, 1994), vol. 2, p. 181.
44. Y. Ichibangase, *100-Year Tokyo Borough Almshouse* (Tokyo, 1973), cited in Y. Ichibangase, 'Introduction to Tokyo Borough Almshouse History', *Journal of History of Social Work*, 1 (1973), in Ichibangase, *Historical Sources for Social Welfare*, vol. 2, p. 183.
45. For example, A. Digby, *Madness, Morality and Medicine: A Study of the York Retreat 1796–1914* (Cambridge: Cambridge University Press, 1985); J. Crammer, *Asylum History: Buckinghamshire County Pauper Lunatic Asylum – St. John's* (London: Gaskell, 1990); J. Andrews, A. Briggs, R. Porter, P. Tucker and K. Waddington, *The History of Bethlem* (London: Routledge, 1997).
46. For example, Y. Okada, *Matsuzawa Hospital: A Private History, 1879–1980* (Tokyo: Iwasaki-gakujutsu-shuppan-sha, 1981); Superintendent D. H. Clark, *The Story of a Mental Hospital, Fulbourn 1853–1983* (London: Process Press, 1996). Note: Work by non-historians is arguably said to be anecdotal, judgemental and partisan.
47. K. Imura, *History of Old People's Almshouses in Japan* (Tokyo: Gakubun-sha, 2005), p. 1.
48. Ibid., p. 2.
49. G. Esping-Andersen, *The Three Worlds of Welfare Capitalism* (Cambridge: Polity, 1990), Japanese translation available.
50. G. Esping-Andersen, *Social Foundations of Postindustrial Economics* (Oxford: Oxford University Press, 1999).
51. A. Cochrane, J. Clarke and S. Gewitz, 'Introduction', in A. Cochrane, J. Clarke and S. Gewitz (eds), *Comparing Welfare States*, 2nd edn (London: Sage in association with the Open University, 2001), pp. 2–27, on p. 19.
52. I. Peng, 'A Fresh Look at the Japanese Welfare State', *Social Policy and Administration*, 34:1 (2000), pp. 87–114, on p. 87; R. Goodman and I. Peng, 'The East Asian Welfare States', in G. Esping-Andersen (ed.), *Welfare States in Transition: National Adaptations in Global Economies* (London: Sage, 1996), pp. 192–224, on p. 193.
53. G. Esping-Andersen, 'Hybrid or Unique?', *Journal of European Social Policy*, 7:3 (1997), pp. 179–89; C. Jones, 'The Pacific Challenge: Confucian Welfare States', in C. Jones (ed.), *New Perspectives on the Welfare State in Europe* (London: Routledge, 1993), pp. 198–217; G. White and R. Goodman, 'Welfare Orientalism and the Search for an East Asian Welfare Model', in R. Goodman, G. White and H. Kwan (eds), *The East Asian Welfare Model* (London; New York: Routledge, 1998), pp. 1–24.
54. For example, A. Gould, *Capitalist Welfare Systems: A Comparison of Japan, Britain and Sweden* (London: Longman, 1993), Japanese translation available; M. Izuhara (ed.), *Comparing Social Policies: Exploring New Perspectives in Britain and Japan* (Bristol: Policy Press, 2003); P. Alcock and G. Craig (eds), *International Social Policy: Welfare Regimes in the Developed World*, 2nd edn (Basingstoke: Palgrave Macmillan, 2009); Y. Fukuchi and Y. Shimizu (eds), *International Comparison in Social Policy for the Elderly* (Tokyo: Daiichi-hoki-shuppan, 1993); S. Abe and T. Ioka (eds), *International Comparison in Social Welfare* (Tokyo: Yuhikaku, 2000); T. Uzuhashi (ed.), *The Welfare State in Comparative Perspective* (Kyoto: Minerva, 2003).
55. For example, R. R. Friedmann, N. Gilbert and M. Sherer (eds), *Modern Welfare States: A Comparative View of Trends and Prospects* (Brighton: Wheatsheaf, 1987); P. Close (ed.), *The State and Caring* (Basingstoke: Macmillan, 1992); N. Onizaki, M. Masuda and H. Inagawa (eds), *Long-Term Care in the World* (Tokyo: Chuo-hoki-shuppan, 2002); and

A. Gunji (ed.), *Role and Limitations of a Medical and Welfare Market: British Experiences and Japanese Problems* (Ageo City: Seigakuin University Press, 2004).

56. S. O. Long (ed.), *Caring for the Elderly in Japan and the US: Practices and Policies* (London: Routledge, 2000).

57. Similar shortcomings of transnational comparison between East and West are noted in R. Goodman, G. White and H. Kwan, 'Editors' Preface', in R. Goodman, G. White and H. Kwan (eds), *The East Asian Welfare Model*, pp. xiv–xvii, on pp. xiv–xv.

58. For details of the research materials employed, including oral testimony, see M. Hayashi, 'Residential Care for the Elderly in England and Japan in the Twentieth Century: Local Authority Provision in the County of Norfolk and Gifu Prefecture' (PhD dissertation, University of East Anglia, 2010), pp. 14–22.

59. S. Cherry, 'Medicine and Rural Health Care in 19th Century Europe', in J. L. Barona and S. Cherry (eds), *Health and Medicine in Rural Europe* (Valencia: University of Valencia, 2005), pp. 19–61, on p. 20.

60. S. Rowbotham, *Hidden from History: 300 Years of Women's Oppression and the Fight against It* (London: Pluto Press, 1973); R. Perks and A. Thomson, 'Introduction', in R. Perks and A. Thomson (eds), *The Oral History Reader* (London: Routledge, 1998), pp. ix–xiii, on p. ix.

61. P. Thompson, *The Voice of the Past* (Oxford: Oxford University Press, 2000), pp. 6–9.

62. R. Perks and A. Thomson, 'Part I Critical Developments: Introduction', in Perks and Thomson (eds), *The Oral History Reader*, pp. 1–8, on p. 2.

1 The English Context

1. For a summary, see Thane, *Old Age in English History*, pp. 95–118; and Townsend, *The Last Refuge*, pp. 12–19.

2. B. Abel-Smith, *The Hospitals, 1800–1948: A Study in Social Administration in England and Wales* (London: Heinemann, 1964), pp. 1–15, 46–65.

3. N. Longmate, *The Workhouse: A Social History* (London: Pimlico, 2003), p. 13.

4. S. Fowler, *Workhouse: The People, the Places, the Life behind Doors* (Kew: National Archives, 2007), pp. 7–9.

5. P. Slack, *The English Poor Law, 1531–1782* (Cambridge: Cambridge University Press, 1995), pp. 9–13; P. Slack, *Poverty and Policy in Tudor and Stuart England* (London: Longman, 1988), pp. 113–61. In Japanese, see e.g. S. Takashima, *History of British Welfare Development* (Kyoto: Minerva, 1979), pp. 207–29.

6. Extracts from the 1601 Act, in A. E. Bland, P. A. Brown and R. H. Tawney (eds), *English Economic History: Select Documents* (London: Bell, 1914), p. 380.

7. J. S. Taylor, 'The Unreformed Workhouse 1776–1834', in E. W. Martin (ed.), *Comparative Development in Social Welfare* (London: Allen & Unwin, 1972), pp. 57–84, on p. 61.

8. G. Taylor, *The Problem of Poverty 1660–1834* (Harlow: Longman, 1969), pp. 51–2.

9. Cited in Thane, *Old Age in English History*, p. 148.

10. M. Neuman, 'Speenhamland in Berkshire', in Martin (ed.), *Comparative Development in Social Welfare*, pp. 85–127.

11. K. Williams, *From Pauperism to Poverty* (London: Routledge & Kegan Paul, 1981), pp. 148–55.

12. J. R. Poynter, *Society and Pauperism: English Ideas on Poor Relief, 1795–1834* (London: Routledge & Kegan Paul, 1969), p. 189.

13. S. King, 'Sickness and Old Age', in S. King, T. Nutt and A. Tomkins, *Narratives of the Poor in Eighteenth-Century Britain*, 5 vols (London: Pickering & Chatto, 2006), vol. 1, pp. 1–125, on p. 3.

14. Williams, *From Pauperism to Poverty*, p. 40; Thane, *Old Age in English History*, p. 150.

15. S. R. Ottaway, 'Providing for the Elderly in Eighteenth-Century England', *Continuity and Change*, 13:3 (1998), pp. 391–418, on pp. 402–3; R. M. Smith, 'Ageing and Well-Being in Early Modern England', in Johnson and Thane (eds), *Old Age from Antiquity to Post-Modernity*, pp. 64–95.

16. S. Webb and B. Webb, *English Poor Law History Part 1* (1910; London: Frank Cass & Co., 1963), p. 396; J. D. Marshall, *The Old Poor Law, 1795–1834*, 2nd edn (Basingstoke: Macmillan, 1985), p. 38.

17. G. W. Oxley, *Poor Relief in England and Wales 1601–1834* (Newton Abbot: David & Charles, 1974), p. 102.

18. M. Blaug, 'The Poor Law Report Reexamined', *Journal of Economic History*, 24:2 (1964), pp. 229–45, on p. 229; Thane, *Old Age in English History*, p. 147.

19. D. Thomson, 'The Decline of Social Security: Falling State Support for the Elderly since Early Victorian Times', *Ageing and Society*, 4 (1984), pp. 451–82, esp. pp. 452–4; P. Thane, 'Old People and their Families in the English Past', in M. Daunton (ed.), *Charity, Self-Interest and Welfare in the English Past* (London: UCL Press, 1996), pp. 113–38, on pp. 120–2.

20. Great Britain Poor Law Commissioners, *The Poor Law Report of 1834*, ed. and intro. S. G. Checkland and E. O. A. Checkland (Harmondsworth: Penguin, 1974), p. 335.

21. Ibid., pp. 375, 419.

22. Ibid., p. 386.

23. M. A. Crowther, *The Workhouse System 1834–1929* (London: Batsford Academic and Educational, 1981), p. 270.

24. G. Nicholls, *A History of the English Poor Law*, 3 vols (London, 1904), vol. 2, pp. 289–314.

25. Williams, *From Pauperism to Poverty*, p. 220.

26. Ibid., pp. 158, 223. For a discussion, see A. Digby, 'The Rural Poor Law', in D. Fraser (ed.), *The New Poor Law in the Nineteenth Century* (London: Macmillan, 1976), pp. 149–70, esp. pp. 157–63; M. E. Rose, 'The Allowance System under the New Poor Law', *Economic History Review* (19 December 1966), pp. 607–20, on p. 607. In Japanese, see S. Ito, *History of Social Security: Comparative Research on Britain and Japan* (Tokyo: Aoki-shoten, 1994), pp. 87–8.

27. Great Britain Poor Law Commissioners, *The Poor Law Report of 1834*, pp. 429–30.

28. Ibid.

29. *Report of the Royal Commission on the Poor Laws (Minority Report): 'Break Up the Poor Law and Abolish the Workhouse' being Part I of The Minority Report of the Poor Law Commission, printed for the Fabian Society* (1909), p. 5.

30. *Report of the Royal Commission on the Poor Laws (Majority Report)*, Cmd 4499 (1909), para. 329, p. 169.

31. D. Thomson, 'Welfare and the Historians', in L. Bonfield, R. M. Smith and K. Wrightson (eds), *The World We Have Gained* (Oxford: Blackwell, 1986), pp. 355–78, on p. 374.

32. L. G. C. Money, *Riches and Poverty* (London: Methuen & Co., 1905), pp. 264–5.

33. *Report of the Royal Commission on the Aged Poor*, Cmd 7684 (1895), pp. xii–xiii, cited in B. Harris, *The Origins of the British Welfare State: Society, State, and Social Welfare in England and Wales, 1800–1945* (Basingstoke and New York: Palgrave Macmillan, 2004), p. 57.

34. C. Booth, *The Aged Poor in England and Wales* (London and New York: Macmillan & Co., 1894), pp. 53–4.

35. C. Booth, *Poor Law Reform* (1910), p. 37, cited in J. Macnicol, *The Politics of Retirement in Britain, 1878–1948* (Cambridge: Cambridge University Press, 1998), p. 79.

36. C. Booth, *Pauperism and the Endowment of Old Age* (London: Macmillan & Co., 1892), p. 148.

37. For example, C. Booth (ed.), *Life and Labour of the People in London*, 17 vols (London: Macmillan & Co., 1902–3); B. S. Rowntree, *Poverty: A Study of Town Life* (London: Macmillan & Co., 1901). For a summary, see E. R. Michael, *The Relief of Poverty 1834–1914* (London: Macmillan, 1972). In Japanese, see e.g. T. Fujimoto, *A History of Poverty in Britain* (Tokyo: Shin-nihon-shuppan-sha, 2000).

38. For a summary, see P. Thane, *Foundations of the Welfare State*, 2nd edn (Harlow: Longman, 1996), pp. 31–7, Japanese translation available; M. E. Rose, *The English Poor Law 1780–1930* (Newton Abbot: David & Charles, 1971), pp. 283–320.

39. L. Clarke, *Domiciliary Services for the Elderly* (Beckenham: Croom Helm, 1984), pp. 3–5; MoH, *Circular 179/44: Domestic Help* (14 December 1944).

40. S. Cherry, *Medical Services and the Hospitals in Britain, 1860–1939* (Cambridge: Cambridge University Press, 1996), p. 63.

41. E. P. Hennock, *British Social Reform and German Precedents: The Case of Social Insurance 1880–1914* (Oxford: Clarendon, 1987), p. 111.

42. Brown, 'The Development of Local Authority Welfare Services', pp. 9–10.

43. B. B. Gilbert, *British Social Policy 1914–1939* (London: B. T. Batsford, 1970), pp. 229, 235.

44. Townsend, *The Last Refuge*, p. 17.

45. Ministry of Health (hereafter MoH), *Persons in Receipt of Poor-Law Relief, England and Wales* (London: HMSO, May 1927), pp. 19, 22–3; Williams, *From Pauperism to Poverty*, pp. 161, 205.

46. Crowther, *The Workhouse System*, pp. 54–87.

47. B. Bosanquet, *Rich and Poor* (London and New York: Macmillan & Co., 1896), p. 177.

48. Booth, *The Aged Poor in England and Wales*, pp. 330–1.

49. See e.g. the Norwich wartime experience, p. 71.

50. Means and Smith, *From Poor Law to Community Care*, p. 21.

51. R. M. Titmuss, *Problems of Social Policy* (London: HMSO, 1950), p. 451.

52. Ibid., p. 501; Nuffield Foundation, *Old People: Report of a Survey Committee on the Problems of Ageing and the Care of Old People* (London: Oxford University Press, 1947), pp. 67–8.

53. *Summary Report by the Ministry of Health*, Cmd 6340 (February 1942), p. 36; Cmd 6394 (October 1942), p. 14.

54. E. D. Samson, *Old Age in the New World* (London: Pilot Press, 1944), p. 46.

55. Ibid., p. 47.

56. Nuffield Foundation, *Old People*, p. 64.

57. National Archives, CAB 134/698, *Report of the Committee on the Break-up of the Poor Law*, enclosed in the Minutes of the Seventh Meeting of the Social Services Committee, 12 July 1946. I am grateful to Professor Robin Means for sending me a copy. See also a summary given to the Parliamentary Medical Group by Lord Amulree and E. L. Sturdee, 'Care of the Chronic Sick and of the Aged', *British Medical Journal*, 1:20 (April 1946), pp. 617–19.

58. Parliamentary Debates (Hansard), *House of Commons 444* (24 November 1947), col. 1608.

59. Hansard, *House of Commons 448* (5 March 1948), cols 754–5; Hansard, *House of Lords 154* (6 April 1948), col. 1097.

60. Hansard, *House of Commons 444*, col. 1631.

61. National Assistance Act (1948), Part I, section 1.

62. National Assistance Act, Part III, section 21.

63. Hansard, *House of Commons 444*, col. 1609.

64. National Assistance Act, Part III, section 22.

65. Hansard, *House of Commons 444*, col. 1603.

66. J. Phillips, *Private Residential Care: The Admission Process and Reactions of the Public Sector* (Aldershot: Avebury, 1992), p. 19.

67. *The Times*, 1 November 1947; *Eastern Daily Press*, 1 November 1947.

68. S. K. Ruck, 'A Policy for Old Age', *Political Quarterly*, 31 (1960), pp. 120–31, on p. 120.

69. National Assistance Act, Part III, sections 29, 31.

70. National Health Service Act (1946), sections 25, 29.

71. J. Parker, *Local Health and Welfare Services* (London: George Allen & Unwin, 1965), p. 106.

72. Nuffield Foundation, *Old People*, p. 96.

73. Means and Smith, *From Poor Law to Community Care*, p. 147.

74. P. Townsend, 'The Structured Dependency of the Elderly: A Creation of Social Policy in the Twentieth Century', *Ageing and Society*, 1 (1981), pp. 5–28, on p. 22.

75. Hansard, *House of Commons 444*, col. 1609.

76. Parker, *Local Health and Welfare Services*, p. 108.

77. Figures from MoH, *Report of the Ministry of Health for the Year Ended 31st March 1949*, Cmd 7910 (London: HMSO, 1950) (*hereafter MoH Report*), p. 370; Townsend, *The Last Refuge*, pp. 20–1.

78. *MoH Report 1949*, p. 311.

79. Ibid., pp. 311–12.

80. *MoH Report 1950*, p. 150.

81. B. Davies, *Social Needs and Resources in Local Services: A Study of Variations in Standards of Provision of Personal Social Services between Local Authority Areas* (London: Michael Joseph, 1968), p. 92.

82. B. E. Shenfield, *Social Policies for Old Age: A Review of Social Provision for Old Age in Great Britain* (London: Routledge & Kegan Paul, 1957), p. 159.

83. J. A. G. Griffith, *Central Departments and Local Authorities* (London: George Allen & Unwin, 1966), p. 515.

84. Means and Smith, *From Poor Law to Community Care*, p. 157.

85. Davies, *Social Needs and Resources in Local Services*, p. 92. See e.g. the five-year local plans (schemes) of Norfolk and Norwich councils, p. 77 and p. 78 respectively.

86. MoH, *Report of the Committee of Enquiry into the Cost of the National Health Service*, Cmd 9663 (London: HMSO, 1956) (hereafter *Guillebaud Report*), p. 217.

87. *MoH Report 1954*, p. 138; *MoH Report 1955*, p. 139. See also a comment by R. Thompson, Parliamentary Secretary to Minister of Health, Hansard, *House of Commons 582* (12 February 1958), col. 535.

88. P. Townsend and D. Wedderburn, *The Aged in the Welfare State: The Interim Report of a Survey of Persons Aged 65 and Over in Britain, 1962 and 1963* (London: G. Bell & Sons, 1965), p. 69.

89. *MoH Report 1952*, p. 90; Davies, *Social Needs and Resources in Local Services*, pp. 72–81.

90. T. N. Rudd, 'Basic Problems in Social Welfare of the Elderly', *Almoner*, 10:10 (1958), pp. 348–51, on pp. 348–9.

91. C. H. Wright and L. Roberts, 'The Place of the Home-Help Service in the Care of the Aged', *Lancet*, 1:7014 (1958), pp. 254–6.

92. Hansard, *House of Commons 522* (14 December 1953), col. 167.

93. Davies, *Social Needs and Resources in Local Services*, p. 66.

94. MoH, *Circular 3/55: Residential Accommodation for Old People, Homes for the More Infirm* (25 February 1955).

95. *The Times*, 10 April 1951.

96. Hansard, *House of Commons 512* (6 March 1953), col. 710.

97. *Report of the Committee on the Economic and Financial Problems of the Provision for Old Age*, Cmd 9333 (London: HMSO, 1954) (hereafter *Phillips Report*), pp. 73–4.

98. Lord Amulree, 'Proper Use of the Hospital in Treatment of the Aged Sick', *Lancet*, 260:1 (1951), pp. 123–6, on p. 125.

99. MoH, *Survey of Services Available to the Chronic Sick and Elderly 1954–55* (London: HMSO, 1957) (hereafter *Boucher Report*), pp. 13, 36, 51. Note: There were then 56,000 hospital and 69,000 residential beds.

100. *MoH Report 1954*, p. 13.

101. Hansard, *House of Commons 578* (29 November 1957), cols 1492–9, esp. col. 1495.

102. MoH, *Boucher Report*, pp. 46–7.

103. *Royal Commission on the Law Relating to Mental Illness and Mental Deficiency*, Cmnd 169 (London: HMSO, 1957), pp. 214–16.

104. Hansard, *House of Commons 512* (6 March 1953), col. 716.

105. Shenfield, *Social Policies for Old Age*, p. 164.

106. Viz. MoH, *Circular 14/57: Local Authority Services for the Chronic Sick and Infirm* (7 October 1957); MoH, *HM(57)86: Geriatric Services and the Care of the Chronic Sick* (7 October 1957). For a summary, see MoH, *Guillebaud Report*, pp. 216–17; MoH, *Boucher Report*, p. 55.

107. M. Davies, 'Swopping [*sic*] the Old Around', *Community Care*, 296 (1979), pp. 16–17.

108. Shenfield, *Social Policies for Old Age*, p. 164.

109. Townsend, *The Last Refuge*, p. 20.

110. Ibid., p. 29.

111. Ibid., p. 21.

112. Ibid., p. 29.

113. Ibid., p. 34.

114. Ibid., p. 33.

115. *MoH Report 1958*, p. 239; MoH, *Health and Welfare: The Development of Community Care*, Cmnd 1973 (London: HMSO, 1963) (hereafter *Community Care Plan*), p. 21.

116. Townsend, *The Last Refuge*, p. 209.

117. Ibid.

118. Ibid.

119. *Report of the Working Party on Social Workers in the Local Authority Health and Welfare Services* (London: HMSO, 1959) (hereafter *Younghusband Report*), p. 95.

120. Ibid., pp. 271–2.

121. *MoH Report 1960*, p. 113.

122. Townsend, *The Last Refuge*, pp. 37–9.

123. G. Sumner and R. Smith, *Planning Local Authority Services for the Elderly* (London: George Allen & Unwin, 1969), p. 41.

124. MoH, *A Hospital Plan for England and Wales*, Cmnd 1604 (London: HMSO, 1962) (hereafter *Hospital Plan*), p. 9.

125. MoH, *Community Care Plan*, p. 2.

126. MoH, *Hospital Plan*, p. iii.

127. MoH, *Community Care Plan*, p. 21.

128. MoH, *Community Care Plan*, p. iii.

129. Ibid., p. 21. See also MoH, *Health and Welfare: The Development of Community Care: Revision to 1973–4 of Plans for the Health and Welfare Services of the Local Authorities in England and Wales*, Cmnd 3022 (London, HMSO, 1964).

130. J. Hanson, 'Challenge in the Welfare Services', *Municipal Review*, 36:431 (November 1965), p. 666; N. Bosanquet, *A Future for Old Age* (London: Temple Smith/New Society, 1978), p. 110.

131. Sumner and Smith, *Planning Local Authority Services for the Elderly*, p. 210.

132. DHSS, *Health and Personal Social Services Statistics for England 1982* (London: HMSO, 1982), p. 101; MoH, *Community Care Plan*, p. 21.

133. Department of Health and Social Security (hereafter DHSS), *Department of Health and Social Security Annual Report for 1970*, Cmnd 4714 (London: HMSO, 1971) (hereafter *DHSS Report 1970*), p. 216.

134. Figures for 1951–71 Censuses, referring to England and Wales.

135. Bosanquet, *A Future for Old Age*, p. 7; *DHSS Report 1970*, p. 216. Note: Figures from 1951–71 Censuses, referring to England and Wales.

136. DHSS, *Health and Personal Social Services Statistics for England 1982*, p. 101.

137. *MoH Report 1960*, p. 112.

138. *MoH Report 1958*, p. 239.

139. *MoH Report 1961*, p. 91; *MoH Report 1958*, p. 239.

140. *MoH Report 1952*, p. 118; *DHSS Report 1970*, p. 24.

141. *Caring for People, Staffing Residential Homes: Report of the Committee of Enquiry* (London: Allen & Unwin, 1967) (hereafter *Williams Report*), pp. 189–92.

142. E. Younghusband, *Social Work in Britain 1950–1975: A Follow-up Study*, 2 vols (London: Allen & Unwin, 1978), vol. 2, p. 184.

143. Townsend, *The Last Refuge*, p. 190.

144. D. Cole and J. E. G. Utting, *The Economic Circumstances of Old People* (Welwyn: Codicote Press, 1962), p. 98; P. Alcock, *Poverty and State Support* (London: Longman, 1987), p. 61.

145. M. Brown, 'A Welfare Service Not a Welfare Department', *Social Services Quarterly*, 39:3 (December 1965–February 1966), pp. 91–4, on p. 92.

146. Means and Smith, *From Poor Law to Community Care*, p. 207.

147. A. Hunt, *The Home Help Service in England and Wales* (London: HMSO, 1970), p. 25.

148. A. Butler, C. Oldman and J. Greve, *Sheltered Housing for the Elderly* (London: Allen & Unwin, 1983), p. 59; Townsend, *The Last Refuge*, p. 201; Bosanquet, *A Future for Old Age*, p. 98.

149. Thomson, 'Workhouse to Nursing Home', pp. 65, 67.

150. Bosanquet, *A Future for Old Age*, pp. 107, 109.

151. Jones, 'The Development of Institutional Care', pp. 290–1; Means and Smith, *From Poor Law to Community Care*, p. 208.

152. Comments by local authority welfare officers (M. Beglin and M. Speed respectively), cited in Means and Smith, *From Poor Law to Community Care*, p. 210.

153. *Williams Report*, p. 114.

154. A. I. Harris, *Social Welfare for the Elderly*, vol. 1, pp. 49–50.

155. Younghusband, *Social Work in Britain 1950–1975*, vol. 1, p. 199.
156. R. M. Titmuss, *Essays on 'The Welfare State'*, 2nd edn (London: Unwin University Books, 1963), p. 56, Japanese translation available.
157. *Report of the Committee on Local Authority and Allied Personal Social Services*, Cmnd 3703 (London: HMSO, 1968) (hereafter *Seebohm Report*), p. 44.
158. D. V. Donnison, 'Seebohm: The Report and its Implications', *Social Work* (Britain), 25:4 (1968), pp. 3–8, on p. 3; P. Townsend, 'The Objectives of the New Local Social Service', in P. Townsend et al., *The Fifth Social Service: A Critical Analysis of the Seebohm Proposals* (London: Fabian Society, 1970), pp. 7–22, on p. 7.
159. R. G. S. Brown, *Reorganising the National Health Service: A Case Study in Administrative Change* (Oxford: Blackwell, 1979), p. 22. For a summary, see C. Webster, *The National Health Service: A Political History* (Oxford: Oxford University Press, 2002), pp. 107–9.
160. National Health Service Reorganisation Act (1973), sections 10–12.
161. R. Adams, *The Personal Social Services: Clients, Consumers or Citizens?* (London and New York: Longman, 1996), p. 40; M. Hill, 'Origins of the Local Authority Social Services', in M. Hill (ed.), *Local Authority Social Services: An Introduction* (Oxford: Blackwell, 2000), pp. 22–37, on p. 32.
162. F. Gould and B. Roweth, 'Public Spending and Social Policy: The United Kingdom 1950–1977', *Journal of Social Policy*, 9:3 (1980), pp. 337–57, on p. 353.
163. P. Townsend, 'Social Planning and Treasury', in N. Bosanquet and P. Townsend (eds), *Labour and Equality: A Fabian Study of Labour in Power 1974–79* (London: Heinemann Educational, 1980), pp. 3–23, on p. 11.
164. DHSS, *Priorities for Health and Personal Social Services in England* (London: DHSS/HMSO, 1976), p. 83.
165. DHSS, *Circular 35/72: Local Authority Social Services Ten Year Development Plans 1973–1983* (31 August 1972). In Japanese, see K. Hiraoka, *Welfare and Social Policy in Britain* (Kyoto: Minerva, 2003), pp. 5–23.
166. A. Webb, 'The Personal Social Services', in N. Bosanquet and P. Townsend (eds), *Labour and Equality: A Fabian Study of Labour in Power 1974–79* (London: Heinemann Educational, 1980), pp. 279–95, on p. 288.
167. Viz. DHSS, *Priorities for Health and Personal Social Services in England*; DHSS, *The Way Forward: Priorities in the Health and Social Services* (London: HMSO, 1977).
168. J. Wright and F. Sheldon, 'Health and Social Services Planning', *Social Policy and Administration*, 19:3 (1985), pp. 258–72. See local example of Norfolk, p. 89.
169. A. Webb and G. Wistow, *Planning, Need and Scarcity: Essays on the Personal Social Services* (London: Allen & Unwin, 1986), pp. 33, 41.
170. A. Webb and G. Wistow, 'The Personal Social Services: Incrementalism, Expediency or Systematic Social Planning?', in A. Walker (ed.), *Public Expenditure and Social Policy: An Examination of Social Spending and Social Priorities* (London: Heinemann Educational, 1982), pp. 137–64, on pp. 154–5.
171. Ibid., p. 155.
172. Cited in Norfolk County Council Social Services Committee Minutes 1974–80, held at Norfolk County Hall, Norfolk (hereafter NCCSSCM), 17 December 1975, p. 907. See p. 88 in this volume.
173. Bosanquet, *A Future for Old Age*, p. 109.

174. DHSS, *Health and Personal Social Services Statistics for England 1982*, pp. 101–2: Viz. 168,000 residential places in England – 102,000 direct local authority (61 per cent); 15,000 local authority-supported (9 per cent); 25,000 voluntary (15 per cent); and 26,000 private places (15 per cent).

175. A. C. Bebbington, 'Changes in the Provision of Social Services to the Elderly in the Community over Fourteen Years', *Social Policy and Administration*, 13:2 (1979), pp. 111–23, on pp. 120–2.

176. A. Fleiss, *Home Ownership Alternatives for the Elderly* (London: HMSO, 1985), p. 1.

177. Butler, Oldman and Greve, *Sheltered Housing for the Elderly*, pp. 64, 67; R. Wheeler, 'Staying Put: A New Development in Policy?', *Ageing and Society*, 2 (1982), pp. 299–329, on p. 310. In Japanese, see S. Takegawa, *Welfare State and Civil Society* (Kyoto: Horitsu-bunka-sha, 1992), pp. 67–91.

178. A. J. Willcocks (ed.), *The Care and Housing of the Elderly in the Community: A Report of a Seminar Held at the University of Nottingham on 19–21 September 1979* (Stafford: Hempits, 1981), pp. 38–41.

179. Butler, Oldman and Greve, *Sheltered Housing for the Elderly*, p. 62.

180. Wheeler, 'Staying Put', p. 310.

181. MoH, *Hospital Plan*, p. iii.

182. A. Walker, 'The Meaning and Social Division of Community Care', in A. Walker (ed.), *Community Care: The Family, the State and Social Policy* (Oxford: Blackwell, 1982), pp. 13–39, on p. 19.

183. Bosanquet, *A Future for Old Age*, pp. 120–1.

184. Hansard, *House of Commons 77, Written Answers* (17 April 1985), cols 215–20.

185. G. Davies and D. Piachaud, 'Social Policy and the Economy', in H. Glennerster (ed.), *The Future of the Welfare State: Remaking Social Policy* (London: Heinemann, 1983), pp. 40–60, on pp. 46–7.

186. Conservative Party, *Conservative Manifesto 1979* (London: Conservative Central Office, 1979), p. 7.

187. DHSS, *Growing Older*, Cmnd 8173 (London: HMSO, 1981), p. 3; HM Treasury, *Public Expenditure Analyses to 1993–94* (London: HMSO, 1991), p. 12.

188. R. Robinson, 'Restructuring the Welfare State: An Analysis of Public Expenditure 1979/80–1984/85', *Journal of Social Policy*, 15:1 (1986), pp. 1–21, on pp. 3–4.

189. W. Laing, *Financing Long-Term Care* (London: Age Concern England, 1993), p. 27. See Social Security Act (1980), para. 9.9/10.

190. Laing, *Financing Long-Term Care*, p. 27.

191. Department of Health, *Health and Personal Social Services Statistics for England 1993 edition* (London: HMSO/Stationery Office, 1993), p. 76.

192. Laing & Buisson, *Care of Elderly People: UK Market Survey 2003* (London: Laing & Buisson, 2003) (hereafter *Laing Survey* 2003), p. 141.

193. S. Player and A. M. Pollock, 'Long-Term Care: From Public Responsibility to Private Good', *Critical Social Policy*, 21:2 (2001), pp. 231–55, on p. 234.

194. *Laing Survey 2008*, p. 23.

195. Robinson, 'Restructuring the Welfare State', p. 19.

196. R. Parker, 'Care and the Private Sector', in I. Sinclair, R. Parker, D. Leat and J. Williams, *The Kaleidoscope of Care: A Review of Research on Welfare Provision for Elderly People* (London: HMSO, 1990), pp. 291–361, on p. 302.

197. Audit Commission, *Making a Reality of Community Care* (London: HMSO, 1986), pp. 43–8.

198. A. Walker, 'Community Care: Past, Present and Future', in S. Lliffe and J. Munro (eds), *Healthy Choices: Future Options for the NHS* (London: Lawrence & Wishart, 1997), pp. 178–200, on p. 185.

199. B. J. Bradshaw, 'Financing Private Care for the Elderly', in S. Baldwin, G. Parker and R. Walker (eds), *Social Security and Community Care* (Aldershot: Avebury, 1988), pp. 175–87, on p. 179.

200. House of Commons Health Committee, *Public Expenditure on Health and Personal Social Services, Session 1992–93* (London: HMSO, 1993), p. 29.

201. A. Tinker, *The Care of Frail Elderly People in the United Kingdom* (London: HMSO, 1994), pp. 14, 21.

202. Laing, *Financing Long-Term Care*, p. 29.

203. Tinker, *The Care of Frail Elderly People*, p. 16; House of Commons Health Committee, *Public Expenditure on Health and Personal Social Services, Session 1992–93*, p. 29.

204. D. R. Phillips, J. A. Vincent and S. Blacksell, 'Petit Bourgeois Care: Private Residential Care for the Elderly', *Policy and Politics*, 14:2 (1986), pp. 189–208, on pp. 193, 204–5.

205. For example, speeches by the Parliamentary Under-Secretaries for Health and Social Security (Ray Whitney and John Major), cited respectively in Hansard, *House of Commons 94* (27 March 1986), col. 1136; Hansard, *House of Commons 97* (14 May 1986), col. 831.

206. S. Biggs, 'Quality of Care and the Growth of Private Welfare for Old People', *Critical Social Policy*, 20:7 (1987), pp. 74–82, on p. 79; T. Weaver, D. Willcocks and L. Kellaher, *The Business of Care: A Study of Private Residential Homes for Old People* (London: Polytechnic of North London, 1985), p. 31.

207. H. Bartlett and R. B. Ross, 'Terms of a Contract', *Community Care*, 592 (1986), pp. 14–15.

208. J. A. Vincent, A. D. Tibbenham and D. R. Phillips, 'Choice in Residential Care: Myths and Realities', *Journal of Social Policy*, 16:4 (1987), pp. 435–60, on p. 459.

209. Parker, 'Care and the Private Sector', p. 357.

210. H. Glennerster, J. Falkingham and M. Evandrow, 'How Much Do We Care?', *Social Policy and Administration*, 24:2 (1990), pp. 93–103, on p. 97; A. Walker, 'Dependent Relativities', *The Times Higher Education Supplement*, 22 April 1988, p. 17.

211. Biggs, 'Quality of Care', p. 75.

212. Ibid., p. 81.

213. Viz. Centre for Policy on Ageing, *Home Life: A Code of Practice for Residential Care* (London: Centre for Policy on Ageing, 1984); National Association of Health Authorities, *Registration and Inspection of Nursing Homes: A Handbook for Health Authorities* (Birmingham: National Association of Health Authorities, 1985).

214. R. B. Ross, 'Keeping the Register Up to Date', *Social Services Insight*, 15:22 (March 1986), pp. 13–15, on p. 15.

215. Centre for Policy on Ageing, *Home Life*, p. 15.

216. D. Carson, 'Registering Homes: Another Fine Mess?', *Journal of Social Welfare Law* (March 1985), pp. 67–84, on pp. 68–70.

217. R. B. Ross, 'Ways of Keeping Standards High', *Social Services Insight*, 5:12 (April 1986), pp. 14–15; R. B. Ross, 'Registered Homes and Residents' Well-Being', *Social Work Today*, 19:13 (1987), pp. 12–13.

218. R. B. Ross, 'Regulation of Residential Homes for the Elderly', *Journal of Social Welfare Law* (March 1985), pp. 85–95.

219. B. Holmes, *The Realities of Home Life* (Birmingham: National Union of Public Employees, 1986), pp. 3–13; *The Times*, 29 April 1986.

220. B. Holmes and A. Johnson, *Cold Comfort: The Scandal of Private Rest Homes* (London: Souvenir Press, 1988), pp. 32–6, 116–17.

221. *Eastern Evening News*, 24 May 1987; *Guardian*, 29 April 1986; *Daily Telegraph*, 30 October 1986.

222. ITV broadcast, 6 October 1987; *Guardian*, 8 October 1987.

223. For example, speeches by Willie W. Hamilton and Ray Whitney, cited in Hansard, *House of Commons 94* (27 March 1986), cols 1131–6.

224. T. Booth, 'Camden Shows the Way', *Community Care*, 649 (1987), pp. 16–17, on p. 16. For each case, see J. Gibbs, M. Evans and S. Rodway, *Report of the Inquiry into Nye Bevan Lodge* (London: London Borough of Southwark, 1987); *The Times*, 22 and 23 July 1987; and D. Clough, *Independent Review of Residential Care for the Elderly within the London Borough of Camden* (London: London Borough of Camden, 1987).

225. Booth, 'Camden Shows the Way', p. 16.

226. G. Wagner, *Residential Care: A Positive Choice* (London: HMSO, 1988), pp. 1, 3, 7–9.

227. J. Lewis and H. Glennerster, *Implementing the New Community Care* (Buckingham: Open University Press, 1996), p. 8. In Japanese, see e.g. T. Tabata, *The Making and Development of Community-Based Social Services in Britain* (Tokyo: Yuhikaku, 2003), pp. 177–212.

228. D. Kenny and P. Edwards, *Community Care Trends: The Impact of Funding on Local Authorities* (London: Local Government Management Board, 1996), p. 6; N. Valios, 'Services Cut to Balance Books', *Community Care*, 1117 (1996), p. 3.

229. *Laing Survey 2008*, p. 160.

230. Ibid., p. 23.

231. L. Easterbrook, *Moving On from Community Care: The Treatment, Care and Support of Older People in England* (London: Age Concern Books, 2003), pp. 98–103; *Laing Survey 2003*, p. 26.

232. S. O'Kell, 'Short Changed', *Community Care*, 1115 (1996), pp. 26–7, on p. 27.

233. *Laing Survey 2003*, p. 31; B. Hardy, R. Young and G. Wistow, 'Dimensions of Choice in the Assessment and Care Management Process: The Views of Older People, Carers and Care Managers', *Health and Social Care in the Community*, 7:6 (1999), pp. 483–91, on p. 484.

234. Player and Pollock, 'Long-Term Care', p. 241.

235. Means, Morbey and Smith, *From Community Care to Market Care*, p. 27.

236. R. Warburton and J. McCracken, 'An Evidence-Based Perspective from the Department of Health on the Impact of the 1993 Reforms on the Care of Frail, Elderly People', in *Report by the Royal Commission on Long Term Care: With Respect to Old Age*, Cm 4192-I, II/1-3 (London: Stationery Office, 1999) (hereafter *Sutherland Report*), vol. II/3, pp. 25–36, on p. 25.

237. M. Knapp, B. Hardy and J. Forder, 'Commissioning for Quality: Ten Years of Social Care Markets in England', *Journal of Social Policy*, 30:2 (2001), pp. 283–306, on p. 285.

238. *Laing Survey 2008*, pp. 23, 106–7, 160.

239. D. Wanless, *Securing Good Care for Older People: Taking a Long-Term View* (London: King's Fund, 2006) (hereafter *Wanless Report*), p. 98.

240. *Laing Survey 2008*, pp. 129, 138, 140.

241. Ibid., pp. 129, 138.

242. *Wanless Report*, p. 98; *Laing Survey 2008*, p. 169.

243. *Wanless Report*, p. 98.

244. *Laing Survey 2008*, p. 57.

245. Ibid., pp. 76, 82.

246. H. Land, 'Future Expectations of Care in Old Age', in J. Robinson (ed.), *Towards a New Social Compact for Care in Old Age* (London: King's Fund, 2001), pp. 47–65, on p. 64.

247. H. Lewis, G. Wistow, S. Abbott and L. Cotterill, 'Continuing Health Care: The Local Development of Policies and Eligibility Criteria', *Health and Social Care in the Community*, 7:6 (1999), pp. 455–63, on p. 456.

248. Ibid.

249. G. Dalley and M. Mandelstam, *Assessment Denied?: Council Responsibilities Towards Self-Funders Moving into Care* (London: Relatives & Residents Association, 2008), p. 9.

250. National Health Service and Community Care Act (1990), sections 48, 50.

251. Centre for Policy on Ageing, *A Better Home Life* (London: Centre for Policy on Ageing, 1996), pp. x–xi, 1, Japanese translation available.

252. Department of Health, *Care Homes for Older People: National Minimum Standards and the Care Homes Regulations 2001*, 3rd edn (London: Stationery Office, 2003), pp. 24–5.

253. *Laing Survey 2008*, p. 38.

254. *Wanless Report*, p. 225.

255. Ibid., p. xxx; M. Samuel, 'Poorer People May Not Feel Benefit of Wanless Funding Vision', *Community Care*, 1617 (2006), pp. 16–17.

256. G. Carson, 'Call for Free Minimum Level of Care', *Community Care*, 1616 (2006), p. 6.

257. Viz. HM Government, White Paper, *Building the National Care Service*, Cm 7854 (Norwich: Stationery Office, 2010); Commission on Funding of Care and Support (Dilnot Commission), *Fairer Care Funding*.

258. 'Andrew Lansley: Elderly will be Able to Opt in to Social Care Insurance Scheme', *Guardian*, 11 July 2012, at http://www.guardian.co.uk/society/2012/jul/11/andrew-lansley-social-care-insurance/print [accessed 10 August 2012].

259. L. Buckner and S. Yeandle, *Valuing Carers 2011: Calculating the Value of Carers' Support* (London: Carers UK, 2011): cf. the annual cost of the NHS was £98.8 billion in the year 2009–10.

260. HM Government, Green Paper: *Shaping the Future of Care Together*, Cm 7673 (Norwich: Stationery Office, 2009), pp. 38–9.

261. A. Charlesworth and R. Thorlby, *Reforming Social Care: Options for Funding* (London: Nuffield Trust, May 2012), pp. 2, 4, at http://www.nuffieldtrust.org.uk/sites/files/nuffield/publication/120529_reforming-social-care-options-funding_0.pdf [accessed 10 August 2012]; Carson, 'Call for Free Minimum Level of Care', p. 6.

2 The Japanese Context

1. For a summary, see Y. Ikeda, *History of Japanese Social Welfare* (Kyoto: Horitsu-bunka-sha, 1986), pp. 61–5; T. Momose, *History of Elderly Welfare in Japan* (Tokyo: Chuo-hoki-shuppan, 1997), pp. 8–10.

2. K. Yoshida, *New Edition: History of Japanese Social Services* (Tokyo: Keiso-shobo, 2004), pp. 60–110. Christian-run charitable infirmaries first appeared in the early sixteenth century, their development interrupted by the early seventeenth-century 'closed-door policy', pp. 94–7.

3. Y. Ikeda and Y. Doi (eds), *Comprehensive Chronology of Social Welfare in Japan* (Kyoto: Horitsu-bunka-sha, 2000), pp. 12–21; T. Seki, 'History of Institutions', in K. Imura and M. Fujiwara (eds), *Modern History of Japanese Social Welfare* (Tokyo: Keiso-shobo, 2007), pp. 113–22, on pp. 115–16; Y. Ogasawara, 'Research on Pre-War Social Welfare

Institutions', in Social Welfare Survey Research Council (ed.), *Pre-War Social Work Survey in Japan* (Tokyo: Keiso-shobo, 1983), pp. 354–68, on pp. 356–8, 366–7.

4. Bethel, 'Life on Obasuteyama', p. 112.

5. Bethel, 'Alienation and Reconnection', p. 131.

6. Fukazawa, *Ballad of Oak Mountain*.

7. M. Izuhara, 'Care and Inheritance: Japanese and English Perspectives on the "Generational Contract"', *Ageing and Society*, 22:1 (2002), pp. 61–77, on p. 63. Viz. Article 4 of the 1950 New National Assistance Act, see Chapter 2, p. 47. See also Peng, 'A Fresh Look at the Japanese Welfare State', p. 91.

8. Plath, 'Japan: The After Years', p.133; Bethel, 'Life on Obasuteyama', p. 109.

9. R. Goodman, 'The "Japanese-Style Welfare State" and the Delivery of Personal Social Services', in R. Goodman, G. White and H. Kwon (eds), *The East Asian Welfare Model* (London and New York: Routledge, 1998), pp. 139–58, on pp. 139–42; Y. Ikeda, *History of Welfare in Japan* (Kyoto: Horitsu-bunka-sha, 1994), pp. 12–43.

10. T. Fukutake, *The Structure of Japanese Society*, 2nd edn (Tokyo: Tokyo University Press, 1987), pp. 25–32; M. Izuhara, *Family Change and Housing in Post-War Japanese Society* (Aldershot: Ashgate, 2000), pp. 20–3.

11. M. Izuhara, 'Ageing and Intergenerational Relations in Japan', in Izuhara (ed.), *Comparing Social Policies*, pp. 73–94, on p. 85.

12. W. G. Beasley, *The Rise of Modern Japan* (London: Weidenfeld & Nicolson, 1995), pp. 54–69.

13. D. Fraser, *The Evolution of the British Welfare State: A History of Social Policy since the Industrial Revolution* (Basingstoke: Palgrave Macmillan, 2003), pp. xxiv–xxxviii; R. Pinker, *Social Theory and Social Policy* (London: Heinemann Educational, 1971), pp. 52–4. Note: However, an active role of the state in economic and social efforts was seen in Germany. See e.g. R. Lowe, 'The State and the Development of Social Welfare', in M. Pugh (ed.), *A Companion to Modern European History 1871–1945* (Oxford: Blackwell, 1997), pp. 45–69, on pp. 56–9, 68–9.

14. H. K. Lee, 'The Japanese Welfare State in Transition', in Friedmann, Gilbert and Sherer (eds), *Modern Welfare States*, pp. 243–63, on p. 244; Ito, *History of Social Security*, p. 157.

15. Lee, 'The Japanese Welfare State in Transition', p. 246.

16. R. Pinker, 'Social Welfare in Japan and Britain', in E. Øyen (ed.), *Comparing Welfare States and their Futures* (Aldershot: Gower, 1986), pp. 114–28, on p. 122.

17. Ito, *History of Social Security*, p. 169. See also T. Ishida, *Political Culture and Language Symbolism in Modern Japan* (Tokyo: Tokyo University Press, 1983), pp. 182–4.

18. K. Adachi, 'The Development of Social Welfare Services in Japan', in Long (ed.), *Caring for the Elderly in Japan and the US*, pp. 191–205, on p. 192.

19. Poor Relief Order (1874), No. 162, Introduction. See Ministry of Health and Welfare Fifty-Year Historical Editorial Board (ed.), *Fifty–Year History of Ministry of Health and Welfare, Description* (Tokyo: Chuo-hoki-shuppan, 1988) (hereafter MoHW Board, *Fifty-Year History*), pp. 241–2.

20. R. Komatsu, 'The State and Social Welfare in Japan', in Close (ed.), *The State and Caring*, pp. 128–47, on p. 134.

21. Yoshida, *New Edition: History of Japanese Social Services*, pp. 162, 203; M. E. Rose, *The Relief of Poverty: 1834–1914* (London: Macmillan, 1972), p. 53. In England and Wales there were 801,000 Poor Law relief recipients in 1875 and 916,000 in 1910.

22. K. Yoshida, 'A History of Poverty in Japan', in Social Welfare Survey Research Council (ed.), *Pre-War Social Work Survey in Japan* (Tokyo: Keiso-shobo, 1983), pp. 3–26, on p. 10.

23. N. Noguchi, 'Residential Care for the Elderly in Japan: History and Issues' (PhD dissertation, Nihon Fukushi University, 2003), p. 123.

24. M. Ogawa, 'Poor Relief System, 1912–26', in Japan University of Social Work (ed.), *Poor Law System in Japan* (Tokyo: Keiso-shobo, 1960), pp. 153–222, on p. 206.

25. Ogasawara, '100-Year History', p. 17.

26. Y. Ogasawara, *Basics and Theory of Nursing Care: Function and Living Assistance of Old People's Homes* (Tokyo: Chuo-hoki-shuppan, 1995), pp. 4–5.

27. E. Miyazaki, 'Survey of the Elderly', in Social Welfare Survey Research Council (ed.), *Pre-War Social Work Survey in Japan* (Tokyo: Keiso-shobo, 1983), pp. 336–52, on p. 345; Statistics Bureau, *Population Estimates of Japan 1920–2000* (Tokyo: Japan Statistical Association, 2003), pp. 16–33. Note: Population data below derive from the latter source, unless otherwise stated.

28. B. Takahashi, 'Youikusha Old People's Almshouse', in Central Charity Association (ed.), *Historical Sources for the Old-Age Pension System and Almshouse* (Tokyo: Central Charity Association, 1937), repr. in Y. Ogasawara (ed.), *Basic Historical Sources for Old Age Research* (hereafter *Historical Sources*), 29 vols (Tokyo: Ozora-sha, 1990–2), vol. 3, pp. 1–8, on p. 2.

29. NCSW, *Cheerful Elderly Welfare* (Tokyo: NCSW, 1953), repr. in Ogasawara (ed.), *Historical Sources*, vol. 29, p. 18.

30. Cited in Imura, *History of Old People's Almshouses*, p. 28.

31. Cited in Ikeda, *History of Japanese Social Welfare*, p. 338.

32. Komatsu, 'The State and Social Welfare in Japan', p. 134.

33. Ogasawara, '100-Year History', p. 47. See also Momose, *History of Elderly Welfare in Japan*, pp. 50–3.

34. Y. Ichibangase, '100-Year History of Tokyo Borough Almshouse', in Tokyo Borough Almshouse Committee (ed.), *127–Year History of Tokyo Borough Almshouse* (Tokyo: Hobun-sha, 1999), pp. 164–78, on p. 165.

35. Ibid., pp. 173, 177; Ogasawara, '100-Year History', p. 10.

36. H. Yabe, 'History and Life of Tokyo Borough Almshouse 1872–1975', in Tokyo Borough Almshouse Committee (ed.), *127–Year History of Tokyo Borough Almshouse* (Tokyo: Hobun-sha, 1999), pp. 217–58, on p. 220.

37. Ogasawara, '100-Year History', pp. 11–12.

38. Poor Law, No. 39 (1929), Article 7. See MoHW Board, *Fifty-Year History*, pp. 258–9. Note: In Japan, since 1925 only males aged 25 or over, paying a minimum level of tax, were enfranchised.

39. Y. Washiya, 'The Wartime Poor Relief System', in Japan University of Social Work (ed.), *Poor Law System in Japan* (Tokyo: Keiso-shobo, 1960), pp. 223–68, on pp. 250–3.

40. Miyazaki, 'Survey of the Elderly', p. 341.

41. T. Terawaki, 'Survey of Poor Relief Recipients and Eligible People', in Social Welfare Survey Research Council (ed.), *Pre-War Social Work Survey in Japan* (Tokyo: Keiso-shobo, 1983), pp. 94–143, on p. 109.

42. Y. Aida (ed.), *The Third National Survey of Institutional Care Provision for the Elderly* (Tokyo: Zenkoku-yoro-jigyo-kyokai, 1940), repr. in Ogasawara (ed.), *Historical Sources*, vol. 4, p. 1; T. Okamoto, 'Wartime History of Institutional Care for the Elderly', *Social Gerontology*, 21 (1984), pp. 84–95, p. 94.

43. Ogasawara, '100-Year History', p. 85.

44. Ibid., pp. 84–6.
45. Cited in Imura, *History of Old People's Almshouses*, p. 47.
46. Ogasawara, '100-Year History', p. 90.
47. Y. Aida (ed.), *The Second National Survey of Institutional Care Provision for the Elderly* (Tokyo: Zenkoku-yoro-jigyo-kyokai, 1936), repr. in Ogasawara (ed.), *Historical Sources*, vol. 4, pp. 14–15.
48. Y. Ogasawara, 'History and Remnants of Old People's Home', in NCSW and NCEH (eds), *Annual Report on Elderly Welfare 1982* (Tokyo: NCSW, 1982), pp. 140–55, on pp. 149–55.
49. Ibid., p. 155.
50. Note: The main aim of the English COS was to avoid multiplication of charity organizations, whereas that of the Japanese CCA was to promote charitable work. See Chapter 1, p. 17.
51. Ogasawara, '100-Year History', pp. 67–9.
52. Ibid., pp. 70–7. The first week-long staff training event was held in *Rakufuen* (Tokyo) in 1937, cited in *Journal of Social Work for the Elderly*, 18 (1937), repr. in Ogasawara (ed.), *Historical Sources*, vol. 11, pp. 36–42. Note: The Association later became the National Council of Elderly Homes (NCEH).
53. For a summary, see Goodman, 'The "Japanese-Style Welfare State"', pp. 141–2; and Adachi, 'The Development of Social Welfare Services in Japan', pp. 197–8.
54. Ito, *History of Social Security*, pp. 167–8.
55. T. Kimura, *A History of Social Services in Modern Japan* (Kyoto: Minerva, 1964), p. 133.
56. Ikeda, *History of Japanese Social Welfare*, p. 696.
57. Cited in Ichibangase, '100-Year History of Tokyo Borough Almshouse', p. 172.
58. Cited in *Journal of Social Work for the Elderly*, 24 (1943), pp. 32–3, repr. in Ogasawara (ed.), *Historical Sources*, vol. 12, p. 32.
59. Ogasawara, '100-Year History', p. 98.
60. Yabe, 'History and Life of Tokyo Borough Almshouse 1872–1975', p. 205.
61. Cited in M. Ogawa, 'Social Work in Wartime', in Tokyo Borough Almshouse Committee (ed.), *127-Year History of Tokyo Borough Almshouse* (Tokyo: Hobun-sha, 1999), pp. 179–201, on p. 194.
62. Ogasawara, '100-Year History', pp. 107–8.
63. Viz. the 1937 Military Relief Act; the 1937 Mother and Baby Relief Act; the 1941 Health Relief Act; and the 1942 Wartime Disaster Assistance Act. In 1944 there were 2.5 million recipients under the 1937 Act and 1.2 million under the 1942 Act, compared with 143,000 under the 1929 Poor Law, in MoHW Board, *Fifty-Year History*, p. 477.
64. Ikeda, *History of Japanese Social Welfare*, p. 778.
65. Speech by Minister of Health Koichi Kido in 1938, cited in Ikeda, *History of Japanese Social Welfare*, p. 774.
66. D. Maeda, 'The Socioeconomic Context of Japanese Social Policy for Aging', in Long (ed.), *Caring for the Elderly in Japan and the US*, pp. 28–51, on p. 31.
67. Gould, *Capitalist Welfare Systems*, p. 35.
68. N. Maruo, 'The Development of the Welfare Mix in Japan', in R. Rose and R. Shiratori (eds), *The Welfare State East and West* (Oxford: Oxford University Press, 1986), pp. 64–79, on p. 65.
69. Adachi, 'The Development of Social Welfare Services in Japan', pp. 191–2; K. Tamai, 'Development of Social Policy in Japan', in Izuhara (ed.), *Comparing Social Policies*, pp. 35–47, p. 37.

70. Lee, 'The Japanese Welfare State in Transition', p. 247.

71. Ministry of Health and Welfare (hereafter MoHW), *Annual Report of Health and Welfare 1998–9: Social Security and National Life* (Tokyo: Japan International Corporation of Welfare Services, 1999), p. 13.

72. MoHW, *White Paper on Health and Welfare 1956/7* (Tokyo: Toyokezai-shinpo-sha, 1956) (hereafter *MoHW Report 1956/7*), pp. 2–3.

73. T. Kida, 'History of Post-War National Assistance System Part 1', in Japan University of Social Work (ed.), *Poor Law System in Japan* (Tokyo: Keiso-shobo, 1960), pp. 299–342, on pp. 304–7.

74. National Assistance Act, No. 17 (1946), Article 2. See T. Momose, *History of the Welfare System in Japan* (Kyoto: Minerva, 1997), pp. 112–13; MoHW Board, *Fifty-Year History*, p. 585.

75. Yoshida, *New Edition: History of Japanese Social Services*, p. 290; M. Iwata, 'Survey of Public Assistance Recipients', in Social Welfare Survey Research Council (ed.), *Pre-War Social Work Survey in Japan* (Tokyo: Keiso-shobo, 1983), pp. 144–54, on p. 147.

76. *MoHW Report 1956/7*, p. 25.

77. Ibid., p. 32.

78. Y. Ogasawara, *Old People's Home as a 'Place for Living'* (Tokyo: Chuo-hoki-shuppan, 1999), p. 107.

79. Dowaen, *50-Year History of Dowaen* (Kyoto: Dowaen, 1971), pp. 77–8, cited in Ogasawara, *Old People's Home as a 'Place for Living'*, p. 106.

80. Constitution of Japan (1946), Article 25. Other important legislation included the 1947 Child Welfare Act and the 1949 Welfare for the Physically Disabled Persons Act, each offering specific services, distinct from the 1950 National Assistance Act.

81. New National Assistance Act, No. 144 (1950), Articles 64–9. See MoHW Board, *Fifty-Year History*, pp. 611–13.

82. New National Assistance Act, Articles 30, 38.

83. MoHW Board, *Fifty-Year History*, p. 610.

84. Social Services Reform Act, No. 45 (1951). See MoHW Board, *Fifty-Year History*, pp. 748–54.

85. Noguchi, 'Residential Care for the Elderly in Japan', p. 125.

86. *MoHW Report 1956/7*, p. 32; Ogasawara, *Basics and Theory of Nursing Care*, pp. 15–16.

87. H. Tsuruta, *Analysis of Old People's Institution Survey* (Tokyo: Shakai-fukushi-shisetsu-kenkyu-kai, 1956), repr. in Ogasawara (ed.), *Historical Sources*, vol. 9, pp. 162–3.

88. M. Mori, *Theory of the Old People's Home* (Osaka: Rojin-seikatsu-kenkyu-jo, 1978), pp. 41–2.

89. Tsuruta, *Analysis of Old People's Institution Survey*, p. 156.

90. Ibid., pp. 26, 62.

91. New National Assistance Act (1950), Articles 46, 48. See MoHW (ed.), *Welfare Institutions in Japan* (Tokyo: Shakai-fukushi-chosa-kai, 1981), pp. 266–7.

92. Tsuruta, *Analysis of Old People's Institution Survey*, pp. 157–8.

93. O. Kawabata, K. Atsumi and S. Shimamura, *Daily Chronology of Older People 1925–2000* (Tokyo: Nihon Editor School Press, 2001) (hereafter *Chronology*), p. 22.

94. Y. Okamoto, *Medical Care and Welfare for the Elderly* (Tokyo: Iwanami-shinsho, 1996), pp. 36–8.

95. *MoHW Report 1956/7*, p. 25. In English, see MoHW, *Annual Report of Health and Welfare 1998–9: Social Security and National Life*, p. 17.

96. Maeda, 'The Socioeconomic Context', p. 31. See also Fukutake, *The Structure of Japanese Society*, pp. 181–2.

97. T. Momose, *The Establishment of 'Social Welfare'* (Kyoto: Minerva, 2002), p. 238.

98. *MoHW Report 1981/2*, pp. 550–2.

99. *MoHW Report 1956/7*, pp. 8–10, 18.

100. Cited in Momose, *The Establishment of 'Social Welfare'*, p. 220.

101. *MoHW Report 1957/8*, pp. 178, 190.

102. *MoHW Report 1956/7*, pp. 169–70.

103. J. C. Campbell, *How Policies Change: The Japanese Government and the Aging Society* (Princeton, NJ and Oxford: Princeton University Press, 1992), p. 358, Japanese translation available.

104. *MoHW Report 1961/2*, p. 178; Kawabata et al., *Chronology*, pp. 27, 32–3.

105. Seikatsu-kagaku-chosa-kai (ed.), *Research on the Old Age Problem* (Tokyo: Ishiyaku-shuppan, 1961), pp. 68–70.

106. *MoHW Report 1960/1*, p. 118.

107. Ibid., pp. 118–21.

108. Seikatsu-kagaku-chosa-kai (ed.), *Research on the Old Age Problem*, pp. 190–1.

109. *Asahi Newspaper*, 18 February 1955; *Asahi Evening Newspaper*, 17, 19 and 20 February 1955.

110. Kawabata et al., *Chronology*, p. 36.

111. MoHW, *A Code of Practice for Assessed Institutions* (Tokyo: Seikatsu-fukushi-shisetsu-kenkyu-kai, 1957), repr. in Ogasawara (ed.), *Historical Sources*, vol. 6, pp. 36–7.

112. Noguchi, 'Residential Care for the Elderly in Japan', p. 130; Tsuruta, *Analysis of Old People's Institution Survey*, p. 165.

113. Tsuruta, *Analysis of Old People's Institution Survey*, p. 53.

114. Mori, *Theory of the Old People's Home*, p. 116.

115. *MoHW Report 1962/3*, pp. 55–6; *MoHW Report 1963/4*, p. 174.

116. *MoHW Report 1962/3*, p. 42.

117. Seikatsu-kagaku-chosa-kai (ed.), *Research on the Old Age Problem*, pp. 127, 130.

118. *MoHW Report 1963/4*, p. 174.

119. Kawabata et al., *Chronology*, pp. 29, 33.

120. Campbell, *How Policies Change*, p. 109.

121. *MoHW Report 1963/4*, p. 169.

122. Elderly Welfare Act, No. 133 (1963), Articles 11, 14. See Shakai-fukushi-jigyo-shinko-kai (ed.), *The New Old People's Home* (Tokyo: Shakai-fukushi-shinko-kenkyu-kai, 1964), repr. in Ogasawara (ed.), *Historical Sources*, vol. 9, pp. 99–103. Note: Unless otherwise stated, home figures are from MoHW, *Summary of the Year 1975/6 Social Welfare Facilities Survey*, 2 vols (Tokyo: MoHW Statistics Bureau, 1975 and successive years).

123. *MoHW Report 1963/4*, p. 175.

124. MoHW, *Ten-Year History of Elderly Welfare* (Tokyo: MoHW, 1974), p. 76.

125. Maeda, 'The Socioeconomic Context', p. 37; Campbell, *How Policies Change*, p. 112.

126. M. Mori, *A New Evolution of the 'Aged Theory': Criticism of Current Gerontology* (Higashimurayama: Kirisutokyo-tosho-shuppan, 1995), p. 99.

127. S. Tanaka, 'The Institutional Care System in Japan', in H. Asano and S. Tanaka (eds), *Institutional Care in Japan* (Tokyo: Chuo-hoki-shuppan, 1993), pp. 245–85, on p. 262.

128. H. Hashimoto, 'The Margin of Welfare for the Aged in "The Law for the Welfare of the Aged"', in S. Nasu and Y. Yuzawa (eds), *A Sociological Study on Family Help for the Aged* (Tokyo: Kakiuchi-shuppan, 1973), pp. 311–52, on pp. 347–9.

129. T. Okamoto, *Establishment of the Elderly Welfare Act* (Tokyo, Seishin-shobo, 1993), p. 181.
130. Campbell, *How Policies Change*, p. 358.
131. Maeda, 'The Socioeconomic Context', p. 37.
132. *MoHW Report 1969/70*, p. 386; Kawabata et al., *Chronology*, pp. 49, 51.
133. Cited in Campbell, *How Policies Change*, p. 117.
134. Kokumin-seikatsu-shingikai-chosabu-rojin-mondai-shoiinkai, *Report on the Growing Old Age Problem* (Tokyo: MoHW, 15 September 1968). Full text available at National Institute of Population and Social Security Research website: http://www.ipss.go.jp/publication/j/shiryou/no.13/data/shiryou/syakaifukushi/23.pdf [accessed 10 August 2012].
135. *MoHW Report 1969/70*, pp. 385, 387.
136. U. Mori, *Long-Term Care Insurance Reform in Contemporary Japan* (Kyoto: Horitsu-bunka-sha, 2008), pp. 25–33.
137. Central Committee of Social Welfare, *Comprehensive Programmes to Respond to Old Age Problem* (Tokyo: MoHW, 25 November 1970). Full text available at the National Council of Population and Social Security Research website, at http://www.ipss.go.jp/publication/j/shiryou/no.13/data/shiryou/syakaifukushi/46.pdf [accessed 10 August 2012].
138. S. Harada, 'The Aging Society, the Family, and Social Policy', *University of Tokyo Institute of Social Science Occasional Papers in Law and Society*, 8 (March 1996), pp. 1–70, on pp. 21–2; Kawabata et al., *Chronology*, p. 60.
139. *MoHW Report 1981/2*, pp. 472–3, 552, 556–7.
140. MoHW Board, *Fifty-Year History*, p. 1519.
141. *MoHW Report 1981/2*, p. 472.
142. Ibid., p. 552.
143. Kawabata et al., *Chronology*, p. 59.
144. MoHW Board, *Fifty-Year History*, p. 1180.
145. Viz. 71,500 nursing home places and 70,800 old people's home places in 1979.
146. MoHW (ed.), *Welfare Institutions in Japan*, pp. 271–2, 276.
147. M. Mori, *Old People in Japan and the World* (Tokyo: Shakai-hoken-shuppan-sha, 1974), pp. 179–80.
148. Mori, *Theory of the Old People's Home*, p. 8.
149. S. Tanikawa, 'A Modern Reading of "Ballad of Oak Mountain"', in NCSW and NCEH (eds), *Annual Report on Elderly Welfare 1976* (Tokyo: NCSW, 1976), pp. 50–6, on p. 51.
150. S. Ariyoshi, *Man in Rapture* (Tokyo: Shincho-bunko, 1972). Note: This was translated as *The Twilight Years* in 1984 and made into a powerful film.
151. Plath, 'Japan: The After Years', p. 137.
152. Kawabata et al., *Chronology*, p. 62.
153. MoHLW, *Patient Survey 2002*, 2 vols (Tokyo: MoHLW, 2004), vol. 1, pp. 92–3, 100. Cf. England and Wales had sixteen hospital beds and twenty-four residential home places per 1,000 older population in 1975.
154. *MoHW Report 1984/5*, p. 93; MoHLW, *Patient Survey 2002*, vol. 1, p. 112.
155. *MoHW Report 1985/6*, p. 45.
156. J. C. Campbell, 'Changing Meaning of Frail Old People and the Japanese Welfare State', in Long (ed.), *Caring for the Elderly in Japan and the US*, pp. 82–97, on p. 88.
157. Hayashi, 'The Care of Older People in Japan'.
158. Comments by Katsuo Iwata, Chair of National Council of Elderly Homes, cited in NCSW and NCEH (eds), *Annual Report on Elderly Welfare 1980* (Tokyo: NCSW, 1980), p. 19.

159. N. Otsuka, 'Current Situation and Reforms of Old People's Hospitals: Problems of Social Hospitalization', in H. Asano and S. Tanaka (eds), *Institutional Care in Japan* (Tokyo: Chuo-hoki-shuppan, 1993), pp. 200–22, on p. 203.

160. Cited in Tanaka, 'The Institutional Care System in Japan', p. 259.

161. Mori, *Theory of the Old People's Home*, p. 139; NCEH (ed.), *The Fourth National Survey of Elderly Homes* (Tokyo: NCEH, 1993), p. 36.

162. NCEH (ed.), *The Fourth National Survey of Elderly Homes*, p. 166.

163. S. Kinoshita, 'Living Space of the Elderly', in S. Nasu and M. Masuda (eds), *Japanese Elderly People*, 3 vols (Tokyo: Kakiuchi-shuppan, 1972), vol. 3, pp. 331–51, on p. 334.

164. For example, N. Hidaka, *Old People's Home Diary* (Tokyo: Asahi-shinbun-sha, 1979); T. Yoshida, *Old People's Home Now* (Kyoto: Minerva, 1980). See also local institutional studies in Chapter 6.

165. N. Ebie, 'Current Situation and Problem of the Nursing Home', in H. Asano and S. Tanaka (eds), *Institutional Care in Japan* (Tokyo: Chuo-hoki-shuppan, 1993), pp. 28–51, on pp. 38–40.

166. Mori, *Theory of the Old People's Home*, p. 153.

167. J. Sakai, 'Problems of Institutional Care', in NCSW and NCEH (eds), *Annual Report on Elderly Welfare 1980*, pp. 67–71, on p. 69.

168. NCEH (ed.), *The Fourth National Survey of Elderly Homes*, p. 81.

169. Ibid., p. 83.

170. Tanikawa, 'A Modern Reading of "Ballad of Oak Mountain"', p. 54; M. Kato, 'Elderly Women in Old People's Homes', in NCSW and NCEH (eds), *Annual Report on Elderly Welfare 1980*, pp. 105–10, on p. 106.

171. Mori, *Theory of the Old People's Home*, p. 171.

172. Ibid., p. 102.

173. Cited in Kawabata et al., *Chronology*, p. 57.

174. Tanikawa, 'A Modern Reading of "Ballad of Oak Mountain"', p. 53.

175. Quoted by R. Shiratori, 'The Future of the Welfare State', in R. Rose and R. Shiratori (eds), *The Welfare State East and West* (Oxford: Oxford University Press, 1986), pp. 193–206, on p. 198.

176. Cited in Kawabata et al., *Chronology*, p. 94.

177. Y. Okamoto, *History of Long-Term Care Insurance System* (Kyoto: Minerva: 2009), pp. 77–9.

178. *MoHW Report 1991/2*, pp. 268–9.

179. Viz. The combined places (228,000) in old people's homes and nursing homes in 1990 represented 15.4 per 1,000 older population, compared to 14.1 per 1,000 (151,000) a decade earlier, in *MoHW Report 1991/2*, pp. 268–9.

180. *MoHW Report 1991/2*, p. 269: Cf. 5 per 1,000 in the USA (1987), 6 in the UK (1988) and 12 in France (1987).

181. MoHLW, *Patient Survey 2002*, vol. 1, pp. 92–3, 101, 113; N. Ikegami, B. E. Fries, Y. Takagi, S. Ikeda and T. Ibe, 'Applying RUG-III in Japanese Long-Term Care Facilities', *Gerontologist*, 34:5 (1994), pp. 628–39, on p. 629.

182. Ikegami et al., 'Applying RUG–III in Japanese Long-Term Care Facilities', p. 629; M. W. Ribbe et al., 'Nursing Homes in 10 Nations: A Comparison between Countries and Settings', *Age and Aging*, 26:52 (1997), pp. 3–12.

183. Cited in Tanaka, 'The Institutional Care System in Japan', pp. 279–80.

184. S. Nishimura, 'Financing of Health Care for the Elderly in Japan', *Japan and the World Economy* (1993), pp. 107–20, on p. 117; *MoHW Report 1992/3*, p. 277.

185. Campbell, *How Policies Change*, p. 308.
186. Kawabata et al., *Chronology*, pp. 127, 134. Note: By then there were 772,000 elderly inpatients in hospitals, with 635,000 unable to be discharged, having nowhere to go; ibid., p. 175.
187. *MoHW Report 1991/2*, pp. 72–3.
188. *MoHW Report 1995/6*, pp. 110–11.
189. Cited in *MoHW Report 1993/4*, pp. 91–2.
190. T. K. Uzuhashi, 'Japan: Bidding Farewell to the Welfare Society', in Alcock and Craig (eds), *International Social Policy*, pp. 104–23, on pp. 122–3.
191. Campbell, 'Changing Meaning of Frail Old People', p. 90.
192. K. Adachi, J. E. Lubben and N. Tsukada, 'Expansion of Formalized In-Home Services for Japan's Aged', *Journal of Aging and Social Policy*, 8:2–3 (1996), pp. 147–59, on p. 156.
193. Izuhara, *Family Change and Housing*, p. 69; T. Kimura, 'From Transfer to Social Service: A New Emphasis on Social Policies for the Aged in Japan', *Journal of Aging and Social Policy*, 8:2–3 (1996), pp. 177–89, on p. 186. Note: The state subsidy for health care facilities was 30 per cent, compared to 50 per cent for nursing homes.
194. Maeda, 'The Socioeconomic Context', pp. 47–8.
195. M. Miyazaki, 'Welfare for the Elderly', in N. Sanada, K. Miyata, S. Kato and K. Kawai (eds), *Illustration: Social Welfare in Japan* (Kyoto: Horitsu-bunka-sha, 2004), pp. 92–109, on p. 103.
196. *Asahi Newspaper*, 19 December 1994.
197. M. Kono, 'The Welfare Mix in the Care of Older People in Japan' (PhD dissertation, University of Sheffield, 1997), p. 193; Kimura, 'From Transfer to Social Service', p. 181.
198. N. Ikegami, 'Public Long-Term Care Insurance in Japan', *Journal of the American Medical Association*, 278:16 (1997), pp. 1310–14, on p. 1311.
199. NCEH (ed.), *The Third National Survey of Elderly Homes* (Tokyo: NCSW and NCEH, 1988), p. 139; Y. Ogasawara et al., *For Whom Are Old People's Homes?* (Tokyo: Akebi-shobo, 1985), p. 168; I. Homma, *Fact of Life in a Nursing Home* (Tokyo: Akebi-shobo, 1995), p. 20.
200. NCEH (ed.), *The Third National Survey of Elderly Homes*, pp. 61–2, 135; Ogasawara et al., *For Whom Are Old People's Homes?*, p. 171.
201. Ogasawara et al., *For Whom Are Old People's Homes?*, p. 199.
202. NCEH (ed.), *The Third National Survey of Elderly Homes*, p. 141.
203. Ibid., pp. 74–8, 97.
204. Ibid., pp. 112–14.
205. MoHW (ed.), *A Code of Practice for Welfare Institutions*, 3 vols (Tokyo: NCSW, 1989); MoHW (ed.), *Revised Version: A Code of Practice for Welfare Institutions*, 3 vols (Tokyo: NCSW, 1994). For *Home Life*, see Chapter 1, p. 34.
206. Cited in Kawabata et al., *Chronology*, p. 142.
207. S. Hoshino, 'Paying for the Health and Social Care of the Elderly', *Journal of Aging and Social Policy*, 8:2–3 (1996), pp. 37–55, on p. 38.
208. Cabinet Office, *White Paper on the Ageing Society 2011/12* (Tokyo: Insatsu-tsuhan, 2011), pp. 2–3.
209. *MoHW Report 1997/8*, p. 111; MoHLW, *White Paper on Health, Labour and Welfare 2003/4* (Tokyo: Gyosei, 2003) (hereafter *MoHLW Report 2003/4*), p. 15.
210. *MoHW Report 1997/8*, p. 110 ; Kawabata et al., *Chronology*, pp. 140, 145.
211. H. Asano, 'Elderly Welfare Services', in Y. Ogasawara, Y. Hashimoto and H. Asano (eds), *Elderly Welfare*, 2nd edn (Tokyo : Yuhikaku, 2003), pp. 95–117, on p. 123; R.

Nakamura, 'Nursing Problems', in Y. Ogasawara, Y. Hashimoto and H. Asano (eds), *Elderly Welfare*, 2nd edn (Tokyo: Yuhikaku, 2003), pp. 41–57, on pp. 52–3. In English, see Y. Uehara, *Group Homes in Japan: Approaches to Dementia Care* (Ann Arbor, MI: Proquest, 2006).

212. *Asahi Newspaper*, 13 November 1994.
213. J. C. Campbell and N. Ikegami, 'Japan's Radical Reform of Long-Term Care', *Social Policy and Administration*, 37:1 (February 2003), pp. 21–34, on p. 24.
214. T. Tsutsui and N. Muramatsu, 'Care-Needs Certification in the Long-Term Care Insurance System of Japan', *International Health Affairs*, 53 (2005), pp. 522–7, on p. 523.
215. For a summary of LTCI, see K. Hiraoka, 'Long-Term Care Insurance in Japan', in H. Yoon and J. Hendricks (eds), *Handbook of Asian Aging* (New York: Baywood Publishing Co., 2006), pp. 123–46; and J. C. Campbell, N. Ikegami and S. Kwon, 'Policy Learning and Cross-National Diffusion in Social Long-Term Care Insurance: Germany, Japan and the Republic of Korea', *International Social Security Review*, 62:4 (2009), pp. 63–80.
216. Cited in N. Okitoh, *Can Long-Term Care Insurance Guarantee Old Age?* (Tokyo: Iwanami-shoten), p. 2.
217. For a summary, see Kosei-tokei-kyokai (ed.), *Illustration: Long-Term Care Insurance Statistics 2008* (Tokyo: Kosei-tokei-kyokai, 2008), pp. 10–23.
218. MoHLW, *The 2000 Survey of Long-Term Care Insurance Residential Facility Providing Agencies* (Tokyo: Kosei-tokei-kyokai, 2002), p. 56.
219. *Yomiuri Newspaper*, 28 January 2005; Tsutsui and Muramatsu, 'Care-Needs Certification', p. 527.
220. *MoHW Report 2000/1*, pp. 168–73.
221. *MoHLW Report 2005/6*, p. 248; MoHLW, *Summary of the Long-Term Care Insurance Act Reform* (Tokyo, MoHLW, March 2006), p. 2, at http://www.mhlw.go.jp/topics/kaigo/topics/0603/dl/data.pdf [accessed 10 August 2012].
222. *MoHLW Report 2005/6*, p. 249.
223. Y. Yuki, *Long-Term Care: Analysis from Grassroots Evidence* (Tokyo: Iwanami-shinsho, 2008), p. 31; Okamoto, *History of the Long-Term Care Insurance System*, pp. 173–4.
224. *Asahi Newspaper*, 5 February 2003.
225. *MoHLW Report 2003/4*, pp. 257–8.
226. MoHLW, *Summary of the Long-Term Care Insurance Act Reform*, pp. 2, 23.
227. Tsutsui and Muramatsu, 'Care-Needs Certification', p. 527.
228. See MoHLW, *Summary of the Long-Term Care Insurance Act Reform*.
229. Okitoh, *Can Long-Term Care Insurance Guarantee Old Age?*, p. 64.
230. MoHLW, *Annual Report on the Year 2010/11 Long-Term Care Insurance Scheme*, pp. 5, 8, 10, at http://www.mhlw.go.jp/topics/kaigo/osirase/jigyo/10/dl/h22_gaiyou.pdf [accessed 10 August 2012]; Tamiya et al., 'Population Ageing and Wellbeing', pp. 1184–5, 1188.
231. Y. Hashimoto, 'Long-Term Care Insurance System', in Y. Ogasawara, Y. Hashimoto and H. Asano (eds), *Elderly Welfare*, 2nd edn (Tokyo: Yuhikaku, 2003), pp. 119–58, on pp. 153–5.
232. Asano, 'Elderly Welfare Services', p. 111.
233. Introduced in 1987 and raised to 30 per cent from 2004; R. Hojo, 'Comfortable Living Environments', in K. Hara and M. Oshima (eds), *Explore Future of Facilities for the Elderly* (Kyoto: Minerva, 2005), pp. 130–60, on p. 140.
234. MoHLW, *Summary of the Long-Term Care Insurance Act Reform*, p. 23.
235. *MoHLW Report 2003/4*, pp. 79–83.
236. MoHLW, *The 2000 Survey of Long-Term Care Insurance Residential Facility Providing Agencies*, p. 64. For a summary of the group home, see H. Murota, 'Residential Care', in

T. Ota (ed.), *Introduction to Welfare for the Elderly*, 3rd edn (Tokyo: Koseikan, 2005), pp. 117–36, on pp. 128–31.

237. T. Toyama, 'The Necessity in Single Rooms as Living Space', in W. Omori (ed.), *New-Style Nursing Homes* (Tokyo: Chuo-hoki-shuppan, 2002), pp. 44–73, on pp. 63–7.

238. S. Ito, 'Long-Term Care Insurance Scheme', in N. Sanada, K. Miyata, S. Kato and K. Kawai (eds), *Illustration: Social Welfare in Japan* (Kyoto: Horitsu-bunka-sha, 2004), pp. 164–77, on p.168; A. Kumon, 'Pensions', in N. Sanada, K. Miyata, S. Kato and K. Kawai (eds), *Illustration: Social Welfare in Japan* (Kyoto: Horitsu-bunka-sha, 2004), pp. 178–91, on p. 182.

239. M. Izuhara, 'Social Inequality under a New Social Contract: Long-Term Care in Japan', *Social Policy and Administration*, 37:4 (2003), pp. 395–410, on p. 408.

240. Okitoh, *Can Long-Term Care Insurance Guarantee Old Age?*, pp. 31–93; Yuki, *Long-Term Care*, pp. 63–71.

241. *Japan Financial Newspaper*, 4 April 2012.

242. A. Konuma, 'Issue Brief: Restructuring Long-Stay Hospital Beds', *Research and Information*, 590 (7 June 2007), pp. 1–10, on pp. 1, 10, held at National Diet Library; also at http://www.ndl.go.jp/jp/data/publication/issue/0590.pdf [accessed 10 August 2012].

243. Cabinet Office, *White Paper on the Ageing Society 2011/12*, p. 5.

244. *MoHLW Report 2005/6*, p. 12.

245. *MoHLW Report 2003/4*, p. 57.

246. Cabinet Office, *White Paper on the Ageing Society 2011/12*, p. 19.

247. MoHLW, *Summary of the Long-Term Care Insurance Act Reform and Philosophy of Comprehensive Community Care* (Tokyo: MoHLW, 2012), at http://www.mhlw.go.jp/stf/shingi/2r98520000026b0a–att/2r98520000026b4b.pdf [accessed 10 August 2012].

3 The Norfolk Experience

1. A. Digby, 'Poor Law Unions and Workhouses 1834–1930', in T. Ashwin and A. Davison (eds), *An Historical Atlas of Norfolk*, 3rd edn (Chichester: Phillimore, 2005), pp. 148–9; K. Morrison, *The Workhouse: A Study of Poor Law Buildings in England* (Swindon: Royal Commission on the Historical Monuments of England, 1999), pp. 207–8.

2. F. W. S. Craig (ed.), *British Parliamentary Election Results* (hereafter *BPER*) *1918–49*, 3rd edn (Chichester: Parliamentary Research Services, 1983), pp. 431–5; Craig (ed.), *BPER 1950–73* (1983), pp. 454–9; Craig (ed.), *BPER 1974–83* (1984), pp. 190–1.

3. Figures from 1931 and 1991 Censuses, referring to England and Wales.

4. B. M. Doyle, 'Politics, 1835–1945', in C. Rawcliffe and R. Wilson (eds), *Norwich Since 1550* (London and New York: Hambledon & London, 2004), pp. 343–60; Craig (ed.), *BPER, 1918–49*, p. 206; Craig (ed.), *BPER, 1950–73*, pp. 224–5; Craig (ed.), *BPER 1974–83*, p. 194.

5. Norfolk Record Office (hereafter NRO), N/TC31/1/1–5, Norwich City Council Public Assistance Committee Minutes 1929–39 (hereafter Norwich PACM), 27 November 1929, pp. 2–3.

6. E. R. Kelly (ed.), *Kelly's Directory of Norfolk*, 20th edn (London: Kelly's Directories, 1933), p. 303; D. Humphreys, *Born Poor: Records, Porter's Lodge and Tramps' Quarters*, privately printed for Age Concern, Norwich, 1990, p. 6, held at Norfolk Heritage Centre; A. Digby, *Pauper Palaces* (London: Routledge & Kegan Paul, 1978), p. 69.

7. S. Cherry, 'Medical Care since 1750', in C. Rawcliffe and R. Wilson (eds), *Norwich since 1550* (London and New York: Hambledon & London, 2004), pp. 271–93, on p. 291;

W. G. Savage, C. Frankau and B. Gibson, *Hospital Survey: The Hospital Services of the Eastern Area* (London: HMSO, 1945), p. 4.

8. NRO, C/SS1/32, House Classification List 1916–42, pp. 111–17.
9. Norfolk Heritage Centre, N361.6, Norwich City Council Public Assistance Committee Reports 1930–9 (hereafter Norwich PAC Reports), 14 December 1932, p. 7.
10. Norwich PAC Report, 5 December 1930, p. 9.
11. Norfolk Heritage Centre, L614, Norwich City Council Medical Officer of Health Annual Reports, 1938–55 (hereafter Norwich MOHA Reports), 1938, p. 21.
12. Norwich PACM, 23 February 1931, p. 55.
13. Humphreys, *Born Poor*, p. 9.
14. Norwich PAC Report, 14 December 1932, p. 9.
15. Humphreys, *Born Poor*, p .10.
16. House Classification List 1916–42, pp. 111–17.
17. Norwich PACM, 13 September 1939, p. 395.
18. Norwich PACM, 9 October 1940, p. 587.
19. Norwich PACM, 10 January 1940, p. 472.
20. Norwich PACM, 8 November 1939, p. 440.
21. NRO, N/TC31/1/6–8, Norwich City Council Social Welfare Committee Minutes 1939–48 (hereafter Norwich SWCM), 13 May 1942, p. 738.
22. Ibid.
23. Norwich SWCM, 10 September 1941, p. 665.
24. Norwich SWCM, 13 May 1942, p. 738.
25. Norwich SWCM, 26 May 1942, p. 744.
26. Norwich SWCM, 22 June 1942, pp. 753, 756.
27. Norwich SWCM, 28 September 1942, p. 807; NRO, C/SS1/27, Indoor Relief List 1942–9, pp. 1–20.
28. Savage, Frankau and Gibson, *Hospital Survey*, p. 17.
29. Norwich SWCM, 26 February 1943, p. 862.
30. Norwich SWCM, 9 June 1943, pp. 24–5; 10 November 1943, p. 88; 9 February 1944, p. 109.
31. Norwich SWCM, 10 January 1945, p. 190; 23 July 1945, p. 246; 12 November 1947, p. 56; 9 June 1948, p. 159.
32. Norwich SWCM, 12 November 1947, p. 56; 9 June 1948, p. 159.
33. Norwich SWCM, 1 March 1948, p. 118.
34. Norwich SWCM, 27 January 1947, p. 429.
35. Norfolk Heritage Centre, L614, Norfolk County Council Medical Officer of Annual Reports 1929–50 (hereafter Norfolk MOA Report), 1929, p. 8.
36. Local Government Act (1929), Part 1: Approval of Administrative Scheme, enclosed in NRO, C/C10/452, Norfolk County Council Public Assistance Advisory Committee Minutes 1929–30, 30 November 1929, #41.
37. NRO, C/C10/453–461, Norfolk County Council Public Assistance Sub-Committee Minutes 1930–48 (hereafter Norfolk PASCM), 9 October 1935, #1542.
38. Savage, Frankau and Gibson, *Hospital Survey*, p. 21.
39. Norfolk MOA Report, 1930, p. 19.
40. Norfolk PASCM, 1 January 1933, #789; 14 February 1934, #1073. Cf. 1,534 Norfolk PAI residents in total, in the 1931 Census.
41. Norfolk MOA Report, 1930, pp. 10–11, 14.
42. Norfolk MOA Report, 1934, p. 13.

43. Norfolk MOA Report, 1930, p. 10.
44. Norfolk MOA Report, 1934, p. 13.
45. Norfolk PASCM, 14 October 1931, #419.
46. S. Cherry, *Mental Health Care in Modern England: The Norfolk Lunatic Asylum/St Andrew's Hospital, c. 1810–1998* (Woodbridge: Boydell, 2003), pp. 176–7; Norfolk PASCM, 9 July 1930, #84.
47. Norfolk PASCM, 13 December 1933, #1030; Norfolk MOA Report, 1932, p. 11; Norfolk MOA Report, 1933, pp. 10–11.
48. Cherry, *Mental Health Care in Modern England*, pp. 180–1; Norfolk PASCM, 19 November 1930, #166.
49. Norfolk PASCM, 13 July 1932, #65.
50. Norfolk MOA Report, 1930, p.18.
51. Norfolk PASCM, 14 February 1934, #1073; Norfolk MOA Report, 1934, p. 14.
52. Norfolk PASCM, 14 February 1934, #1073.
53. Norfolk PASCM, 11 July 1934, #1179.
54. Norfolk PASCM, 6 September 1939, #2785.
55. Norfolk PASCM, 5 January 1944, #4023.
56. F. Meeres, *Norfolk in the Second World War* (Chichester: Phillimore, 2006), p. 82; A. Serreau, *Times and Years: A History of the Blofield Union Workhouse at Lingwood in the County of Norfolk* (Bungay: Morrow & Co., 2000), p. 222.
57. Norfolk PASCM, 5 January 1944, #4023; 13 February 1946, #4588.
58. Norfolk PASCM, 5 April 1944, #4087.
59. Norfolk PASCM, 1 March 1944, #4066.
60. Norfolk PASCM, 26 June 1944, #4156.
61. MoH, *Circular 49/47: The Care of the Aged in Public Assistance Homes and Institutions* (6 June 1947), enclosed in Norfolk PASCM, 7 May 1947, #425, Item 15.
62. Norfolk PASCM, 10 September 1947, #551; 8 October 1947, #577:4.
63. Norfolk PASCM, 11 June 1947, #481; 7 January 1948, #666.
64. Norfolk PASCM, 9 December 1931, #450.
65. S. Pope, *Gressenhall Farm and Workhouse* (Cromer: Poppyland, 2006), p. 85.
66. Norwich MOHA Report, 1948, p. 23; Norwich MOHA Report, 1951, p. 15.
67. Norwich Scheme (Norwich five-year local plan), enclosed in NRO, N/TC31/1/9–14, Norwich City Council Welfare Committee Minutes 1948–70 (hereafter Norwich WCM), 17 February 1949, p. 238.
68. N/TC31/1/9–14, Norwich City Council Hostels Sub-Committee Minutes 1948–70 (hereafter Norwich HSCM), 20 June 1949, p. 284; 7 January 1949, p. 224. Note: These are included within Norwich WCM.
69. Norwich HSCM, 29 March 1951, p. 497.
70. *Eastern Daily Press*, 22 March 1952; 5 March 1954.
71. Norwich MOHA Report, 1955, p. 42.
72. For example, Drayton Wood with thirty-eight acres of land and The Lawn with two acres, in Norwich WCM, 13 September 1965, p. 39.
73. Norwich WCM, 24 November 1952, p. 178; Norwich HSCM, 19 November 1951, p. 67; Norwich WCM, 28 March 1955, p. 444.
74. Norwich WCM, 26 October 1959, p. 411; Norwich HSCM, 21 February 1955, p. 434.
75. Norwich WCM, 23 March 1959, p. 349.
76. Norwich WCM, 26 October 1959, p. 411; 5 January 1961, p. 66.
77. Norwich HSCM, 21 January 1957, p. 125; Norwich WCM, 5 January 1961, p. 66.

78. Norwich WCM, 5 January 1961, p. 66.
79. Norwich WCM, 8 January 1962, p. 194.
80. Norwich HSCM, 7 January 1949, p. 224.
81. Norwich Scheme (Norwich five-year local plan), enclosed in Norwich WCM, 17 February 1949, p. 238; Norwich WCM, 16 March 1949, p. 248.
82. Norwich WCM, 1 June 1950, p. 402; 9 March 1959, p. 345.
83. Norwich WCM, 26 October 1959, p. 411.
84. Norwich WCM, 21 July 1955, p. 478.
85. Norwich WCM, 27 June 1955, p. 474.
86. Norwich WCM, 27 July 1959, p. 390.
87. Norwich WCM, 8 January 1962, p. 193.
88. Norwich WCM, 11 July 1960, p. 6; 24 October 1960, p. 44.
89. MoH, *Community Care Plan*, pp. 150, 366.
90. Norwich WCM, 22 October 1962, p. 291.
91. Ibid.
92. MoH, *Community Care Plan*, pp. 150, 366.
93. Norfolk PASCM, 10 March 1948, #745.
94. Norfolk PASCM, 24 January 1948, #693.
95. NRO, C/C10/675–683, Norfolk County Council Welfare Committee Minutes 1948–70 (hereafter Norfolk WCM), 16 July 1958, #6:5.
96. Norfolk WCM, 21 July 1948, #17.
97. Norfolk Scheme (Norfolk five-year local plan), enclosed in Norfolk WCM, 9 March 1949, #178.
98. Ibid.
99. Ibid.
100. Ibid.
101. Norfolk WCM, 11 October 1950, #545:2; Norfolk MO Report 1950, p. 58.
102. Norfolk WCM, 13 September, 1950, #526:5.
103. Norfolk WCM, 10 September 1952, #945:4.
104. Norfolk WCM, 11 October 1950, #545:2.
105. Ibid.
106. Ibid.
107. Norfolk WCM, 10 September 1952, #945:4.
108. Norfolk WCM, 4 November 1953, #1212:12(a).
109. Norfolk WCM, 16 July 1958, #6:5; 10 September 1952, #945:4.
110. Norfolk WCM, 9 February 1949, #161:5; 9 March 1949, #178:3, #182:7.
111. Norfolk WCM, 10 January 1951, #597.
112. Norfolk WCM, 5 September 1962, #4:4.
113. Norfolk WCM, 16 July 1958, #6:5. Note: It was later sold and became the 3-star Sea Marge Hotel; see *Eastern Daily Press*, 2 February 1998.
114. Norfolk WCM, 13 September 1950, #526:5.
115. Norfolk WCM, 13 October 1954, #1433:2.
116. Norfolk WCM, 17 July 1957, #2025:10A.
117. Norfolk WCM, 13 October 1954, #1433:2.
118. *Eastern Daily Press*, 31 December 1953.
119. Norfolk WCM, 13 March 1957, #1930:2; 14 July 1954, #1395:4.
120. *Eastern Daily Press*, 16 November 1957.
121. Norfolk WCM, 13 March 1957, #1930:2; 14 July 1954, #1395:4.

122. Ibid.
123. Norfolk WCM, 12 June 1957, #2000:2. See Chapter 5, p. 123.
124. Norfolk WCM, 10 September 1958, #15:14; 12 November 1958, #15:13.
125. *Eastern Daily Press*, 12 January 1962. Note: Westfields was used to replace Eastgate House. See Chapter 5, p. 127.
126. *Eastern Daily Press*, 26 May 1960. Note: It was formerly a private home built in 1759, later used as a school.
127. Norfolk WCM, 15 April 1959, #17:16. This reflected MoH, *Circular 3/55*. See Chapter 1, p. 201 n. 94.
128. Norfolk WCM, 9 September 1959, #12.
129. Ibid.
130. Norfolk WCM, 11 May 1960, #4:2.
131. *Eastern Daily Press*, 31 August 1962.
132. Norfolk WCM, 4 December 1963, #3:5.
133. Norfolk WCM, 21 May 1958, #10:9.
134. MoH, *Community Care Plan*, pp. 146, 366; Norfolk WCM, 5 September 1962, #4:4. Note: All figures in this paragraph are from these sources.
135. Norwich WCM, 10 December 1962, p. 1; 9 December 1963, p. 118.
136. Norwich WCM, 9 March 1964, p. 49.
137. Ibid.; Norwich WCM, 10 January 1966, p. 95.
138. Norwich WCM, 12 September 1966, p. 163.
139. The forty represented 2.4 per 1,000 Norwich over-65s population, compared to 6.4 per 1,000 nationally, in Norwich WCM, 12 October 1964, p. 206.
140. Norwich WCM, 12 October 1964, p. 206.
141. Norwich WCM, 12 September 1966, p. 162.
142. Ibid.
143. Booklet, enclosed in Norwich WCM, 10 May 1965, p. 286.
144. Norwich WCM, 11 May 1964, pp. 163, 165.
145. Annual Report of the Chief Welfare Officer for 1966, pp. 15, 31, enclosed in Norwich WCM, 12 December 1966, p. 275.
146. Annual Report of the Chief Welfare Officer for 1966, pp. 10, 32.
147. Norwich HSCM, 13 December 1971, p. 83.
148. Norwich HSCM, 13 March 1972, p. 113; 8 January 1973, p. 47. See below, p. 223 n. 207.
149. Norwich WCM, 27 May 1963, p. 53; 14 September 1964, p. 196. See Chapter 5, p. 129.
150. Norwich WCM, 21 December 1967, p. 38.
151. Norwich WCM, 2 October 1969, p. 122.
152. Ibid.
153. Ibid.
154. Pamphlet: Norwich Social Services 1971–3, p. 15, enclosed in NRO, N/TC31/5/1–3, Norwich City Council Social Services Committee Minutes 1970–4 (hereafter Norwich SSCM), 27 March 1973.
155. Norwich WCM, 2 October 1969, p. 122.
156. Norwich WCM, 21 September 1970, p. 154.
157. Norwich SSCM, 31 January 1972, p. 98.
158. Norwich WCM, 14 December 1970, p. 165; Norwich SSCM, 11 January 1971, p. 7.
159. Pamphlet: Norwich Social Services 1971–3, p. 15.

160. Pamphlet: Norwich Social Services 1971–3, p. 15; Norwich SSCM, 4 September 1972, p. 155.
161. Pamphlet: Norwich Social Services 1971–3, p. 15.
162. Norwich SSCM, 11 June 1973, p. 93.
163. Norwich Ten Year Development Plan 1973–83, enclosed in Norwich SSCM, 27 February 1973, p. 63. Note: Figures in this paragraph are from this source.
164. Norwich SSCM, 10 December 1973, p. 36.
165. Norfolk WCM, 3 November 1965, #21.
166. MoH, *Hospital Plan*, pp. 82–7.
167. Norfolk WCM, 2 September 1964, #9:7.
168. Norfolk WCM, 1 September 1965, #17:16.
169. Norfolk WCM, 3 November 1965, #21; 21 September 1966, #28:22.
170. Norfolk WCM, 10 February 1965, #13:1.
171. Norfolk WCM, 14 April 1965, #9:8; 29 September 1965, #3:2.
172. Norfolk WCM, 3 November 1965, #21; 18 May 1966, #9:7.
173. Norfolk WCM, 15 March 1967, #6:4.
174. Norfolk WCM, 19 July 1967, #8:8; 10 July 1968, #5:4.
175. Norfolk WCM, 15 March 1967, #6:4; 30 September 1970, #4:2.
176. Norfolk WCM, 10 July 1968, #5:4; 9 December 1970, #17:17.
177. Norfolk WCM, 30 September 1970, #4:2; 9 December 1970, #17:17.
178. Ibid.
179. Norfolk WCM, 19 October 1966, #5.
180. Norfolk WCM, 30 September 1970, #4:2. See Chapter 3, p. 86.
181. Norfolk WCM, 20 September 1967.
182. Norfolk WCM, 18 December 1968, #4; 15 December 1971, #144. See also Chapter 5, p. 135.
183. Norfolk WCM, 21 September 1966, #28.
184. Norfolk WCM, 3 November 1965, #21; 14 June 1967, #19:18.
185. NRO, C/C10/610–611, Norfolk County Council Social Services Committee Minutes 1970–4 (hereafter Norfolk SSCM), 20 June 1973, #11:11.
186. For example, Priormead (Thetford, 1971) and Clere House (Ormesby, 1973). See Table 3.2, p. 94.
187. Norfolk WCM, 15 November 1967, #4.
188. *Eastern Daily Press*, 5 May and 14 October 1965.
189. Norfolk WCM, 21 January 1970, #12.
190. Norfolk WCM, 16 November 1966, #15:14.
191. *Eastern Daily Press*, 17 October 1971; Norfolk WCM, 21 January 1970, #12:12; Norfolk SSCM, 20 June 1973, #11:11.
192. Norfolk WCM, 20 September 1967, #7:5(c); 18 February 1970, #4:4(c); Norfolk SSCM, 14 February 1973, #2.
193. Norfolk WCM, 13 May 1970, #12; 30 September 1970, #4.
194. Norfolk SSCM, 17 October 1973, #3.
195. Ibid.
196. Norfolk SSCM, 21 April 1971, #10; 15 September 1971, #20.
197. Norfolk SSCM, 6 September 1972, #6.
198. Norfolk WCM, 9 December 1970, #17.
199. Norfolk Ten Year Development Plan 1973–83, enclosed in Norfolk SSCM, 14 February 1973.

200. Ibid.
201. Norfolk SSCM, 15 September 1971, #20; 5 September 1973, #4.
202. NCCSSCM, 27 June 1975, pp. 745, 767.
203. NCCSSCM, 21 March 1974, pp. 185, 229. Note: Beech House was later converted into the Norfolk Rural Life Museum; see *Eastern Daily Press*, 22 September 1975; Pope, *Gressenhall Farm and Workhouse*, pp. 90–1.
204. NCCSSCM, 23 June 1976, p. 291.
205. NCCSSCM, 12 February 1975, pp. 652–3; 27 June 1975, p. 812.
206. NCCSSCM, 11 September 1974, p. 411; 28 April 1976, p. 226.
207. NCCSSCM, 23 June 1976, p. 291.
208. NCCSSCM, 24 July 1979, p. 153.
209. NCCSSCM, 27 June 1975, p. 769; 14 September 1977, p. 910.
210. NCCSSCM, 15 September 1976, p. 422.
211. NCCSSCM, 23 June 1976, p. 292; 14 December 1977, p. 1014.
212. NCCSSCM, 23 June 1976, p. 262; 30 July 1976, p. 391.
213. NCCSSCM, 17 December 1975, p. 907.
214. NCCSSCM, 11 September 1974, p. 411; 14 December 1977, p. 1014; 12 December 1979, p. 333.
215. NCCSSCM, 27 June 1975, p. 808.
216. Ibid., p. 810.
217. NCCSSCM, 31 May 1977, p. 751; 26 July 1978, pp. 1424–5.
218. NCCSSCM, 15 September 1976, p. 426.
219. NCCSSCM, 14 December 1977, p. 986; 20 February 1980, p. 420.
220. NCCSSCM, 25 April 1978, p. 1361.
221. NCCSSCM, 4 July 1979, pp. 129–39; 10 December 1980, p. 802.
222. NCCSSCM, 4 October 1979, p. 25.
223. NCCSSCM, 18 June 1979, p. 155.
224. NCCSSCM, 31 May 1977, p. 745.
225. NCCSSCM, 18 September 1978, p. 1480.
226. NCCSSCM, 15 September 1976, pp. 401, 420; DHSS, *Priorities for Health and Personal Social Services in England*, p. 2.
227. NCCSSCM, 31 May 1977, pp. 745–6.
228. NCCSSCM, 18 December 1978, pp. 1480–1.
229. NCCSSCM, 20 July 1977, p. 807; *Eastern Daily Press* and *Eastern Evening News*, 26 and 30 July 1977.
230. NCCSSCM, 18 September 1978, p. 1449.
231. *Eastern Daily Press*, 15 February 1978.
232. *Eastern Daily Press*, 2 August 1977.
233. NCCSSCM, 4 October 1979, pp. 255–6.
234. NCCSSCM, 12 December 1979, p. 333.
235. NCCSSCM, 20 February 1980, p. 420.
236. NCCSSCM, 23 June 1976, p. 292; 10 December 1980, p. 792.
237. NCCSSCM, 18 September 1978, p. 1481; 9 June 1980, p. 526.
238. NCCSSCM, 9 June 1980, p. 526.
239. NCCSSCM, 13 December 1978, p. 1612.
240. Ibid., p. 1616; NCCSSCM, 24 July 1979, p. 177; Weaver, Willcocks and Kellaher, *The Business of Care*, p. 14.

241. NCCSSCM, 14 December 1977, p. 1025; 18 September 1978, p. 1460; 10 December 1980, pp. 801, 811.
242. NCCSSCM, 28 April 1976, p. 522.
243. Ibid., p. 521.
244. NCCSSCM, 15 December 1976, p. 516; 13 December 1978, p. 1616.
245. NCCSSCM, 18 December 1978, p. 1481; 18 June 1979, pp. 153–4.
246. Weaver, Willcocks and Kellaher, *The Business of Care*, p. 14.
247. Ibid., p. 29.

4 The Gifu Experience

1. Gifu Prefecture Statistics Division (ed.), *Data Gifu Prefecture 2007–8* (Gifu: Gifu Prefecture, 2008), p. 2.
2. Ibid., pp. 4–6; Statistics Bureau, *Population Estimates of Japan 1920–2000*, pp. 148–59, 278–90; Y. Asai and S. Miwa, 'Research on the Aged in Gifu Prefecture: Ageing Demographical Trends and Reforms', *Gifu Woman's University Journal*, 11 (1993), pp. 27–43, on pp. 29–41. Note: Population data below derive from these sources, unless otherwise stated.
3. Figures from Y. Aida (ed.), *The First National Survey of Institutional Care Provision for the Elderly* (Tokyo: Zenkoku-yoro-jigyo-kyokai, 1933), repr. in Ogasawara (ed.), *Historical Sources*, vol. 4, p. 4; Aida (ed.), *The Second National Survey*, p. 4; Aida (ed.), *The Third National Survey*, p. 7.
4. S. Umemura, 'History of Yamamoto Relief Institution', *Gifu Local History Journal*, 14 (1976), pp. 13–17, on p. 13. Note: In 1868 Japan had just thirty such facilities, including this; W. Omata, *History of Psychiatry* (Tokyo: Daisan-bunmei-sha, 2005), pp. 115–16.
5. S. Kure, *Contemporary Institutions for the Insane in Japan* (publisher unknown, 1920), pp. 125–6, National Diet Library Digital Archive Portal, at http://kindai.ndl.go.jp [accessed 10 August 2012]; Umemura, 'History of Yamamoto Relief Institution', p. 17.
6. Gifu Prefecture (ed.), *History of Gifu Prefecture, Modern*, 3 vols (Gifu: Gifu Prefecture, 1967), vol. 1, pp. 1052–5; Central Charity Association, *National Directory of Social Services 1937/8*, 2 vols (Tokyo: Central Charity Association, 1938), vol. 1, repr. in Shakai-fukushi-chosa-kenkyu-kai (ed.), *Historical Sources for the Pre-War Social Services*, 20 vols, 2nd edn (Tokyo: Nihon-tosho-senta, 1996), vol. 12, p. 387.
7. Gifu Prefecture Statistics Division (ed.), *Digital Archives Gifu Prefecture Statistics 1874–2011* (hereafter *Gifu Statistics*) *1925*, p. 3, at http://www.pref.gifu.lg.jp/kensei-unei/tokeijoho/gifuken-tokeisho/mainendeta [accessed 10 August 2012].
8. *Gifu Statistics 1925*, p. 3; *Gifu Statistics 1928*, p. 6.
9. *Gifu Statistics 1935*, p. 1.
10. *Gifu Statistics 1928*, pp. 6, 27–8; *Gifu Statistics 1930*, p. 6.
11. Aida (ed.), *The Third National Survey*, pp. 1–4.
12. Gifu Prefecture (ed.), *Plain History of Gifu Prefecture* (Gifu: Gifu Prefecture, 2001), pp. 416–19. Note: In Japan, since 1925 only males aged 25 or over, paying a minimum level of taxation, were enfranchised. Thus just 42,000 (5 per cent of the prefecture population) were eligible at the first local election in 1879, and 10,000 at the 1890 first national election.
13. Gifu Prefecture (ed.), *History of Gifu Prefecture, Modern*, vol. 3, p. 1335.
14. K. Yoshida, 'Poor Relief System, 1868–1911', in Japan University of Social Work (ed.), *Poor Law System in Japan* (Tokyo: Keiso-shobo, 1960), pp. 49–100, on p. 88.
15. Gifu Prefecture (ed.), *History of Gifu Prefecture, Modern*, vol. 3, p. 1341.

16. Ibid.; 'The Recent Earthquake in Japan', *The Times*, 8 December 1891, p. 5.
17. Gifu Prefecture (ed.), *History of Gifu Prefecture, Modern*, vol. 3, p. 1341.
18. *Gifu-nichinichi Newspaper*, 26 November 1917.
19. Gifu Prefecture (ed.), *History of Gifu Prefecture, Modern*, vol. 3, pp. 1334, 1356.
20. Gifu Old People's Almshouse Annual Report 1933, privately printed *c*. 1933, held at Gifu Public Library (hereafter GAR 1933).
21. Ibid.
22. Ibid.; Gifu City Welfare Division, *Directory of Welfare Work in Gifu City for 1940* (Gifu: Gifu City, 1940), pp. 40–2.
23. Gifu City Welfare Division, *Directory of Welfare Work in Gifu City for 1940*, p. 42.
24. S. Umemura 'A Short History of Gifu Prefecture Social Work', *Journal of Chubu Woman's Junior College*, 13 (1983), pp. 53–69, on pp. 60–7. See also Chapter 2, p. 44.
25. Umemura, 'A Short History of Gifu Prefecture Social Work', pp. 65–7.
26. Takayama City (ed.), *Reprinted: History of Takayama City*, 2 vols (1952–3; Takayama: Takayama-insatsu Co., 1981), vol. 2, pp. 869–71.
27. Takayama City (ed.), *History of Takayama City*, 3 vols (Takayama: Takayama-insatsu Co., 1983), vol. 1, p. 64.
28. Gifu Prefecture (ed.), *History of Gifu Prefecture, Modern*, vol. 1, p. 1084; Gifu Prefecture (ed.), *Plain History of Gifu Prefecture*, p. 433.
29. Yorokaen History Draft, *c*. 1970. Information in this paragraph from this source. Note: *Yorokaen* documents held at the premises, unless otherwise specified.
30. Yorokaen Annual Financial Statements 1923–58 (hereafter YAFS), 1930–3.
31. YAFS, 1925, 1938.
32. YAFS, 1933, 1927–39.
33. YAFS, 1931, 1933; Aida (ed.), *The Second National Survey*, p. 72.
34. YAFS, 1939–45.
35. Yorokaen Registers of Deaths and Discharges 1926–95 (hereafter YRDD).
36. Gifu Prefecture (ed.), *History of Gifu Prefecture, Modern*, vol. 3, p. 1124; Gifu Prefecture (ed.), *History of Gifu Prefecture, Post-Contemporary* (Gifu: Gifu Prefecture, 2003), p. 4.
37. Aida (ed.), *The Second National Survey*, pp. 28–9, 36–41.
38. GAR 1933.
39. Ibid.; YRDD.
40. YAFS, 1926–45.
41. Gifu City Relief Division, *Directory of Welfare Work in Gifu City for 1932* (Gifu: Gifu City, 1932), pp. 22–3.
42. Takayama City (ed.), *History of Takayama City*, vol. 1, p. 64.
43. Aida (ed.), *The Second National Survey*, pp. 10, 72–3.
44. GAR 1933.
45. Takayama City (ed.), *Reprinted: History of Takayama City*, vol. 2, p. 871.
46. Aida (ed.), *The Second National Survey*, pp. 68, 72–4.
47. Ibid.
48. Gifu City (ed.), *A History of Gifu City, Contemporary* (Gifu: Gifu City, 1981), p. 742; Gifu Record Office (hereafter GRO), 5.02-S38-2, Hino Home File 1950–63; Ogaki City (ed.), *History of Ogaki City*, 3 vols (1968; Kyoto: Rinkawa-shoten, 1987), vol. 2, pp. 827–8.
49. Zenkoku-yoro-jigyo-kyokai *National Survey of Elderly Institutions 1949* (Tokyo: Zenkoku-yoro-jigyo-kyokai, 1950), repr. in Ogasawara, *Historical Sources*, vol. 29, p. 36.

50. Gifu City Welfare Division, *Directory of Welfare Work in Gifu City for 1940*, p. 41; Gifu Times (ed.), *Gifu Yearbook for 1949* (Gifu: Gifu Times, 1948), p. 179.

51. Gifu Times (ed.), *Gifu Yearbook for 1951* (Gifu: Gifu Times, 1950), p. 201; Gifu Prefecture (ed.), *History of Gifu Prefecture, Modern*, vol. 2, pp. 1117–18; Gifu Prefecture (ed.). *History of Gifu Prefecture, Post-Contemporary*, p. 5.

52. Gifu Prefecture (ed.), *History of Gifu Prefecture, Modern*, vol. 2, p. 1126.

53. Gifu Times (ed.), *Gifu Yearbook for 1949*, p. 176; Gifu Times (ed.), *Gifu Yearbook for 1950* (Gifu: Gifu Times, 1949), p. 159.

54. Gifu Times (ed.), *Gifu Yearbook for 1949*, pp. 179–80; *Gifu Yearbook for 1950*, p. 162; GRO, 5.02-S21-1, Plans for Emergency Relief Institutions 1946–48.

55. Gifu Times (ed.), *Gifu Yearbook for 1950*, p. 154; Gifu Prefecture (ed.), *Plain History of Gifu Prefecture*, p. 546. See also Chapter 2, p. 46.

56. Gifu Times (ed.), *Gifu Yearbook for 1951*, p. 207.

57. Tajimi City (ed.), *History of Tajimi City*, 2 vols (Tajimi: Tajimi City, 1987), vol. 2, p. 1023; GRO, 5.02-S38-2, Tajimi Home File 1950–63.

58. Gifu Times (ed.), *Gifu Yearbook for 1955* (Gifu: Gifu Times, 1954), pp. 169–70.

59. Seki City Educational Board (ed.), *Revised Version: History of Seki City, Post-modern* (Seki: Seki City, 1999), p. 1294; *Asahi Newspaper*, 3 February 1951.

60. GRO, 5.02-S38-3, Seki Home File 1952–63. For the 1957 Code of Practice, see Chapter 2, p. 51.

61. Yamato Town (ed.), *History of Yamato Town*, 2 vols (Yamato Town, Gifu: Yamato Town, 1988), vol. 2, p. 238; GRO, 5.02-S38-3, Gujo Home File 1952–63; *Asahi Newspaper*, 11 August 1954.

62. Ibigawa Town (ed.), *History of Ibigawa Town* (Ibigawa Town, Gifu: Ibigawa Town, 1971), p. 535; *Mainichi Newspaper*, 25 January 1951.

63. GRO, 5.02-S38-3, Ibigawa Home File 1952–63.

64. GRO, 5.02-S38-3, Nakatsugawa Home File 1952–63; Tarui Town History Editorial Board (ed.), *History of Tarui Town* (Tarui Town, Gifu: Tarui Town Mayor Mr Yagino, 1969), p. 630; GRO, 5.02-S38-4, Tarui Home File 1952–63; *Asahi Newspaper*, 2 February 1951; *Mainichi Newspaper*, 4 July 1951.

65. *Asahi Newspaper*, 12 December 1952; GRO, 5.02-S38-4, Takayama Home File 1952–63.

66. Takayama City (ed.), *Reprinted: History of Takayama City*, vol. 1, p. 682. Data from the home plan enclosed in GRO, 5.02-S39-8, Takayama Home Annual Home Inspection Report (hereafter AHIR), 1964.

67. *Gifu Times Newspaper*, 18 January 1955.

68. Zenkoku-yoro-jigyo-kyokai, *National Directory of Old People's Institutions 1952* (Tokyo: Zenkoku-yoro-jigyo-kyokai, 1952), repr. in Ogasawara, *Historical Sources*, vol. 29, p. 25.

69. Ibid., pp. 9–10.

70. Tsuruta, *Analysis of Old People's Institution Survey*, p. 21.

71. Zenkoku-yoro-jigyo-kyokai, *National Directory of Old People's Institutions 1952*, p. 8.

72. Data from *Gifu Statistics 1952*, pp. 24–34; Asai and Miwa, 'Research on the Aged in Gifu Prefecture', pp. 29–41.

73. *Gifu Times Newspaper*, 9 January 1953.

74. *Gifu Statistics 1948*, p. 388; *Gifu Statistics 1953*, p. 339.

75. *Mainichi Newspaper*, 12 January 1954.

76. *Mainichi Newspaper*, 15 September 1953; *Chunichi Newspaper*, 11 May 1955.

77. *Gifu Times Newspaper*, 9 January 1953.

78. *Mainichi Newspaper*, 12 January 1954.

79. *Chunichi Newspaper*, 22 June 1955.
80. *Mainichi Newspaper*, 9 February 1955.
81. *Gifu Statistics 1962*, p. 316.
82. Seikatsu-kagaku-chosa-kai (ed.), *Research on the Old Age Problem*, appendix, p. 188.
83. Ibid., pp. 190–1.
84. Respectively, *Gifu Newspaper*, 16 September 1977; 24 September 1975; *Chunichi Newspaper*, 10 November 1971.
85. *Gifu Statistics 1974*, p. 322. Note: The rural fifty-place Ibigawa and Nakatsugawa Homes still had a handful of spare places, however; GRO, 5.02-S47-5, Ibigawa Home AHIR 1972; GRO, 5.02-S47-6, Nakatsugawa Home AHIR 1972.
86. *Chunichi Newspaper*, 26 April 1973; 20 March 1974; Sakahogi Town Educational Board (ed.), *History of Sakahogi Town* (Sakahogi Town, Gifu: Sakahogi Town, 2005), pp. 380–1.
87. *Gifu Statistics 1975*, p. 365; Gifu Prefecture, *Gifu Prefecture First Comprehensive Plan 1966–76* (Gifu: Gifu Prefecture, 1966), p. 207.
88. GRO, 5.02-S38-1, Gifu Home File 1957–63; *Gifu Times Newspaper*, 17 May 1956.
89. Gifu Prefecture, *Journal of Gifu Prefecture 1966* (Gifu: Gifu Prefecture, 1966) (hereafter *Gifu Journal*), p. 207.
90. *Mainichi Newspaper*, 5 June 1959; Tajimi Home File 1950–63.
91. Ena City Historical Editorial Board (ed.), *History of Ena City*, 5 vols (Ena: Ena City, 1993), vol. 4, pp. 643–4; *Gifu Newspaper*, 28 March 1972; *Gifu Journal 1966*, p. 208; *Gifu Newspaper*, 22 March 1968; Mitaka Town Historical Editorial Board (ed.), *History of Mitaka Town*, 2 vols (Mitaka Town, Gifu: Mitaka Town, 1992), vol. 2, p. 236.
92. *Gifu Journal 1963*, p. 160; *Chunichi Newspaper*, 27 February 1969.
93. *Gifu Statistics 1962*, p. 316; *Gifu Statistics 1973*, p. 324.
94. GRO, 5.02-S47-5, Gifu Home AHIR 1972; GRO, 5.02-S38-9, Tarui Home AHIR 1963.
95. Gifu Home AHIR 1972.
96. Tarui Home AHIR 1963.
97. For example, Ena Home, in GRO, 5.02-S42-8, Ena Home AHIR 1967.
98. *Gifu Newspaper*, 28 March 1972.
99. *Asahi Newspaper*, 13 June 1975.
100. *Gifu Newspaper*, 28 March 1972; *Mainichi Newspaper*, 21 November 1973.
101. Motosu Town (ed.), *History of Motosu Town* (Motosu Town, Gifu: Motosu City, 1975), pp. 629–31.
102. Ibid., p. 631. See also the Yorokaen Home, in Chapter 6, p. 157.
103. Motosu Town (ed.), *History of Motosu Town*, p. 631.
104. Kagamihara City Educational Board (ed.), *History of Kagamihara City, Contemporary* (Kagamihara: Kagamihara City, 1987), pp. 617, 870; *Mainichi Newspaper*, 25 April 1974.
105. *Chunichi Newspaper*, 6 April 1975.
106. Ibid.
107. *Mainichi Newspaper*, 12 April 1994: the first such was built by Seki City authority.
108. Kagamihara City Educational Board (ed.), *Historical Source for Kagamihara City, Contemporary* (Kagamihara: Kagamihara City, 1986), p. 567. See also the location map of the prefecture old people's and nursing homes in 1977, in T. Yamagiwa, 'The 1978 Survey of Elderly Welfare', *Think-Tank Gifu Journal*, 23 (November 1979), pp. 3–13, on p. 7.
109. *Asahi Newspaper*, 6 December 1971.
110. *Gifu Newspaper*, 29 March 1968; Gifu Prefecture (ed.), *Historical Sources for Gifu Prefecture, Post-Contemporary*, 2 vols (Gifu: Gifu Prefecture, 1999), vol. 1, pp. 452–5.

111. Gifu Prefecture, *Gifu Prefecture Second Comprehensive Plan 1972–80* (Gifu: Gifu Prefecture, 1972), p. 126.

112. GRO, 5.02-S49-2, Gifu Prefecture Comprehensive Plan 1974.

113. GRO, 5.02-S45-5, Survey of Prefecture Elderly People Living Alone 1970; *Gifu Statistics 1973*, p. 325.

114. GRO, 5.02-S50-6, Petitions to the Gifu Prefecture Social Welfare Division 1975.

115. *Gifu Newspaper*, 15 December 1967.

116. Gifu Prefecture (ed.), *Historical Sources for Gifu Prefecture, Post-Contemporary*, vol. 1, p. 533.

117. GRO, 5.02-S44-7, Elderly Welfare Files 1969; *Gifu Newspaper*, 18 August 1992.

118. Gifu Prefecture, *Gifu Prefecture First Comprehensive Plan 1966–76*, p. 193. Also 234 doctors and 1,200 nurses short.

119. Ibid., p. 191.

120. Gifu City (ed.), *A History of Gifu City, Contemporary*, p. 696.

121. Mr K., psychiatric nursing assistant (1985–9), interview, 20 May 2008.

122. *Mainichi Newspaper*, 15 December 1979.

123. Petitions to the Gifu Prefecture Social Welfare Division 1975; GRO, 5.02-S47-11, Gifu Comprehensive Plan 1972.

124. *Gifu Journal 1973*, p. 100; Gifu Council of Elderly Homes, History of Gifu Council of Elderly Homes (Gifu: Gifu Council of Elderly Homes, 1996), p. 15, held at the Kusunokien nursing home, Ogaki City.

125. GRO, 5.02-S49-19, Petitions to the Gifu Prefecture Social Welfare Division 1974; *Mainichi Newspaper*, 11 April 1974; 15 September 1981. See above, p. 227 n. 86.

126. *Gifu Journal 1976*, p. 395; *Gifu Statistics 1980*, p. 344.

127. *Gifu Newspaper*, 18 December 1976.

128. Gifu Prefecture, *Gifu Prefecture Third Comprehensive Plan 1977–85* (Gifu: Gifu Prefecture, 1977), p. 151; GRO, 5.02-S53-15, Petitions to the Gifu Prefecture Social Welfare Division 1978; Gifu Prefecture, *Gifu Prefecture Fourth Comprehensive Plan 1984–95* (Gifu: Gifu Prefecture, 1984), p. 187; *Gifu Statistics 1992*, p. 366.

129. Gifu Prefecture, *Gifu Prefecture Fifth Comprehensive Plan 1994–98* (Gifu: Gifu Prefecture, 1994), p. 87; Gifu Prefecture, *Gifu Prefecture Health and Welfare Plan for Older People 1994–2000* (Gifu: Gifu Prefecture, 1994) (hereafter *Gifu Welfare Plan 1994–2000*), p. 77; *Gifu Statistics 2002*, p. 188.

130. *Chunichi Newspaper*, 20 December 1995; Mahoroba (ed.), *Directory of Elderly Welfare Facilities in Japan 2000/1* (Tokyo: Daiichi-hoki-shuppan, 2001), pp. 6–8.

131. Mahoroba (ed.), *Directory of Elderly Welfare Facilities in Japan 2000/1*, pp. 6–8; *Gifu Statistics 2004*, p. 356.

132. MoHLW, *The 2004 Survey of Long-term Care Insurance Residential Facility Providing Agencies* (Tokyo: MoHLW, 2004), pp. 81, 106.

133. *Gifu Welfare Plan 1994–2000*, p. 19.

134. GRO, 5.02-S56-12, Survey Files 1981; *Gifu Welfare Plan 1994–2000*, pp. 33, 64.

135. *Gifu Welfare Plan 1994–2000*, p. 33.

136. Ibid., pp. 35, 64.

137. Ibid., p. 53; *Gifu Newspaper*, 20 May 1993; Ogaki City, *Ogaki City Health and Welfare Plan 1994–2000* (Ogaki: Ogaki City, 1994), p. 18; MoHLW, *The 2000 Survey of Long-term Care Insurance Residential Facility Providing Agencies*, p. 160.

138. *Gifu Welfare Plan 1994–2000*, pp. 24, 26; Gifu Prefecture, *Gifu Prefecture Fourth Comprehensive Plan 1984–95*, p. 184. Note: Co-residency rates in Gifu were 72 per cent

(cf. 64 per cent nationally) in 1986 and 65 per cent (50 per cent) in 1998; Juroku Bank Research Team, 'Nursing Care Market Trends in Gifu Prefecture', *Monthly Financial Report*, 564 (June 2001), pp. 1–23, on p. 4.

139. Gifu Prefecture, *Report on the Health and Life of the Prefecture Elderly 1984* (Gifu: Gifu Prefecture, 1985), p. 43; T. Takagi and Y. Takama, 'Living Situation in Homes for the Elderly in Gifu Prefecture, Compared to National Trends', *Journal of Tokai Woman's Junior College*, 27 (2001), pp. 25–36, on p. 35.

140. *Gifu Welfare Plan 1994–2000*, p. 24.

141. *Gifu Newspaper*, 15 September 1992.

142. *Gifu Newspaper*, 16 September 1977; 9 February 1975.

143. Gifu Prefecture, *Report on the Health and Life of the Prefecture Elderly 1984*, pp. 67–8.

144. *Gifu Newspaper*, 1 September 1992.

145. *Gifu Newspaper*, 16 September 1977.

146. MoHW, *National Directory of Elderly Welfare Facilities 1990* (Tokyo: Daiichi-hoki-shuppan, 1990), p. 2.

147. Ibid., pp. 174–6.

148. Survey Files 1981; *Gifu Statistics 1982*, p. 336.

149. Gifu City (ed.), *A History of Gifu City, Contemporary*, p. 744; MoHW, *National Directory of Elderly Welfare Facilities 1990*, p. 178.

150. *Chunichi Newspaper*, 29 September 1972.

151. *Chunichi Newspaper*, 7 April 1973; MoHW, *National Directory of Elderly Welfare Facilities 1990*, p. 77.

152. *Gifu Newspaper*, 27 February 1964.

153. *Chunichi Newspaper*, 19 April 1974.

154. Gifu Prefecture Social Welfare Division, *Report on the Conditions of the Prefecture Elderly 1977* (Gifu: Gifu Prefecture Social Welfare Division, 1978), pp. 57–8.

155. Ibid., p. 58.

156. *Mainichi Newspaper*, 24 April 1991.

157. Gifu Prefecture Social Welfare Corporation, *20-Year History* (Gifu: Gifu Prefecture Social Welfare Corporation, 1987), p. 56.

158. Ibid., p. 63.

159. Ibid., p. 57; *Mainichi Newspaper*, 28 March 1969.

160. Gifu Prefecture Social Welfare Corporation, *20-Year History*, p. 58.

161. Ibid., p. 64; *Gifu Newspaper*, 27 February 1972.

162. *Gifu Newspaper*, 4 April 1976.

163. Ibid.; *Mainichi Newspaper*, 30 March 1973; *Gifu Journal 1968*, p. 99.

164. *Asahi Newspaper*, 27 July 1975; M. Ishihara, *Glad to Be Alive* (Kyoto: Minerva, 1986), pp. 11–16.

165. Ikeda Town (ed.), *History of Ikeda Town* (Ikeda Town, Gifu: Ikeda Town, 1978), p. 585.

166. Hakuju-kai, *Ten-Year History of Ibukien* (privately printed, 1991), pp. 18–29, held at Kusunokien. See also *Gifu Journal 1981*, p. 350; *Asahi Newspaper*, 20 June 1981.

167. Hakuju-kai, *Ten-Year History of Ibukien*, pp. 29, 32.

168. *Gifu Journal 1979*, p. 317.

169. Chiyoda-kai, *Fifteen-Year History of Kikujuen* (privately printed, 1994), p. 15, held at Kusunokien.

170. *Gifu Journal 1980*, p. 67.

171. MoHW, *National Directory of Elderly Welfare Facilities 1990*, p. 173.

172. Gifu Prefecture Social Welfare Corporation, *20-Year History*, p. 60.

173. GRO, 5.02-S45-4, Elderly Welfare Training Files 1970.
174. GRO, 5.02-S38-9, Furukawa Home AHIR 1963; 5.02-S38-9, Hashima Home AHIR 1963; *Mainichi Newspaper*, 7 February 1984.
175. GRO, 5.02-S47-5, Jurakuen Home AHIR 1973; 5.02-S50-18, AHIR Files 1975 (Hida-Jurakuen Home, etc.).
176. *Asahi Newspaper*, 18 June 1984.
177. Gifu Prefecture, *Report on the Health and Life of the Prefecture Elderly 1984*, p. 84; *Chunichi Newspaper*, 31 March 1984.
178. *Mainichi Newspaper*, 7 February 1984. See Chapter 2, p. 66.
179. *Gifu Journal 1985*, p. 345.
180. *Gifu Journal 1987*, pp. 316, 319; *Chunichi Newspaper*, 15 August 1986.
181. *Gifu Journal 1988*, p. 56; *Mainichi Newspaper*, 10 April 1988.
182. *Gifu Newspaper*, 30 March 1989.
183. *Gifu Journal 1990*, p. 73; *Mainichi Newspaper*, 19 April 1990. For Kusunokien, see Chapter 6.
184. Prefecture Circular, 1 December 1999, held at Kusunokien.
185. See Chapter 2, p. 67.
186. *Gifu Statistics 1979*, p. 340; *Gifu Statistics 1987*, p. 348.
187. Gifu Prefecture, *Gifu Prefecture Health and Welfare Plan for Older People 2006–15* (Gifu: Gifu Prefecture, 2006), pp. 16–17.
188. GRO, 5.02-S49-4, Petitions to the Prefecture Public Assistance Division 1974.
189. AHIR Files 1975 (Hida-Jurakuen Homes etc.); *Gifu Statistics 1975*, p. 365.
190. GRO, 5.02-S44-13, Jurakuen Home AHIR 1970; Gifu Prefecture Social Welfare Cooperation, *20-Year History*, pp. 61, 68.
191. Elderly Welfare Files 1969.
192. GRO, 5.02-S48-4, Welfare Facilities Files 1973.
193. GRO, 5.20-S51-13, Petitions to the Gifu Prefecture Social Welfare Division 1976.
194. NCEH (ed.), *The Second National Survey on Elderly Homes* (Tokyo: NCEH, 1982), p. 96; NCEH (ed.), *The Fourth National Survey on Elderly Homes*, pp. 129–30, 136–46.
195. Elderly Welfare Training Files 1970.
196. Petitions to the Prefecture Public Assistance Division 1974.
197. Visiting Report by attendant Ms B., 9 March 1995, held at Kusunokien.
198. Ibid.
199. Elderly Welfare Files 1969.
200. *Chunichi Newspaper*, 8 February 1985; *Gifu Journal 1985*, pp. 335–6.
201. *Gifu Journal 1986*, p. 48; *Mainichi Newspaper*, 16 January 1986; *Gifu Newspaper*, 15 September 1987.
202. Gifu Prefecture Social Welfare Division (ed.), *Research Reports by Residential Staff* (Gifu: Gifu Prefecture Social Welfare Division, 1984), p. 718.
203. Ibid. See also various editions, 1988–93.
204. For example, Shinseien and Ibukien, respectively, Ishihara, *Glad to Be Alive*, pp. 42–52; Hakuju-kai, *Ten-Year History of Ibukien*, pp. 73–7.
205. Cited in *Chunichi Newspaper*, 20 December 1995.
206. Report by attendant Ms P., 17 February 1995, held at a prefecture home (unidentified).
207. Cited in *Chunichi Newspaper*, 20 December 1995.
208. See Chapter 2, p. 215 n. 205.
209. Mahoroba (ed.), *Directory of Elderly Welfare Facilities in Japan 2000/1*, pp. 548–51.

5 Residential Life in Norfolk

1. NRO, G/GP9/152–153, Freebridge Lynn Union, Workhouse Completion Orders, 23 May and 2 August 1836. For its site, see NRO, G/GP9/185, Freebridge Lynn Union, the Plan of June 1838. Also see *The Ordnance Survey* (Southampton: Ordnance Survey, 1905), Norfolk Sheet XXXIV 11, held at Norfolk Heritage Centre.
2. R. O'Donnell, 'W. J. Donthorn (1799–1859): Architecture with "Great Hardness and Decision in the Edges"', *Architectural History*, 21 (1978), pp. 83–92, on pp. 84, 89. Note: Donthorn's similar workhouses included his hometown Swaffham (1836), Downham Market (1836), Aylsham (1849) and Erpingham (1851): see Morrison, *The Workhouse*, pp. 207–8.
3. E. R. Kelly (ed.), *Kelly's Directory of Norfolk* (London: Kelly's Directories, 1883), p. 324; P. Higginbotham, *The Workhouse*, at http://www.workhouses.org.uk [accessed 10 August 2012].
4. Digby, *Pauper Palaces*, p. 71; Great Britain Poor Law Commissioners, *The Poor Law Report of 1834*, p. 438.
5. Morrison, *The Workhouse*, p. 53.
6. W. White, *History, Gazetteer and Directory of Norfolk*, 4th edn (Sheffield: William White, 1883), pp. 42, 282.
7. Averages from NRO, C/GP9/71–73, Guardians Committee (Area 9), Gayton PAI House Committee Minutes 1930–41; C/GC8/15, Guardians Committee (Area 8), Gayton PAI House Committee Minutes 1941–8 (hereafter GHCM). See also GHCM, 14 May 1942, 17 September 1942; and Chapter 3, p. 71.
8. NRO, C/SS3/16–17, Eastgate House Management Sub-Committee Minutes 1948–63 (hereafter EMSCM), 29 July 1948. For example, one resident spent forty-four years (1911–56) until her death at the age of 88, in NRO, C/SS10/2, Eastgate House Patient Days List 1955–67, p. 1; EMSCM, 22 March 1956.
9. Norfolk WCM, 16 July 1958, #6:5.
10. EMSCM, July–September 1948; 21 June 1951.
11. National Assistance Act (1948), sections 17, 21.
12. EMSCM, 14 September 1950; January–December 1950.
13. EMSCM, 8 December 1949; 11 October 1951.
14. Figures from EMSCM, January–December 1954; GHCM, January–December 1945.
15. EMSCM, 30 March 1950; 25 May 1950; 14 September 1950.
16. EMSCM, 23 February 1961; 14 September 1961.
17. NRO, C/SS3/6, Burnham Westgate Hall Management Sub-Committee Minutes 1951–7 (hereafter BMSCM), 2 August 1951.
18. Ibid.
19. Ibid. See Chapter 3, pp. 77–9.
20. EMSCM, 1 December 1955; January–December 1960; Eastgate House Patient Days List 1955–67, pp. 1–4, 55–8.
21. Eastgate House Patient Days List 1955–67, pp. 1–4.
22. EMSCM, 3 January 1963.
23. NRO, C/SS3/41, Sidney Dye House Management Sub-Committee Minutes 1957–68 (hereafter SMSCM), 14 January 1958.
24. In 1960 just one of the thirty-six admissions from their own homes was from Gayton, whereas seven were from the Norwich area; EMSCM, January–December 1960.
25. Viz. EMSCM, 1948–63; NRO, C/SS10/28, Woodlands Register of Pensions 1964–7.

26. EMSCM, 1948–51.
27. Woodlands Register of Pensions 1964–7.
28. EMSCM, 1 March 1951.
29. EMSCM, 24 March 1955; 1953–5.
30. NRO, C/SS10/3, Eastgate House Weekly Return of Admissions and Discharges 1960–3; BMSCM, 14 February, 13 March 1952.
31. EMSCM, 19 August 1948; 31 March 1949; 8 December 1949.
32. GHCM, 30 March 1944.
33. GHCM, 28 September 1944.
34. GHCM, 19 February 1942; 8 April 1948.
35. GHCM, 19 August 1943; 19 July 1945; 25 March 1948.
36. Pope, *Gressenhall Farm and Workhouse*, pp. 67, 79.
37. GHCM, 24 October 1946.
38. GHCM, 21 November 1946.
39. GHCM, 19 August 1943; 1 January 1948; EMSCM, 29 March 1951.
40. EMSCM, 11 November 1948; 9 December 1948; Norfolk Scheme (Norfolk five-year local plan), enclosed in Norfolk WCM, 9 March 1949, #178. See also Chapter 3, p. 220 n. 97.
41. EMSCM, 14 October 1948; 2 February 1950.
42. EMSCM, 29 March 1951; 4 December 1952; 24 March 1955.
43. NRO, C/SS10/26, Eastgate House Plan 1955.
44. EMSCM, 2 March 1950.
45. EMSCM, 17 August 1950; 8 October 1953; 16 June 1955; 24 March 1960.
46. EMSCM, 31 January 1952.
47. EMSCM, 28 February 1952.
48. EMSCM, 2 March 1950.
49. EMSCM, 20 July 1950; 19 July 1951; 17 July 1952.
50. EMSCM, 27 April 1950; 28 February 1952.
51. EMSCM, 17 July 1952.
52. EMSCM, 18 June 1953.
53. Ibid.
54. EMSCM, 12 July 1956.
55. EMSCM, 24 March 1955; 9 August 1956.
56. EMSCM, 17 April 1958.
57. EMSCM, 10 September 1959.
58. EMSCM, 2 December 1954; 4 October 1956; 25 April 1957.
59. EMSCM, 4 October 1956; 16 May 1957; 20 February 1958.
60. EMSCM, 16 May 1957.
61. EMSCM, 15 October 1959.
62. Ibid.
63. EMSCM, 23 March 1961.
64. EMSCM, 6 October 1960.
65. EMSCM, 9 November 1961.
66. EMSCM, 3 December 1959; 14 July 1960; 3 November 1960; 1 August 1962.
67. *Eastern Daily Press* (King's Lynn edn), 13 March 1964.
68. EMSCM, 19 July 1962.
69. Norfolk WCM, 12 June 1963; 17 July 1963, #5:4; NRO, C/GP9/189, Transfer of Equipment from Eastgate House to Other County Homes, 1963.

70. Norfolk WCM, 12 June 1963; *Eastern Daily Press*, Lynn edn, 13 March 1964.
71. NRO, C/GP9/193, Printed Sale Catalogue for Eastgate House, 21 April 1964; C/GP9/195, Agreement to the Sale of Eastgate House, 21 April 1964; C/GP9/200, Eastgate House Draft Deed of Purchase, 11 June 1964; *Eastern Daily Press* (King's Lynn edn), 22 April 1964. For example, Walsingham PAI was converted into thirty-five flats; Gressenhall PAI into the Norfolk Rural Life Museum; and Pulham PAI into the Bumbles Hotel.
72. EMSCM, 16 June 1960.
73. EMSCM, 3 November 1960.
74. GHCM, 19 July 1945; 20 November 1947.
75. GHCM, 3 June 1948; 9 August 1948; EMSCM, 29 June 1948.
76. EMSCM, 18 June 1953; 13 August 1953; NRO, C/SS10/16, Eastgate House TV and Comforts Fund Accounts 1953–63; EMSCM, 19 May 1960; 29 December 1960.
77. EMSCM, 4 January 1954.
78. EMSCM, 29 November 1956.
79. EMSCM, 3 January 1952.
80. EMSCM, 4 January 1951; 28 January 1954.
81. For example, a nearby hostel had chiropodist visits only once a year; BMSCM, 1951–3.
82. EMSCM, 2 December 1954; NRO, C/SS10/11, Eastgate House Letters on Entertainments 1956.
83. EMSCM, 24 January 1957; 6 October 1960.
84. For example, a nearby hostel had no voluntary visits in 1951 and just one in 1952; BMSCM, 1951–2.
85. EMSCM, 11 August 1960; 1949–63.
86. EMSCM, 17 July 1952.
87. EMSCM, 19 May 1960; Eastgate House TV and Comforts Fund Accounts 1953–63.
88. EMSCM, 19 April 1956; 17 May 1956.
89. EMSCM, 17 June 1954.
90. EMSCM, 22 April 1954.
91. Matron's grant ceased in 1953; EMSCM, 26 March 1953.
92. EMSCM, 4 January 1962; Chapter 3, p. 82.
93. EMSCM, 23 March 1961; January–December 1962; NRO, C/SS3/36, St Nicholas's House Management Sub-Committee Minutes 1960–8, January–December 1962.
94. EMSCM, 1 August 1962; 11 October 1962.
95. EMSCM, 29 January 1959; NRO, C/SS10/15, Eastgate House Sweet and Tobacco Book 1961–3.
96. EMSCM, 21 April 1960.
97. SMSCM, 10 March 1959; 9 January 1962.
98. Eastgate House TV and Comforts Fund Accounts 1953–63. A Christmas cake was given by the queen in 1960; EMSCM, 26 January 1961.
99. NRO, C/SS3/43, Woodlands Management Sub-Committee Minutes 1963–8 (hereafter WMSCM), 12 November 1963.
100. Eastgate House TV and Comforts Fund Accounts 1953–63.
101. Ibid.; EMSCM, 28 November 1957. Note: the fund's profit in 1959 was lower than that in other county home funds, partly due to 'some petty pilfering ... with regard to the security of the stock'; EMSCM, 3 December 1959.
102. EMSCM, 17 April 1958.
103. EMSCM, 14 July 1960; 11 August 1960; 3 November 1960.
104. EMSCM, 29 December 1960.

105. EMSCM, 28 November 1957.

106. EMSCM, 17 June 1954; 19 April 1956.

107. EMSCM, 29 July 1948.

108. EMSCM, 3 December 1953; 11 September 1958.

109. EMSCM, 29 July 1948.

110. GHCM, 6 August 1942.

111. GHCM, 9 October 1947.

112. GHCM, 23 October 1947.

113. EMSCM, 23 June 1949.

114. EMSCM, 25 May 1950.

115. EMSCM, 4 January 1951.

116. EMSCM, 11 August 1955.

117. EMSCM, 26 January 1956.

118. EMSCM, 1 December 1955; 26 April 1962; 21 June 1962.

119. EMSCM, 10 September 1963; WMSCM, 12 September 1967.

120. EMSCM, 7 December 1950; 29 December 1955; 17 May 1962; WMSCM, 12 September 1967.

121. EMSCM, 29 December 1955.

122. GHCM, 24 April 1947; EMSCM, 28 February 1952.

123. Figures from EMSCM, 1948–52.

124. EMSCM, 6 October 1955.

125. EMSCM, 1 February 1951; 1 March 1951.

126. EMSCM, 23 February 1961.

127. EMSCM, 8 November 1951.

128. EMSCM, 25 February 1954; 1 November 1956.

129. SMSCM, 14 January 1958.

130. EMSCM, 11 September 1958.

131. EMSCM, 6 November 1958.

132. EMSCM, 4 December 1958.

133. EMSCM, 17 July 1958; 6 November 1958.

134. EMSCM, 11 September 1958.

135. EMSCM, 11 July 1957.

136. EMSCM, 28 January 1960.

137. EMSCM, 22 June 1961.

138. EMSCM, 23 February 1961.

139. Between 1968 and 1974 there were only thirty-three superintendents' and eleven visitors' reports for Woodlands: Viz. NRO, C/SS4/7, Area 7 Management Sub-Committee Minutes 1968–70 (hereafter MSCM(7)); and NRO, C/SS5/4, Area 4 Management Sub-Committee Minutes 1970–4 (hereafter MSCM(4)). And no further information after 1974.

140. MSCM(4), 19 April 1971; 31 January 1973; 27 March 1973.

141. WMSCM, 8 October 1963; MSCM(4), 8 August 1972; 22 September 1972; 15 October 1973.

142. MSCM(4), 17 December 1973.

143. WMSCM, 10 September 1963.

144. WMSCM, 14 January 1964; MSCM(7), 11 February 1969; 11 March 1969; MSCM(4), 20 January 1972; 16 April 1973.

145. WMSCM, 10 September 1963.

146. MSCM(4), 20 January 1972; 27 March 1973; 27 April 1973.

147. MSCM(4), 19 April 1971.

148. MSCM(4), 2 March 1972; 27 April 1973.

149. MSCM(7), 14 May 1968; 15 May 1969; 8 June 1970.

150. MSCM(4), 9 October 1972.

151. WMSCM, 9 March 1965; 8 June 1965; 14 September 1965; 12 October 1965.

152. WMSCM, 8 November 1966; 13 December 1966; 14 March 1967.

153. MSCM(7), 14 May 1968; MSCM(4), 19 April 1971; 18 June 1973.

154. WMSCM, 14 March 1967; MSCM(4), 23 August 1971.

155. MSCM(4), 19 June 1973.

156. MSCM(4), 23 August 1971; 19 June 1972.

157. MSCM(4), 19 June 1972; 21 August 1972.

158. MSCM(4), 27 December 1972; 19 February 1973; 25 March 1973.

159. MSCM(4), 16 October 1972; 25 March 1973.

160. MSCM(4), 17 April 1972; 17 December 1973.

161. MSCM(4), 20 August 1973.

162. MSCM(4), 17 April 1972; 1972–4.

163. WMSCM, 8 March 1966; 10 January 1967; MSCM(7), 11 March 1969; 8 April 1969.

164. WMSCM, 12 July 1966; 8 November 1966.

165. WMSCM, 13 June 1967; 12 September 1967; MSCM(7), 8 December 1969.

166. WMSCM, 11 April 1967; 12 September 1967; MSCM(7), 13 May 1969.

167. Respectively, 18.6 and 24.5 per 1,000 Norfolk (including Norwich and Great Yarmouth) elderly population; MoH, *Community Care Plan*, p. 146–50; MoH, *Hospital Plan*, pp. 82–7.

168. The term used by Ms C, Norfolk County Council social worker (1981–3), interview, 15 April 2008.

169. Cherry, *Mental Health Care in Modern England*, pp. 245–6.

170. Ibid., p. 247.

171. Ibid.

172. Viz. from 4,900 beds in 1960 to 2,760 by 1975; MoH, *Hospital Plan*, pp. 86–7.

173. M. Fisher, '"Getting Out of the Asylum": Discharge and Decarceration Issues in Asylum History *c*. 1890–1959' (PhD dissertation, University of East Anglia, 2003), p. 375; Cherry, *Mental Health Care in Modern England*, p. 263.

174. Fisher, '"Getting out of the Asylum"' p. 378; Cherry, *Mental Health Care in Modern England*, pp. 272, 293, 296.

175. For example, designated units in a King's Lynn general hospital opened in 1986; NHS nursing homes for the elderly mentally ill at Rebecca House (North Walsham, 1994) and Cygnet House (Long Stratton, 1998).

176. Viz. twenty-nine local authority and sixty-eight voluntary/private places, in Cherry, *Mental Health Care in Modern England*, p. 279.

177. Mrs S., nurse assistant (1970–82), interview, 15 December 2008.

178. Ms N., student nurse (1972–5), first interview, 30 April 2008.

179. Mrs S., interview, 15 December 2008.

180. Ms N., first interview, 30 April 2008.

181. Ibid.

182. Ibid.

183. Ibid.

184. Ibid.

185. Ibid.
186. Ibid.
187. Ibid.
188. Ibid.
189. Ms N., second interview, 11 November 2008; Fisher, '"Getting out of the Asylum"', p. 363.
190. Ms N., second interview, 11 November 2008.
191. Ibid.
192. Ibid.
193. Ibid.
194. Ibid.
195. Ibid.
196. C. McCall, *Looking Back from the Nineties: An Autobiography* (Norwich: Gliddon Books, 1994), pp. 99–102.
197. Ms D., NHS domiciliary (community) nurse (1976–8), interview, 29 November 2008.
198. Ms N., third interview, 24 November 2008.
199. Ibid.
200. Ibid.
201. Mrs S., interview, 15 December 2008.
202. Ms N., third interview, 24 November 2008.
203. Ms N., first interview, 30 April 2008.
204. Ms A., qualified nurse (1986–8), interview, 1 December 2008.
205. Ibid.
206. Ms N., third interview, 24 November 2008.
207. Mrs S., interview, 15 December 2008.
208. Cherry, *Mental Health Care in Modern England*, pp. 273, 300.
209. Ms N., third interview, 24 November 2008.
210. Ms V., hospital ward sister (1976–8), interview, 8 December 2008.
211. Ibid.
212. Ibid.
213. Ibid.
214. Ms H., charge nurse (1978–85), interview, 22 November 2008.
215. Ibid.
216. Ibid.
217. Ibid.
218. Mrs S., interview, 15 December 2008.
219. Respectively, Ms E. and Ms L., daughters of an incapacitated English private care home resident (2003–7), interview, 17 April 2008; Ms M., Norfolk County Council social worker, working with Norfolk Mental Health team in 2005, interview, 27 November 2008. Note: There are parallels here with 'Scull's Dilemma'. This is discussed in the Conclusion, p. 191.
220. Ms I., deputy matron (1976–8), interview, 13 November 2008.
221. Ibid.
222. Ibid.
223. Ibid.
224. Ibid.
225. Ibid.

226. Respectively, Ms J., Norfolk County Council relief care assistant (1982–5), interview, 30 November 2008; Ms C., interview, 15 April 2008.
227. Ms C., interview, 15 April 2008.
228. Ibid.
229. Ms J., interview, 30 November 2008.
230. Ms C., interview, 15 April, 2008.
231. Ms J., interview, 30 November 2008.
232. Ibid.
233. Ibid.
234. Ibid.
235. Ibid.
236. Ibid.
237. Ibid.
238. Ibid.
239. Ms O., private home care assistant (1991–3), interview, 3 December 2008.
240. Ms J., interview, 30 November 2008.
241. Ibid.
242. Ibid.
243. Ibid.
244. Ibid.
245. Ibid.
246. Ibid.
247. Ibid.
248. Ms C., interview, 15 April 2008.
249. Ibid.
250. Mrs W., private care home resident (1989–), married Mr W., resident in the same home, interview, 25 May 2009.
251. Ms K., private home care assistant (1983–92), interview, 7 December 2008.
252. Mrs G., daughter of a private care home resident (1983–5), interview, 3 June 2008.
253. Ms K., interview, 7 December 2008.
254. Ibid.
255. Ms O., interview, 3 December 2008.
256. Respectively, Ms K., interview, 7 December 2008; Ms Y., private care home nurse (1988–90), interview, 25 October 2008.
257. Mrs R., daughter of the resident (1985–8), interview, 5 June 2008.
258. Ms O., interview, 3 December 2008.
259. Ibid.
260. Ms K., interview, 7 December 2008.
261. Ms T., care assistant in local authority home (1983–6) and private home (1990–5), interview, 12 December 2008.
262. Ibid.
263. Ibid.
264. Ms O., interview, 3 December 2008.
265. Ms Y., interview, 25 October 2008.
266. Ms K., interview, 7 December 2008.
267. Ms F., private care home deputy matron (1989–90), interview, 25 October 2008.
268. Ms E., interview, 17 April 2008.
269. Comment by a colleague, cited in Ms O., interview, 3 December 2008.

270. Ms K., interview, 7 December 2008.
271. Ms T., interview, 12 December 2008.
272. Ms O., interview, 3 December 2008.
273. Ms T., interview, 12 December 2008.
274. Ibid.
275. Mr W., private care home resident (1993–2011), first interview, 25 May 2009.

6 Residential Life in Gifu

1. For the Ogaki Old People's Almshouse (1926–45), see Chapter 4, pp. 98–101.
2. Yokokaen History Draft, *c.* 1970. Note: Yorokaen documents held at the premises, unless otherwise specified. Viz. thirty-four of the forty Yorokaen residents were aged 60 or more in 1949; Zenkoku-yoro-jigyo-kyokai, *National Survey of Elderly Institutions 1949*, p. 36.
3. Yorokaen Relief Institution Files 1950.
4. Yorokaen Registration Files 1952–69, 30 May 1952; Yorokaen Annual Reports 1952–8 (hereafter YAR), 1952–8. For example, the number of over-65s in Ogaki City living alone increased from 3,700 to 5,900 during the 1950s.
5. YAFS, 1950, 1955.
6. Zenkoku-yoro-jigyo-kyokai, *National Survey of Elderly Institutions 1949*, p. 36; YAR, 1958; Yorokaen Brochure, *c.* 1958.
7. YAR, 1958.
8. Yorokaen Regulations, revised 1951, Article 4.
9. YAR, 1952; *Chunichi Newspaper*, 3 April 1992.
10. YAR, 1952.
11. YRDD, 1950–2. See also Chapter 6, p. 159.
12. YAR, 1958.
13. Ibid.
14. YAR; YRDD, 1958.
15. YRDD, 1953–9.
16. YRDD, 1955.
17. YAR, 1957.
18. Zenkoku-yoro-jigyo-kyokai *National Survey of Elderly Institutions 1949*, p. 43. Just 40 per cent of girls and 80 per cent of boys had four years' primary education in 1898.
19. YAR, 1953, 1957.
20. YAFS, 1950–8; YAR, 1952–8.
21. YAR, 1955–7.
22. YRDD, 1955–62.
23. Yorokaen Regulations, revised 1959, Article 33.
24. Yorokaen Plan File, *c.* 1960; GRO, 5.02-S38-2, Yorokaen File 1950–63.
25. YAFS, 1949; Yorokaen Plan File, *c.* 1960.
26. MoHW, *A Code of Practice for Assessed Institutions* (Tokyo: Seikatsu-fukushi-shisetsu-kenkyu-kai, 1957), repr. in Ogasawara (ed.), *Historical Sources*, vol. 6, p. 36.
27. YAFS, 1948; 1949–52; Chapter 4, p. 102.
28. YAFS, 1950–6; Yorokaen Plan File, *c.* 1960.
29. *Mainichi Newspaper*, 14 July 1955.
30. Yorokaen Inventories 1956; Yorokaen Lists of Donations to Ogaki City Council, 1963.
31. Yorokaen Inventories 1956; Yorokaen Lists of Donations to Ogaki City Council, 1963.
32. MoHW, *A Code of Practice for Assessed Institutions*, p. 36.

33. Yorokaen Petition to the Ogaki City Council, 11 September 1961.
34. Photographs held at the premises show damage caused by Typhoon Vera, with 104 deaths and 133,000 victims in Gifu Prefecture alone; see Gifu Prefecture (ed.), *Plain History of Gifu Prefecture*, pp. 578–9.
35. Yorokaen Brochure, *c.* 1958.
36. Yorokaen Regulations, revised 1959, Article 31.
37. Yorokaen Annual Plan for 1951; Yorokaen Brochure, *c.* 1958.
38. Yorokaen Annual Plan for 1951; Yorokaen Brochure, *c.* 1958.
39. Yorokaen Regulations, revised 1951, Article 8. See Chapter 2, p. 211 n. 91.
40. Yorokaen Ministry Home Inspection Report of 1955.
41. Yorokaen Brochure, *c.* 1958.
42. Ibid.
43. Ibid.
44. Yorokaen Regulations, revised 1959, Article 23.
45. Ibid., Article 6.
46. Yorokaen Brochure, *c.* 1958; Yokokaen History Draft, *c.* 1970.
47. YAR, 1952–8.
48. Yorokaen Regulations, revised 1959, Articles 19, 21.
49. Ibid., Article 20.
50. Yorokaen Annual Plan for 1951.
51. Chapter 3, p. 76.
52. Yorokaen Memoranda Files 1952–65, 1 August 1955.
53. YAR, 1952; 1953–8.
54. Yorokaen Memoranda Files 1952–65, 25 August 1956.
55. YAR, 1952; 1954–5: Donations from nearby Christian churches were also received for a number of years.
56. YAFS, 1950.
57. YAR, 1954; Yorokaen Appointment Lists 1952–8. Note: Only one in twenty-three of the prefecture's households had a television even in 1958; see Gifu Prefecture (ed.), *Historical Sources for Gifu Prefecture, Post-Contemporary*, vol. 1, p. 402.
58. Yorokaen Brochure, *c.* 1958.
59. Ibid.
60. YAR, 1954; 1952–8.
61. YAFS, 1947–58.
62. Yorokaen Regulations, revised 1951, Article 9.
63. Yorokaen Regulations, revised 1959, Article 34.
64. YAR, 1952; 1953–8.
65. Yorokaen Brochure, *c.* 1958; YAR, 1952–8.
66. YAFS, 1952–8.
67. YAR, 1958.
68. *Asahi Newspaper*, 21 December 1951; 24 April 1954; Ogaki City (ed.), *History of Ogaki City*, vol. 2, pp. 540–2.
69. Yorokaen Brochure, *c.* 1958.
70. Yorokaen Minutes of the Ogaki Relief Foundation 1930–80 (hereafter YMORF), 22 March 1955.
71. YAR, 1952; 1954.
72. Yorokaen Staff Regulations, 1951.
73. YMORF, 22 March 1955.

74. YRDD, 1950; Yorokaen Appointment Lists 1952–8.
75. Yorokaen Appointment Lists 1952–8.
76. Ibid: Mr H. served for ten years until his resignation on health grounds in 1960.
77. Ibid.; YRDD, 1974.
78. YMORF, 24 December1954; Yorokaen Appointment Lists 1952–8.
79. YMORF, 24 December 1954.
80. YMORF, 12 February 1955; 19 November 1955.
81. YMORF, 27 May 1955; 29 August 1956.
82. Yorokaen Staff Regulations, 1951.
83. Yorokaen Staff Regulations, revised 1956.
84. YMORF, 30 May 1956.
85. Ibid.
86. Yorokaen Staff Regulations, revised 1956.
87. YMORF, 31 October 1958.
88. Viz. a superintendent, two clerks, a welfare supervisor, four orderlies/nurses and three kitchen staff; YAR, 1958.
89. YAFS, 1945–8.
90. Ogaki City (ed.), *History of Ogaki City*, vol. 2, p. 542.
91. Ibid., p. 828; *Gifu Journal 1963*, pp. 160–1.
92. See Chapter 2, p. 53.
93. YMORF, 28 January 1963. Description from Yorokaen Brochure, *c.* 1963, enclosed in GRO, 5.02-S39-6, Yorokaen Home AHIR 1965.
94. Extant years are 1965, 1967, 1968, 1969, 1970 and 1973.
95. GRO, 5.02-S41-4, Yorokaen Home AHIR 1967; GRO, 5.02-S47-6, Yorokaen Home AHIR 1973.
96. Yorokaen Home AHIR 1967; GRO, 5.02-S43-5, Yorokaen Home AHIR 1968.
97. Yorokaen Home AHIR 1967; Yorokaen Home AHIR 1968; Yorokaen Home AHIR 1973.
98. Yorokaen Home AHIR 1967; Yorokaen Home AHIR 1968; Yorokaen Home AHIR 1973; YAR, 1958; YRDD, 1953–72.
99. YRDD, 1954–60; Yorokaen Home AHIR 1973.
100. YAR, 1956–8; Yorokaen Home AHIR 1973.
101. Yorokaen Home AHIR 1973.
102. GRO, 5.02-S38-9, Gujo Home AHIR 1963; GRO, 5.02-S47-6, Gujo Home AHIR 1973.
103. Yokokaen History Draft, *c.* 1970.
104. Yorokaen Home AHIR 1967.
105. GRO, 5.02-S43-5, Yorokaen Home AHIR 1969.
106. Yorokaen Home AHIR 1965.
107. Yorokaen Home AHIR 1973.
108. Yorokaen Home AHIR 1965; Yorokaen Home AHIR 1973.
109. Yorokaen Home AHIR 1973.
110. Yorokaen Regulations, revised 1968, Articles 9–10, enclosed in Yorokaen Home AHIR 1973.
111. Yorokaen Home AHIR 1967.
112. Ibid.; GRO, 5.02-S44-14, Yorokaen Home AHIR 1970.
113. Yorokaen Home AHIR 1973.
114. Yorokaen Home AHIR 1970; Yorokaen Home AHIR 1973.

115. Yorokaen Home AHIR 1970; Yorokaen Home AHIR 1973; Yorokaen Home AHIR 1967.
116. Yorokaen Home AHIR 1968.
117. Yorokaen Home AHIR 1969.
118. Yorokaen Home AHIR 1968.
119. GRO, 5.02-S43-7, Elderly Welfare Files 1968.
120. Yorokaen Regulations, revised 1968, Articles 32, 37.
121. Yorokaen Home AHIR 1967; Yorokaen Home AHIR 1973.
122. See Chapter 3, p. 133.
123. Ogaki City, *Ogaki City First Comprehensive Plan 1970–85* (Ogaki: Ogaki City, 1970), pp. 202–3.
124. Ogaki City, *Ogaki City Second Comprehensive Plan 1986–95* (Ogaki: Ogaki City, 1981), p. 158.
125. *Chunichi Newspaper*, 5 April 1984.
126. *Chunichi Newspaper*, 15 July 1986; 8 and 16 April 1987; *Gifu Journal 1987*, p. 319.
127. *Mainichi Newspaper*, 21 February 1989; 19 April 1990; *Gifu Journal 1990*, p. 73.
128. *Mainichi Newspaper*, 29 December 1990; *Gifu Journal 1991*, p. 421.
129. *Mainichi Newspaper*, 1 March 1990, 21 April 1991; *Gifu Journal 1991*, p. 425.
130. Okachiyama Community Centre Brochure, *c.* 2006, held at Yorokaen.
131. Ogaki City Council Secretariats, *Ogaki City Government History* (Ogaki: Ogaki City, 2001), p. 209.
132. Ms K., Yorokaen attendant (1994–7) and Kusunokien care manager (2003–), first interview, 27 May 2008.
133. Mrs F., attendant of the public institution for disabled adults (1992–4); Yorokaen attendant (1995–8; 2000–2); care house attendant (1998–9); Kusunokien senior attendant (2002–), interview, 28 May 2008.
134. Ibid.
135. Yorokaen Summary Report of 1985, *c.* 1985, held at Ogaki City Library; Ogaki City, *Ogaki City Health and Welfare Plan 1994–2000*, p. 48.
136. Yorokaen Home AHIR 1973; Yorokaen Summary Report of 1985.
137. Ms K., first interview, 27 May 2008.
138. Yorokaen Summary Report of 1985.
139. Mr O., Yorokaen attendant (1996–2001), interview, 28 May 2008.
140. Respectively, Mrs F., interview, 28 May 2008; Mr I., Yorokaen kitchen staff (2000–7), interview, 28 May 2008; Mr O., interview, 28 May 2008.
141. Yorokaen Summary Report of 1985; Yorokaen Brochure, *c.* 1992, held at Ogaki City Library.
142. Yorokaen Summary Report of 1985.
143. Yorokaen Brochure, *c.* 1992.
144. Ms K., first interview, 27 May 2008.
145. Ibid.
146. Ibid.
147. Respectively Ms K., first interview, 27 May 2008; Mrs F., interview, 28 May 2008.
148. Ms C., Yorokaen attendant (1994–8), interview, 25 May 2008.
149. Ms K., first interview, 27 May 2008.
150. Ibid.
151. Ibid.
152. Ibid.

153. Ibid.
154. Ibid.
155. Ibid.
156. *Chunichi Newspaper*, 16 December 1994.
157. Respectively, Ms C., interview, 25 May 2008; Ms K., first interview, 27 May 2008.
158. Ms C., interview, 25 May 2008.
159. Ms K., first interview, 27 May 2008.
160. Ms C., interview, 25 May 2008.
161. Ibid.; Mr O., interview, 28 May 2008.
162. Visits to Mrs H., Yorokaen resident (1980–) on 25 April and 23 December 2007.
163. Mrs H., interview, 25 April 2007.
164. Ibid.
165. Ibid.
166. Mrs F., interview, 28 May 2008.
167. Ibid.
168. Ibid.
169. Cited by Ms K., first interview, 27 May 2008.
170. Ms K., first interview, 27 May 2008.
171. Mr O., interview, 28 May 2008.
172. Ms M., Yorokaen kitchen staff (1998–2007), interview, 3 June 2008.
173. Ms F., interview, 28 May 2008.
174. Ms M., interview, 3 June 2008.
175. Ms B., Yorokaen attendant (2000–7), interview, 29 May 2008.
176. Ms F., interview, 28 May 2008.
177. Ibid.
178. Mr O., interview, 28 May 2008.
179. Ms B., interview, 29 May 2008.
180. Mr I., interview, 28 May 2008.
181. Cited by Ms K., first interview, 27 May 2008.
182. Ms B., interview, 29 May 2008.
183. Ms K., first interview, 27 May 2008.
184. Mrs F., interview, 28 May 2008.
185. Kusunokien Annual Home Inspection Report of 1988, held at Kusunokien.
186. Ms A., Yorokaen attendant (1987–2003) and Kusunokien chief attendant (2003–7), interview, 2 June 2008.
187. Ibid.
188. Ibid.
189. Ibid.
190. Ibid.
191. Ms T., Yorokaen attendant (1995–8) and Kusunokien attendant (1998–), interview, 3 June 2008.
192. Ms W., Kusunokien day care assistant (1991–3) and Kusunokien attendant (1993–), interview, 3 June 2008.
193. Ms T., interview, 3 June 2008.
194. Ibid.
195. Ms D., Kusunokien attendant (1992–), interview, 30 May 2008.
196. Mr Y., Kusunokien volunteer (January–March 1989), Kusunokien qualified attendant (1989–2005) and Kusunokien care supervisor (2005–), first interview, 26 May 2008.

197. Ms A., interview, 2 June 2008.

198. Ibid. Broadly similar sentiments were expressed by Ms T., interview, 3 June 2008; Mr Y., first interview, 26 May 2008.

199. Mr Y., second interview, 30 May 2008.

200. Ms N., Kusunokien qualified nurse (1990–), interview, 29 May 2008.

201. Ms K., first interview, 27 May 2008; Wedge, 'How to Age and Die at Home', *Wedge*, 22:11 (November 2010), pp. 20–8, on pp. 25–6.

202. Ms G., Kusunokien qualified attendant (1990–9) and Kusunokien chief attendant (2005–), interview, 29 May 2008.

203. Ms T., interview, 3 June 2008.

204. Kusunokien Home Manual, privately printed *c*. 2001, held at Kusunokien.

205. Cited by Mr Y., second interview, 30 May 2008.

206. Ms D., interview, 30 May 2008.

207. Ms J., Kusunokien attendant (2003–), interview, 2 June 2008; Ms E., Kusunokien attendant (2007–), interview, 28 May 2008.

208. Ms D., interview, 30 May 2008.

209. Ms W., interview, 3 June 2008. Note: Traditionally the Japanese family provided care and security by confining the mentally ill in a *zashikiro* cell within the house; see A. Suzuki, 'A Brain Hospital in Tokyo, 1926–45', *History of Psychiatry*, 14 (2003), pp. 337–60, on pp. 339–40.

210. Ms N., interview, 29 May 2008.

211. Ms Q., Kusunokien resident (2003–), interview, 28 May 2008.

212. During the first interview with Mr Y. at Kusunokien, 26 May 2008.

213. Ms W., interview, 3 June 2008.

214. Wedge, 'How to Age and Die at Home', p. 25.

215. Ms T., interview, 3 June 2008.

216. Ms P., Kusunokien attendant (1991–), interview, 29 May 2008.

217. Ms N., interview, 29 May 2008.

218. Ibid; Ms S., Kusunokien attendant (2000–), interview, 4 June 2008.

219. Mr U., Kusunokien resident (2006–), interview, 28 May 2008; Ms V., Kusunokien resident (2003–), interview, 28 May 2008.

220. Mr W., English private care home resident (1993–2011), second interview, 11 July 2009.

221. Ms S., interview, 4 June 2008.

222. Ms O., English private home care assistant (1991–3), interview, 3 December 2008. See also observation and conversations with staff at Q voluntary care home, Norfolk, 7 June 2008.

223. Ms N., interview, 29 May 2008.

224. Ms T., interview, 3 June 2008.

225. Ms K., second interview, 4 June 2008.

226. Ms T., interview, 3 June 2008.

227. Ms K., second interview, 4 June 2008.

228. Ms G., interview, 29 May 2008.

229. Ms A., interview, 2 June 2008.

230. Ms T., interview, 3 June 2008.

231. Ms Q., interview, 28 May 2008.

232. Ms T., interview, 3 June 2008.

233. Ms N., interview, 29 May 2008.

234. Ms K., second interview, 4 June 2008.
235. Mr Y., second interview, 30 May 2008.
236. Ms V., interview, 28 May 2008; Ms Q., interview, 28 May 2008.
237. Mr U., interview, 28 May 2008.
238. Ms K., second interview, 4 June 2008.
239. Mr R., Kusunokien attendant (1994–), interview, 2 June 2008.
240. Mr L., Kusunokien attendant (1991–), interview, 2 June 2008.
241. Ms T., interview, 3 June 2008.
242. Ms P., interview, 29 May 2008.
243. Ms N., interview, 29 May 2008; Ms T., interview, 3 June 2008.

Conclusion

1. National Assistance Act (1948), Part III, section 21.
2. Cambridgeshire Record Office, Cambridge County Borough Council Welfare Committee Minutes 1948–70; Brown, 'The Development of Local Authority Welfare Services', pp. 181–95, 207–21. See also Townsend, *The Last Refuge*, p. 209.
3. MoHW, *National Directory of Elderly Welfare Facilities 1990*, p. 2; Chapter 4, p. 111.
4. Ms E. and Ms L., daughters of an incapacitated English private home resident (2003–7), interviews, 17 April 2008. See also A. Gentleman, 'Life in an Old People's Home', *Guardian*, 14 July 2009, *G2*, pp. 5–11; and 'Can Gerry Robinson Fix Dementia Care Homes?: Episodes 1–2', *BBC 2*, broadcast, 8 and 15 December 2009.
5. Ms W., Japanese nursing home attendant (1993–), interview, 3 June 2008; see Chapter 6, p. 243 n. 213.
6. Ms E., interview, 17 April 2008; Ms K., English private care home assistant (1983–92), interview, 7 December 2008.
7. 'Call for Debate on Suicide Laws', *BBC News*, 31 July 2009, at http://news.bbc.co.uk/1/hi/health/8177583.stm [accessed 10 August 2012].
8. 'Britons Die at Dignitas Suicide Clinic in Record Numbers', *Daily Mail*, 17 April 2011, at http://www.dailymail.co.uk/news/article-1377924/Britons-die-Dignitas-suicide-clinic-record-numbers.html#ixzz20cyr1fNv [accessed 10 August 2012].
9. Cabinet Office, *White Paper on the Ageing Society 2012/3*, p. 54.
10. 'State-Funded Elderly Care Declining, Labour Figures Suggest', *BBC News*, 16 May 2012, at http://www.bbc.co.uk/news/health-1802653 [accessed 10 August 2012].
11. Age UK, *Care in Crisis 2012*, p. 1, at http://www.ageuk.org.uk/Documents/EN-GB/Campaigns/care_in_crisis_2012_report.pdf?dtrk=true [accessed 10 August 2012]; Ms M., Norfolk County Council social worker, working with Norfolk Mental Health team in 2005, interview, 27 November 2008.
12. 'It'll Be the End of My World', *Eastern Daily Press*, 15 October 2009, p. 1. See also *Eastern Daily Press*, 27 November 2009.
13. MoHLW, 'Current State of Nursing Home Waiting Lists' (Tokyo: MoHLW, 22 December 2009), at http://www.mhlw.go.jp/stf/houdou/2r98520000003byd.html [accessed 10 August 2012].
14. Ms K., Japanese care manager at the nursing home (2003–), second interview, 4 June 2008.
15. Carers UK, *Policy Briefing: Facts about Carers 2009* (London: Carers UK, June 2009), at http://www.carersuk.org/media/k2/attachments/Facts_about_Carers_2009.pdf [accessed 10 August 2012].

16. The NHS Information Centre for Health and Social Care, *Survey of Carers in Households 2009/10* (London: NHS Information Centre for Health and Social Care, 2010), pp. 7, 10, at http://www.ic.nhs.uk/webfiles/publications/009_Social_Care/carersurvey0910/Survey_of_Carers_in_Households_2009_10_England_NS_Status_v1_0a.pdf [accessed 10 August 2012].

17. T. Doran, F. Drever and M. Whitehead, 'Health of Young and Elderly Informal Carers: Analysis of UK Census Data', *British Medical Journal*, 327:7428 (13 December 2003), p. 1388. See also Carers UK, *Policy Briefing*, and NHS Information Centre for Health and Social Care, *Survey of Carers in Households 2009/10*, pp. 53–68. For an informed discussion (in Japanese) of carers' issues, see K. Mitomi, *Community Care and Carers in the UK: International Development of Support for Carers* (Kyoto: Minerva, 2008).

18. A recent Google search for this term yielded over 6 million hits, demonstrating the scale of the problem.

19. E. Kato, *Care-Giving Murder* (Tokyo: Kuresu-shuppan, 2005), pp. 43–4, 296–313.

20. K. Jones, 'Scull's Dilemma', *British Journal of Psychiatry*, 141 (1982), pp. 221–6; G. E. Langley, 'It May Be "Community" but is it Comprehensive?', *Psychiatric Bulletin*, 7:4 (1983), pp. 67–9.

21. See e.g. my Leverhulme-funded research on 'Voluntary Sector Social Care for Older People in Britain and Japan, 1945–2010', 2012–15; and M. Hayashi, *The Care of Older People in Norfolk: Experiences of Social Engagement, Informal Care and Volunteering* (Norwich: University of East Anglia, 2011).

22. K. Sugimoto, *The Japanese and Ageing* (Tokyo: Nihon-shakai-bunka-kenkyu-kai, 2001), p. 203. Figures from Cabinet Office, *White Paper on the Ageing Society 2011/2*, p. 31; J. Maher and H. Green, *Carers 2000* (London, Office of National Statistics/Stationery Office, 2002), p. 10.

23. Kaigo-rodo-antei-senta, *Result of Care Labour Survey 2010/11* (Tokyo: Kaigorodo-antei-senta, 23 August 2010), at http://www.kaigo-center.or.jp/report/pdf/h22_chousa_kekka.pdf [accessed 10 August 2012].

24. The proportions of male carers to the total numbers of carers were 40 per cent in England (2009–10) and 28 percent in Japan (2007): see, respectively, NHS Information Centre for Health and Social Care, *Survey of Carers in Households 2009/10*, p. 7; and Cabinet Office, *White Paper on the Ageing Society 2011/2*, pp. 33–4.

25. F. Coulmas, *Population Decline and Ageing in Japan* (London: Routledge, 2007), p. 65.

26. Democratic Party of Japan, *The Democratic Party of Japan, Manifesto 2009* (Tokyo: Democratic Party of Japan, 2009), p. 19, at http://www.dpj.or.jp/policies/manifesto2009 [accessed 10 August 2010]; Cabinet Office, *White Paper on the Ageing Society 2011/2*, p. 35.

27. L. Beesley, *Informal Care in England* (London: King's Fund, 2006), p. v.

WORKS CITED

Archival Sources in England

Norfolk Record Office, Norwich

Norwich City Council Committee Minutes

N/TC31/1/1–5, Norwich City Council Public Assistance Committee Minutes 1929–39.

N/TC31/1/6–8, Norwich City Council Social Welfare Committee Minutes 1939–48.

N/TC31/1/9–14, Norwich City Council Welfare Committee Minutes 1948–70; this includes the Norwich City Council Hostels Sub-Committee Minutes.

N/TC31/5/1–3, Norwich City Council Social Services Committee Minutes 1970–4.

Norfolk County Council Committee Minutes

C/C10/452, Norfolk County Council Public Assistance Advisory Committee Minutes 1929–30.

C/C10/453–461, Norfolk County Council Public Assistance Sub-Committee Minutes 1930–48.

C/C10/675–683, Norfolk County Council Welfare Committee Minutes 1948–70.

C/C10/610–611, Norfolk County Council Social Services Committee Minutes 1970–4.

NRO, Norwich Workhouse/Public Assistance Institution Records

C/SS1/27, Indoor Relief List 1942–9.

C/SS1/32, House Classification List 1916–42.

Gayton Workhouse/Public Assistance Institution Records

C/GP9/71–73, Guardians Committee (Area 9), Gayton Public Assistance Institution House Committee Minutes 1930–41.

C/GC8/15, Guardians Committee (Area 8), Gayton Public Assistance Institution House Committee Minutes 1941–8.

G/GP9/152–153, Freebridge Lynn Union, Workhouse Completion Orders, 23 May and 2 August 1836.

G/GP9/185, Freebridge Lynn Union, the Plan of June 1838.

Eastgate House (1948–63) and Woodlands (1963–74) Records

C/SS3/16–17, Eastgate House Management Sub-Committee Minutes 1948–63.

C/SS3/43, Woodlands Management Sub-Committee Minutes 1963–8.

C/SS4/7, Area 7 Management Sub-Committee Minutes 1968–70.

C/SS5/4, Area 4 Management Sub-Committee Minutes 1970–4.

C/SS10/2, Eastgate House Patient Days List 1955–67.

C/SS10/3, Eastgate House Weekly Return of Admissions and Discharges 1960–3.

C/SS10/11, Eastgate House Letters on Entertainments 1956.

C/SS10/15, Eastgate House Sweet and Tobacco Book 1961–3.

C/SS10/16, Eastgate House TV and Comforts Fund Accounts 1953–63.

C/SS10/26, Eastgate House Plan 1955.

C/SS10/28, Woodlands Register of Pensions 1964–7.

C/GP9/189, Transfer of Equipment from Eastgate House to Other County Homes, 1963.

C/GP9/193, Printed Sale Catalogue for Eastgate House, 21 April 1964.

C/GP9/195, Agreement to the Sale of Eastgate House, 21 April 1964.

C/GP9/200, Eastgate House Draft Deed of Purchase, 11 June 1964.

Other Norfolk Residential Home Records

C/SS3/6, Burnham Westgate Hall Management Sub-Committee Minutes 1951–7.

C/SS3/36, St Nicholas's House Management Sub-Committee Minutes 1960–8.

C/SS3/41, Sidney Dye House Management Sub-Committee Minutes 1957–68.

Norfolk County Hall, Norwich

Norfolk County Council Social Services Committee Minutes 1974–80.

Norfolk Heritage Centre, Norwich

N361.6, Norwich City Council Public Assistance Committee Reports 1930–9.

L614, Norwich City Council Medical Officer of Health Annual Reports 1938–55.

L614, Norfolk County Council Medical Officer of Annual Reports 1929–50.

Humphreys, D., *Born Poor: Records, Porter's Lodge and Tramps' Quarters*, privately printed for Age Concern, Norwich, 1990.

The Ordnance Survey (Southampton: Ordnance Survey, 1905), Norfolk Sheet XXXIV 11.

National Archives, Kew

CAB 134/698, *Report of the Committee on the Break-up of the Poor Law*, enclosed in the Minutes of the Seventh Meeting of the Social Services Committee, 12 July 1946.

Cambridgeshire Record Office, Cambridge

Cambridge County Borough Council Welfare Committee Minutes 1948–70.

Archival Sources in Japan

Gifu Record Office (GRO), Gifu

Hogoshisetsu ninka, kosei sewa-ka [Elderly Home Files 1950–63].

5.02-S38-1, Hogoshisetsu ninka, kosei sewa-ka showa 32-nen kara 38-nen (Gifu Yoroin) [Gifu Home File 1957–63].

5.02-S38-2, Hogoshisetsu ninka, kosei sewa-ka showa 25-nen kara 38-nen (Hino Yoroin) [Hino Home File 1950–63].

5.02-S38-2, Hogoshisetsu ninka, kosei sewa-ka showa 25-nen kara 38-nen (Tajimi Yoroin) [Tajimi Home File 1950–63].

5.02-S38-2, Hogoshisetsu ninka, kosei sewa-ka showa 25-nen kara 38-nen (Ogaki Yoroin) [Yorokaen Home File 1950–63].

5.02-S38-3, Hogoshisetsu ninka, kosei sewa-ka showa 27-nen kara 38-nen (Ibi Yoroin) [Ibigawa Home File 1952–63].

5.02-S38-3, Hogoshisetsu ninka, kosei sewa-ka showa 27-nen kara 38-nen (Seki Yoroin) [Seki Home File 1952–63].

5.02-S38-3, Hogoshisetsu ninka, kosei sewa-ka showa 27-nen kara 38-nen (Gujo Yoroin) [Gujo Home File 1952–63].

5.02-S38-3, Hogoshisetsu ninka, kosei sewa-ka showa 27-nen kara 38-nen (Nakatsugawa Yoroin) [Nakatsugawa Home File 1952–63].

5.02-S38-4, Hogoshisetsu ninka, kosei sewa-ka showa 27-nen kara 38-nen (Tarui Sefuen) [Tarui Home File 1952–63].

5.02-S38-4, Hogoshisetsu ninka, kosei sewa-ka showa 27-nen kara 38-nen (Takayama Hiyoen) [Takayama Home File 1952–63].

Rojinfukushi shisetsu shidokansa, kosei sewa-ka [Gifu Prefecture Annual Home Inspection Reports 1963–75].

5.02-S38-9, Rojinfukushi shisetsu shidokansa, kosei sewa-ka showa 38-nendo (Tarui Sefuen) [Tarui Home AHIR 1963].

5.02-S38-9, Rojinfukushi shisetsu shidokansa, kosei sewa-ka showa 38-nendo (Furukawa Wakoen) [Furukawa Home AHIR 1963].

5.02-S38-9, Rojinfukushi shisetsu shidokansa, kosei sewa-ka showa 38-nendo (Hashima Rowaen) [Hashima Home AHIR 1963].

5.02-S38-9, Rojinfukushi shisetsu shidokansa, kosei sewa-ka showa 38-nendo (Gujo Kairakuen) [Gujo Home AHIR 1963].

5.02-S39-6, Rojinfukushi shisetsu shidokansa san-satsu no ichi, kosei sewa-ka, showa 39-nendo (Ogaki Yorokaen) [Yorokaen Home AHIR 1965].

5.02-S39-8, Rojinfukushi shisetsu shidokansa san-satsu no ichi, kosei sewa-ka, showa 39-nendo (Takayama-shi Hiyoen) [Takayama Home AHIR 1964].

5.02-S41-4, Rojinfukushi shisetsu shidokansa ni-satsu no ichi, kosei sewa-ka, showa 41-nendo (Ogaki Yorokaen) [Yorokaen Home AHIR 1967].

5.02-S42-8, Rojinfukushi shisetsu shidokansa ni-satsu no ichi, kosei sewa-ka, showa 42-nendo (Ena Keikoen) [Ena Home AHIR 1967].

5.02-S43-5, Rojinfukushi shisetsu shidokansa ni-satsu no ichi, kosei sewa-ka, showa 42-nendo (Ogaki Yorokaen) [Yorokaen Home AHIR 1968].

5.02-S43-5, Rojinfukushi shisetsu shidokansa ni-satsu no ichi, kosei sewa-ka, showa 43-nendo (Ogaki Yorokaen) [Yorokaen Home AHIR 1969].

5.02-S44-13, Rojinfukushi shisetsu shidokansa san-satsu no ichi, kosei sewa-ka, showa 44-nendo (Jurakuen) [Jurakuen Home AHIR 1970].

5.02-S44-14, Rojinfukushi shisetsu shidokansa san-satsu no ni, kosei sewa-ka, showa 44-nendo (Ogaki Yorokaen) [Yorokaen Home AHIR 1970].

5.02-S47-5, Rojinfukushi shisetsu shidokansa san-satsu no ni, kosei sewa-ka, showa 47-nendo (Gifu Rojinhomu) [Gifu Home AHIR 1972].

5.02-S47-5, Rojinfukushi shisetsu shidokansa san-satsu no ni, kosei sewa-ka, showa 47-nendo (Ibi Showaen) [Ibigawa Home AHIR 1972].

5.02-S47-5, Rojinfukushi shisetsu shidokansa san-satsu no ni, kosei sewa-ka, showa 47-nendo (Jurakuen) [Jurakuen Home AHIR 1973].

5.02-S47-6, Rojinfukushi shisetsu shidokansa san-satsu no san, kosei sewa-ka, showa 47-nendo (Nakatsugawa Seiwaryo) [Nakatsugawa Home AHIR 1972].

5.02-S47-6, Rojinfukushi shisetsu shidokansa san-satsu no san, kosei sewa-ka, showa 47-nendo (Ogaki Yorokaen) [Yorokaen Home AHIR 1973].

5.02-S47-6, Rojinfukushi shisetsu shidokansa san-satsu no san, kosei sewa-ka, showa 47-nendo (Gujo Kairakuen) [Gujo Home AHIR 1973].

5.02-S50-18, Shidokansa fukushi-ka showa 50-nendo (hida-jurakuen hoka) [AHIR Files 1975 (Hida-Jurakuen Home, etc.)].

Other Records

5.02-S21-1, Seikatsuhogo shisetsu keikakusho tsuzuri, kosei-ka showa 21-nendo [Plans for Emergency Relief Institutions 1946–8].

5.02-S43-7, Rojinfukushi: rojin no hi, rojinfukushi taikai, kosei sewa-ka showa 43-nendo [Elderly Welfare Files 1968].

5.02-S44-7, Rojinfukushi sokatsu: gennin kunren (shisetsu, kateihoshi-in), ryokyaku unchin, kosei sewa-ka showa 44-nendo [Elderly Welfare Files 1969].

5.02-S45-4, Rojinfukushi: gennin kunren, kosei sewa-ka showa 45-nendo [Elderly Welfare Training Files 1970].

5.02-S45-5, Shiryo (dokkyo rojin jittai chosa), kosei sewa-ka, showa 45-nendo [Survey of Prefecture Elderly People Living Alone 1970].

5.02-S47-11, Gifu-ken sogo keikaku, kosei sewa-ka showa 47-nendo [Gifu Comprehensive Plan 1972].

5.02-S48-4, Shakaifukushi shisetsu san-satsu no ichi, kosei engo-ka showa 48-nendo [Welfare Facilities Files 1973].

5.02-S49-2, Gifu-ken sogo keikaku, kosei engo-ka showa 49-nendo [Gifu Prefecture Comprehensive Plan 1974].

5.02-S49-4, Chinjo, kosei engo-ka showa 49-nendo [Petitions to the Gifu Prefecture Public Assistance Division 1974].

5.02-S49-19, Chinjo, fukushi-ka showa 49-nendo [Petitions to the Gifu Prefecture Social Welfare Division 1974].

5.02-S50-6, Chinjo, kosei engo-ka showa 50-nendo [Petitions to the Gifu Prefecture Social Welfare Division 1975].

5.20-S51-13, Chinjo, kosei engo-ka showa 51-nendo [Petitions to the Gifu Prefecture Social Welfare Division 1976].

5.02-S53-15, Chinjo (kuni e no) ni-satsu no ichi, kosei engo-ka showa 53-nendo [Petitions to the Gifu Prefecture Social Welfare Division 1978].

5.02-S56-12, Sangiin kyodochosa kenkyu shiryo, fukushi-ka showa 56-nendo [Survey Files 1981].

Ogaki yorokaen shiori [Yorokaen Brochure, *c.* 1963], enclosed in Yorokaen Home AHIR 1965.

Yorokaen secchi jorei kanri kitei kaitei [Yorokaen Regulations, revised 1968], enclosed in Yorokaen Home AHIR 1973.

Gifu Public Library, Gifu

Gifu Yoroin showa hachi-nendo yoroin jigyo gaikyo [Gifu Old People's Almshouse Annual Report 1933], privately printed *c.* 1933.

Ogaki City Library, Ogaki

Yorokaen no gaiyo [Yorokaen Summary Report of 1985], *c.* 1985.

Yorokaen no shiori [Yorokaen Brochure, *c.* 1992].

Kusunokien Nursing Home, On-Site Archives, Ogaki

Showa 63-nendo rojinfukushi shisetsu kansa shiryo [Kusunokien Annual Home Inspection Report of 1988].

Gifu-ken roreifukushi-ka tsutatsu [Prefecture Circular], 1 December 1999.

Hakuju-kai, Tokubetsu rojinhomu ibukien 10-nen no ayumi: nukumori [Ten-Year History of Ibukien], privately printed in 1991.

Chiyoda-kai, Jugo-shunen kinenshi: kagayaki [Fifteen-Year History of Kikujuen], privately printed in 1994.

Shisetsu shisatsu kenshu hokokusho [Visiting Report] by attendant Ms B., 9 March 1995.

Gifu Council of Elderly Homes, Gifu-ken rojinfukushi shisetsu kyogikai no aramashi [History of Gifu Council of Elderly Homes] (Gifu: Gifu Council of Elderly Homes, 1996).

Kusunokien homu no tebiki [Kusunokien Home Manual], privately printed *c.* 2001.

Yorokaen Old People's Home, On-Site Archives, Ogaki

Ogaki-shi hogo kyokai sainyu saisyutsu kessansho [Yorokaen Annual Financial Statements 1923–58].

Taiin shibo tuzuri [Yorokaen Registers of Deaths and Discharges 1926–95].

Ogaki-shi hogo kyokai yakuinkai gijiroku [Yorokaen Minutes of the Ogaki Relief Foundation 1930–80].

Hogoshisetsu ni kansuru tsuzuri [Yorokaen Relief Institution Files 1950].

Showa 31-nendo jigyo keikaku [Yorokaen Annual Plan for 1951].

Yorokaen secchi jorei kanri kitei [Yorokaen Regulations, revised 1951].

Yorokaen shokuin kitei [Yorokaen Staff Regulations, 1951].

Toki shorui tsuzuri [Yorokaen Registration Files 1952–69].

Nenkan jigyo hokokusho [Yorokaen Annual Reports 1952–8].

Jirei bo [Yorokaen Appointment Lists 1952–8].

Bunsho tsuzuri [Yorokaen Memoranda Files 1952–65].

Kosei sho hogoshisetsu kansa showa 30-nen [Yorokaen Ministry Home Inspection Report of 1955].

Tanaoroshi meisai [Yorokaen Inventories 1956].

Yorokaen shokuin kitei kaitei [Yorokaen Staff Regulations, revised 1956].

Ogaki yorokaen shiori [Yorokaen Brochure, *c.* 1958].

Yorokaen secchi jorei kanri kitei kaitei [Yorokaen Regulations, revised 1959].

Ogaki yorokaen gaizu [Yorokaen Plan File, *c.* 1960].

Ogaki-shi eno tangan sho [Yorokaen Petition to the Ogaki City Council, 11 September 1961].

Ogaki-shi eno kifukin meisai [Yorokaen Lists of Donations to Ogaki City Council, 1963].

Ogaki yorokaen rekishi enkaku [Yorokaen History Draft, *c.* 1970].

Okachiyama senta no shiori [Okachiyama Community Centre Brochure, *c.* 2006].

An Unidentified Prefecture Home

Sutaffu kaigi hokokusho [Report] by attendant Ms P., 17 February 1995.

Parliamentary Papers

In England

Censuses 1931–91, referring to England and Wales.

Department of Health and Social Security, *Department of Health and Social Security Annual Report for 1970*, Cmnd 4714 (London: HMSO, 1971).

—, *Circular 35/72: Local Authority Social Services Ten Year Development Plans 1973–1983* (31 August 1972).

—, *Priorities for Health and Personal Social Services in England* (London: Department of Health and Social Security/HMSO, 1976).

—, *The Way Forward: Priorities in the Health and Social Services* (London: HMSO, 1977).

—, *Growing Older*, Cmnd 8173 (London: HMSO, 1981).

Hansard (Parliamentary Debates), *House of Commons 444* (24 November 1947); *448* (5 March 1948); *512* (6 March 1953); *522* (14 December 1953); *578* (29 November 1957); *582* (12 February 1958); *77, Written Answers* (17 April 1985); *94* (27 March 1986); *97* (14 May 1986).

Hansard, *House of Lords 154* (6 April 1948).

HM Government, Green Paper: *Shaping the Future of Care Together*, Cm 7673 (Norwich: Stationery Office, 2009).

HM Government, White Paper: *Building the National Care Service*, Cm 7854 (Norwich: Stationery Office, 2010).

HM Government, White Paper: *Caring for Our Future: Reforming Care and Support*, Cm 8378 (Norwich: Stationery Office, 2012).

HM Treasury, *Public Expenditure Analyses to 1993–94* (London: HMSO, 1991).

House of Commons Health Committee, *Public Expenditure on Health and Personal Social Services, Session 1992–93* (London: HMSO, 1993).

Ministry of Health, *Persons in Receipt of Poor-Law Relief, England and Wales* (London: HMSO, May 1927).

—, *Circular 179/44: Domestic Help* (14 December 1944).

—, *Circular 49/47: The Care of the Aged in Public Assistance Homes and Institutions* (6 June 1947).

—, *Circular 3/55: Residential Accommodation for Old People, Homes for the More Infirm* (25 February 1955).

—, *Circular 14/57: Local Authority Services for the Chronic Sick and Infirm* (7 October 1957).

—, *HM(57)86: Geriatric Services and the Care of the Chronic Sick* (7 October 1957).

—, *A Hospital Plan for England and Wales*, Cmnd 1604 (London: HMSO, 1962).

—, *Health and Welfare: The Development of Community Care*, Cmnd 1973 (London: HMSO, 1963).

—, *Health and Welfare: The Development of Community Care: Revision to 1973–4 of Plans for the Health and Welfare Services of the Local Authorities in England and Wales*, Cmnd 3022 (London: HMSO, 1964).

—, *Report of the Committee of Enquiry into the Cost of the National Health Service*, Cmd 9663 (London: HMSO, 1956).

—, *Survey of Services Available to the Chronic Sick and Elderly 1954–55* (London: HMSO, 1957).

—, *Report of the Ministry of Health for the Year Ended 31st March 1949*, Cmd 7910 (London: HMSO, 1950). Other years consulted: *1950*, Cmd 8342 (1951); *1952*, Cmd 8933 (1953); *1954*, Cmd 9566 (1955); *1955*, Cmd 9857 (1956); *1958*, Cmnd 806 (1959); *1960*, Cmnd 1418 (1961); *1961*, Cmnd 1754 (1962).

Report by the Royal Commission on Long Term Care: With Respect to Old Age, Cm 4192-I, II/1–3 (London: Stationery Office, 1999), vol. II/3.

Report of the Committee on Local Authority and Allied Personal Social Services, Cmnd 3703 (London: HMSO, 1968).

Report of the Committee on the Economic and Financial Problems of the Provision for Old Age, Cmd 9333 (London: HMSO, 1954).

Report of the Royal Commission on the Poor Laws (Majority Report), Cmd 4499 (1909).

Report of the Royal Commission on the Poor Laws (Minority Report): 'Break Up the Poor Law and Abolish the Workhouse' being Part I of The Minority Report of the Poor Law Commission, printed for the Fabian Society (1909).

Report of the Working Party on Social Workers in the Local Authority Health and Welfare Services (London: HMSO, 1959).

Royal Commission on the Law Relating to Mental Illness and Mental Deficiency, Cmnd 169 (London: HMSO, 1957).

Summary Report by the Ministry of Health, Cmd 6340 (February 1942); Cmd 6394 (October 1942).

In Japan

Cabinet Office, *Heisei 23-nenban koureishakai hakusho* [*White Paper on the Ageing Society 2011/12*] (Tokyo: Insatsu-tsuhan, 2011).

Cabinet Office, *Heisei 24-nenban koureishakai hakusho* [*White Paper on the Ageing Society 2012/13*], at http://www8.cao.go.jp/kourei/whitepaper/w-2012/zenbun/24pdf_index.html [accessed 10 August 2012].

Central Committee of Social Welfare, *Rojinmondai ni kansuru sogoteki shoshisaku ni tsuite* [*Comprehensive Programmes to Respond to the Old Age Problem*] (Tokyo: Ministry of Health and Welfare, 25 November 1970). Full text available at the National Council of Population and Social Security Research website, at http://www.ipss.go.jp/publication/j/shiryou/no.13/data/shiryou/syakaifukushi/46.pdf [accessed 10 August 2012].

Kokumin-seikatsu-shingikai-chosabu-rojin-mondai-shoiinkai, *Shinkokuka suru korekara no rojinmondai* [*Report on the Growing Old Age Problem*] (Tokyo: Ministry of Health and Welfare, 15 September 1968). Full text available at the National Institute of Population and Social Security Research website, at http://www.ipss.go.jp/publication/j/shiryou/no.13/data/shiryou/syakaifukushi/23.pdf [accessed 10 August 2012].

Ministry of Health, Labour and Welfare, *Koseirodo hakusho heisei 15-nendo ban* [*White Paper on Health, Labour and Welfare 2003/4*] (Tokyo: Gyosei, 2003). Also consulted: 2005/6.

Ministry of Health and Welfare, *Kosei hakusho showa 31-nendo ban* [*White Paper on Health and Welfare 1956/7*] (Tokyo: Toyokezai-shinpo-sha, 1956). Other years consulted:

1957/8, 1960/1, 1961/2, 1962/3, 1963/4, 1969/70, 1981/2, 1984/5, 1985/6, 1991/2, 1992/3, 1993/4, 1995/6, 1997/8, 2000/1.

— (ed.), *Shakaifukushi shisetsu unei shishin* [*Revised Version: A Code of Practice for Welfare Institutions*], 3 vols (Tokyo: National Council of Social Welfare, 1994).

— (ed.), *Shakaifukushi shisetsu unei shishin* [*A Code of Practice for Welfare Institutions*], 3 vols (Tokyo: National Council of Social Welfare, 1989).

—, *Hogoshisetsu toriatsukai shishin* [*A Code of Practice for Assessed Institutions*] (Tokyo: Seikatsu-fukushi-shisetsu-kenkyu-kai, 1957), repr. in Y. Ogasawara (ed.), *Rojinmondai kenkyu kihonbunken shu (Rekishi bunken)* [*Basic Historical Sources for Old Age Research (Historical Sources)*], 29 vols (Tokyo: Ozora-sha, 1990–2), vol. 6.

—, *Annual Report of Health and Welfare 1998–9: Social Security and National Life* (Tokyo: Japan International Corporation of Welfare Services, 1999).

Major Acts of Parliament

In England

1601   Old Poor Law.
1834   Poor Law Amendment Act (New Poor Law).
1908   Old Age Pensions Act.
1911   National Insurance Act.
1918   Maternity and Child Welfare Act.
1925   Old Age and Widows and Orphans Contributory Pensions Act.
1929   Local Government Act.
1934   Unemployment Act.
1946   National Health Service Act.
1946   National Insurance Act.
1948   Children Act.
1948   National Assistance Act.
1958   Local Government Act.
1959   Mental Health Act.
1962   National Assistance (Amendment) Act.
1968   Health Services and Public Health Act.
1970   Chronically Sick and Disabled Act.
1970   Local Authority Social Services Act.
1973   National Health Service Reorganisation Act.
1980   Social Security Act.
1980   Residential Homes Act.
1984   Registered Homes Act.
1990   National Health Service and Community Care Act.
2000   Care Standards Act.
2001   Health and Social Care Act.

In Japan

1874   Jutsukyu kisoku [Poor Relief Order], No. 162.
1911   Kojo ho [Factory Law], No. 46.

1922 Kenko hoken ho [Health Insurance Act], No. 70.
1929 Kyugo ho [Poor Law], No. 39.
1931 Rodosha saigaifujo ho [Industrial Injury Assistance Act], No. 54.
1937 Boshi hogo ho [Mother and Baby Relief Act], No. 19.
1937 Kaisei gunjifujo ho [Military Relief Act], No. 20.
1938 Shakai jigyo ho [Social Services Charities Act], No. 59.
1938 Kokumin kenko hoken ho [National Health Insurance Act], No. 60.
1941 Iryo hogo ho [Health Relief Act], No. 36.
1941 Rodosha nenkin hoken ho [Workers Pensions Act], No. 60.
1942 Senjisaigai hogo ho [Wartime Disaster Assistance Act], No. 71.
1946 Seikatsu hogo ho [Old National Assistance Act], No. 17.
1946 Nihonkoku kempo [Constitution of Japan].
1947 Jido fukushi ho [Child Welfare Act], No. 164.
1949 Shintai shogaisha fukushi ho [Physically Disabled Persons Act], No. 283.
1950 Shin seikatsu hogo ho [New National Assistance Act], No. 144.
1951 Shakaifukushi jigyo ho [Social Services Reform Act], No. 45.
1958 Kokumin kenko hoken ho [National Health Care Act], No. 192.
1959 Kokumin nenkin ho [National Pensions Act], No. 141.
1963 Rojin fukushi ho [Elderly Welfare Act], No. 133.
1982 Rojin hoken ho [Elderly Health Care Act], No. 80.
1997 Kaigo hoken ho [Long-Term Care Insurance (ITCI) Act], No. 123.

Interviews

In England

A. (Ms), qualified nurse (1986–8), interview, 1 December 2008.

C. (Ms), Norfolk County Council social worker (1981–3), interview, 15 April 2008.

D. (Ms), NHS domiciliary (community) nurse (1976–8), interview, 29 November 2008.

E. (Ms), daughter of an incapacitated private care home resident (2003–7), interview, 17 April 2008.

F. (Ms), private care home deputy matron (1989–90), interview, 25 October 2008.

G. (Mrs), daughter of a private care home resident (1983–5), interview, 3 June 2008.

H. (Ms), charge nurse (1978–85), interview, 22 November 2008.

I. (Ms), deputy matron (1976–8), interview, 13 November 2008.

J. (Ms), Norfolk County Council relief care assistant (1982–5), interview, 30 November 2008

K. (Ms), private home care assistant (1983–92), interview, 7 December 2008.

L. (Ms), daughter of an incapacitated private care home resident (2003–7), interview, 17 April 2008.

M. (Ms), Norfolk County Council social worker, working with Norfolk Mental Health team in 2005, interview, 27 November 2008.

N. (Ms), student nurse (1972–5), first interview, 30 April 2008; second interview, 11 November 2008; third interview, 24 November 2008.

O. (Ms), private home care assistant (1991–3), interview, 3 December 2008.

R. (Mrs), daughter of a private care home resident (1985–8), interview, 5 June 2008.

S. (Mrs), nurse assistant (1970–82), interview, 15 December 2008.

T. (Ms), care assistant in local authority home (1983–6) and private home (1990–5), interview, 12 December 2008.

V. (Ms), hospital ward sister (1976–8), interview, 8 December 2008.

W. (Mr), private care home resident (1993–2011), first interview, 25 May 2009, second interview, 11 July 2009.

W. (Mrs), private care home resident (1989–), first interview, 25 May 2009.

Y. (Ms), private care home nurse (1988–90), interview, 25 October 2008.

In Japan

A. (Ms), Yorokaen attendant (1987–2003) and Kusunokien chief attendant (2003–7), interview, 2 June 2008.

B. (Ms), Yorokaen attendant (2000–7), interview, 29 May 2008.

C. (Ms), Yorokaen attendant (1994–8), interview, 25 May 2008.

D. (Ms), Kusunokien attendant (1992–), interview, 30 May 2008.

E. (Ms), Kusunokien attendant (2007–), interview, 28 May 2008.

F. (Mrs), attendant of a public institution for disabled adults (1992–4); Yorokaen attendant (1995–8; 2000–2); care house attendant (1998–9); Kusunokien senior attendant (2002–), interview, 28 May 2008.

G. (Ms), Kusunokien qualified attendant (1990–9) and Kusunokien chief attendant (2005–), interview, 29 May 2008.

H. (Mrs), Yorokaen resident (1980–), interview, 25 April 2007.

I. (Mr), Yorokaen kitchen staff (2000–7), interview, 28 May 2008.

J. (Ms), Kusunokien attendant (2003–), interview, 2 June 2008.

K. (Ms), Yorokaen attendant (1994–7) and Kusunokien care manager (2003–), first interview, 27 May 2008, second interview, 4 June 2008.

K. (Mr), psychiatric nursing assistant (1985–9), interview, 20 May 2008.

L. (Mr), Kusunokien attendant (1991–), interview, 2 June 2008.

M. (Ms), Yorokaen kitchen staff (1998–2007), interview, 3 June 2008.

N. (Ms), Kusunokien qualified nurse (1990–), interview, 29 May 2008.

O. (Mr), Yorokaen attendant (1996–2001), interview, 28 May 2008.

P. (Ms), Kusunokien attendant (1991–), interview, 29 May 2008.

Q. (Ms), Kusunokien resident (2003–), interview, 28 May 2008.

R. (Mr), Kusunokien attendant (1994–), interview, 2 June 2008.

S. (Ms), Kusunokien attendant (2000–), interview, 4 June 2008.

T. (Ms), Yorokaen attendant (1995–8) and Kusunokien attendant (1998–), interview, 3 June 2008.

U. (Mr), Kusunokien resident (2006–), interview, 28 May 2008.

V. (Ms), Kusunokien resident (2003–), interview, 28 May 2008.

W. (Ms), Kusunokien day care assistant (1991–3) and Kusunokien attendant (1993–), interview, 3 June 2008.

Y. (Mr), Kusunokien volunteer (January–March 1989), Kusunokien qualified attendant (1989–2005) and Kusunokien care supervisor (2005–), first interview, 26 May 2008, second interview, 30 May 2008.

Newspapers and Periodicals

In English

Daily Mail.
Daily Telegraph.
Eastern Daily Press.
Eastern Evening News.
Guardian.
The Times Higher Education Supplement.
The Times.

In Japanese

Asahi shinbun [*Asahi Newspaper*].
Asahi shinbun yukan [*Asahi Evening Newspaper*].
Chunichi shinbun [*Chunichi Newspaper*].
Gifu shinbun [*Gifu Newspaper*].
Gifu taimuzu shinbun [*Gifu Times Newspaper*].
Gifu-nichinichi shinbun [*Gifu-nichinichi Newspaper*].
Mainichi shinbun [*Mainichi Newspaper*].
Nihon keizai shinbun [*Japan Financial Newspaper*].
Yomiuri shinbun [*Yomiuri Newspaper*].

Secondary Sources

In English

Abel-Smith, B., *The Hospitals, 1800–1948: A Study in Social Administration in England and Wales* (London: Heinemann, 1964).

Adachi, K., 'The Development of Social Welfare Services in Japan', in S. O. Long (ed.), *Caring for the Elderly in Japan and the US: Practices and Policies* (London: Routledge, 2000), pp. 191–205.

Adachi, K., J. E. Lubben and N. Tsukada, 'Expansion of Formalized In-Home Services for Japan's Aged', *Journal of Aging and Social Policy*, 8:2–3 (1996), pp. 147–59.

Adams, R., *The Personal Social Services: Clients, Consumers or Citizens?* (London and New York: Longman, 1996).

Age UK, *Care in Crisis 2012*, at http://www.ageuk.org.uk/Documents/EN-GB/Campaigns/care_in_crisis_2012_report.pdf?dtrk=true [accessed 10 August 2012].

Alcock, P., *Poverty and State Support* (London: Longman, 1987).

Alcock, P., and G. Craig (eds), *International Social Policy: Welfare Regimes in the Developed World*, 2nd edn (Basingstoke: Palgrave Macmillan, 2009).

Allen, I., D. Hogg and S. Peace, *Elderly People: Choice, Participation and Satisfaction* (London: Policy Studies Institute, 1992).

Lord Amulree, 'Proper Use of the Hospital in Treatment of the Aged Sick', *Lancet*, 260:1 (1951), pp. 123–6.

Lord Amulree and E. L. Sturdee, 'Care of the Chronic Sick and of the Aged', *British Medical Journal*, 1:20 (April 1946), pp. 617–19.

Andrews, J., A. Briggs, R. Porter, P. Tucker and K. Waddington, *The History of Bethlem* (London: Routledge, 1997).

Audit Commission, *Making a Reality of Community Care* (London: HMSO, 1986).

Bartlett, H., and R. B. Ross, 'Terms of a Contract', *Community Care*, 592 (1986), pp. 14–15.

Barton, R., *Institutional Neurosis* (Bristol: John Wright & Sons, 1959).

BBC News, at http://www.bbc.co.uk/news [accessed 10 August 2012].

Beasley, W. G., *The Rise of Modern Japan* (London: Weidenfeld & Nicolson, 1995).

Bebbington, A. C., 'Changes in the Provision of Social Services to the Elderly in the Community over Fourteen Years', *Social Policy and Administration*, 13:2 (1979), pp. 111–23.

Beesley, L., *Informal Care in England* (London: King's Fund, 2006).

Bethel, D. L., 'Life on Obasuteyama, or, Inside a Japanese Institution for the Elderly', in T. S. Lebra (ed.), *Japanese Social Organization* (Honolulu, HI: University of Hawaii Press, 1992), pp. 109–34.

—, 'Alienation and Reconnection in a Home for the Elderly', in J. J. Tobin (ed.), *Re-made in Japan: Everyday Life and Consumer Taste in a Changing Society* (New Haven, CT and London: Yale University Press, 1992), pp. 126–42.

Biggs, S., 'Quality of Care and the Growth of Private Welfare for Old People', *Critical Social Policy*, 20:7 (1987), pp. 74–82.

Bland, A. E., P. A. Brown and R. H. Tawney (eds), *English Economic History: Select Documents* (London: Bell, 1914).

Blaug, M., 'The Poor Law Report Reexamined', *Journal of Economic History*, 24:2 (1964), pp. 229–45.

Booth, C., *Pauperism and the Endowment of Old Age* (London: Macmillan & Co., 1892).

—, *The Aged Poor in England and Wales* (London and New York: Macmillan & Co., 1894).

Booth, C. (ed.), *Life and Labour of the People in London*, 17 vols (London: Macmillan & Co., 1902–3).

Booth, T., 'Camden Shows the Way', *Community Care*, 649 (1987), pp. 16–17.

Bosanquet, B., *Rich and Poor* (London and New York: Macmillan & Co., 1896).

Bosanquet, N., *A Future for Old Age* (London: Temple Smith/New Society, 1978).

Bradshaw, B. J., 'Financing Private Care for the Elderly', in S. Baldwin, G. Parker and R. Walker (eds), *Social Security and Community Care* (Aldershot: Avebury, 1988), pp. 175–87.

Brown, M., 'A Welfare Service not a Welfare Department', *Social Services Quarterly*, 39:3 (December 1965–February 1966), pp. 91–4.

—, 'The Development of Local Authority Welfare Services from 1948–1965 under Part III of the National Assistance Act 1948' (PhD disseration, University of Manchester, 1972).

Brown, R. G. S., *Reorganising the National Health Service: A Case Study in Administrative Change* (Oxford: Blackwell, 1979).

Buckner, L., and S. Yeandle, *Valuing Carers 2011: Calculating the Value of Carers' Support* (London: Carers UK, 2011).

Butler, A., C. Oldman and J. Greve, *Sheltered Housing for the Elderly* (London: Allen & Unwin, 1983).

Campbell, J. C., *How Policies Change: The Japanese Government and the Aging Society* (Princeton, NJ and Oxford: Princeton University Press, 1992). Japanese translation available.

—, 'Changing Meaning of Frail Old People and the Japanese Welfare State', in S. O. Long (ed.), *Caring for the Elderly in Japan and the US: Practices and Policies* (London: Routledge, 2000), pp. 82–97.

Campbell, J. C., and N. Ikegami, 'Japan's Radical Reform of Long-Term Care', *Social Policy and Administration*, 37:1 (February 2003), pp. 21–34.

Campbell, J. C., N. Ikegami and S. Kwon, 'Policy Learning and Cross-National Diffusion in Social Long-Term Care Insurance: Germany, Japan and the Republic of Korea', *International Social Security Review*, 62:4 (2009), pp. 63–80.

Carers UK, *Policy Briefing: Facts about Carers 2009* (London: Carers UK, June 2009), at http://www.carersuk.org/media/k2/attachments/Facts_about_Carers_2009.pdf [accessed 10 August 2012].

Caring for People, Staffing Residential Homes: Report of the Committee of Enquiry (London: Allen & Unwin, 1967).

Carson, D., 'Registering Homes: Another Fine Mess?', *Journal of Social Welfare Law* (March 1985), pp. 67–84.

Carson, G., 'Call for Free Minimum Level of Care', *Community Care*, 1616 (2006), p. 6.

Centre for Policy on Ageing, *Home Life: A Code of Practice for Residential Care* (London: Centre for Policy on Ageing, 1984).

—, *A Better Home Life* (London: Centre for Policy on Ageing, 1996). Japanese translation available.

Charles, E., *The Twilight of Parenthood: A Biological Study of the Decline of Population Growth* (London: Watts & Co., 1934).

Charlesworth, A., and R. Thorlby, *Reforming Social Care: Options for Funding* (London: Nuffield Trust, May 2012), at http://www.nuffieldtrust.org.uk/sites/files/nuffield/

publication/120529_reforming-social-care-options-funding_0.pdf [accessed 10 August 2012].

Cherry, S., *Medical Services and the Hospitals in Britain, 1860–1939* (Cambridge: Cambridge University Press, 1996).

—, *Mental Health Care in Modern England: The Norfolk Lunatic Asylum/St Andrew's Hospital, c. 1810–1998* (Woodbridge: Boydell, 2003).

—, 'Medical Care since 1750', in C. Rawcliffe and R. Wilson (eds), *Norwich since 1550* (London and New York: Hambledon & London, 2004), pp. 271–93.

—, 'Medicine and Rural Health Care in 19th Century Europe', in J. L. Barona and S. Cherry (eds), *Health and Medicine in Rural Europe* (Valencia: University of Valencia, 2005), pp. 19–61.

Clark, D. H., *The Story of a Mental Hospital, Fulbourn 1853–1983* (London: Process Press, 1996).

Clarke, L., *Domiciliary Services for the Elderly* (Beckenham: Croom Helm, 1984).

Close, P. (ed.), *The State and Caring* (Basingstoke: Macmillan, 1992).

Clough, D., *Independent Review of Residential Care for the Elderly within the London Borough of Camden* (London: London Borough of Camden, 1987).

Cochrane, A., J. Clarke and S. Gewitz, 'Introduction', in A. Cochrane, J. Clarke and S. Gewitz (eds), *Comparing Welfare States*, 2nd edn (London: Sage in association with the Open University, 2001), pp. 2–27.

Cole, D., and J. E. G. Utting, *The Economic Circumstances of Old People* (Welwyn: Codicote Press, 1962).

Commission on Funding of Care and Support (Dilnot Commission), *Fairer Care Funding: The Report of the Commission on Funding of Care and Support* (July 2011), at https://www.wp.dh.gov.uk/carecommission/files/2011/07/Fairer-Care-Funding-Report.pdf [accessed 10 August 2012].

Conservative Party, *Conservative Manifesto 1979* (London: Conservative Central Office, 1979).

Cooper, D. G., *Psychiatry and Anti-Psychiatry* (London: Tavistock, 1967).

Coulmas, F., *Population Decline and Ageing in Japan* (London: Routledge, 2007).

Craig, F. W. S. (ed.), *British Parliamentary Election Results 1918–49*, 3rd edn (Chichester: Parliamentary Research Services, 1983).

— (ed.), *British Parliamentary Election Results 1950–73* (Chichester: Parliamentary Research Services, 1983).

— (ed.), *British Parliamentary Election Results 1974–83* (Chichester: Parliamentary Research Services, 1984).

Crammer, J., *Asylum History: Buckinghamshire County Pauper Lunatic Asylum – St. John's* (London: Gaskell, 1990).

Crowther, M. A., *The Workhouse System 1834–1929* (London: Batsford Academic and Educational, 1981).

Dalley, G., and M. Mandelstam, *Assessment Denied?: Council Responsibilities Towards Self-Funders Moving into Care* (London: Relatives & Residents Association, 2008).

Davies, B., *Social Needs and Resources in Local Services: A Study of Variations in Standards of Provision of Personal Social Services between Local Authority Areas* (London: Michael Joseph, 1968).

Davies, G., and D. Piachaud, 'Social Policy and the Economy', in H. Glennerster (ed.), *The Future of the Welfare State: Remaking Social Policy* (London: Heinemann, 1983), pp. 40–60.

Davies, M., 'Swopping [*sic*] the Old Around', *Community Care*, 296 (1979), pp. 16–17.

Department of Health and Social Security, *Health and Personal Social Services Statistics for England 1982* (London: HMSO, 1982).

Dickie, M., 'A Fiscal Frailty', *Financial Times*, 4 August 2009, p. 7.

Digby, A., 'The Rural Poor Law', in D. Fraser (ed.), *The New Poor Law in the Nineteenth Century* (London: Macmillan, 1976), pp. 149–70.

—, *Pauper Palaces* (London: Routledge & Kegan Paul, 1978).

—, *Madness, Morality and Medicine: A Study of the York Retreat 1796–1914* (Cambridge: Cambridge University Press, 1985).

—, *British Welfare Policy: Workhouse to Workfare* (London: Faber, 1989).

—, 'Poor Law Unions and Workhouses 1834–1930', in T. Ashwin and A. Davison (eds), *An Historical Atlas of Norfolk,* 3rd edn (Chichester: Phillimore, 2005), pp. 148–9.

Department of Health, *Health and Personal Social Services Statistics for England 1993 edition* (London: HMSO/Stationery Office, 1993).

—, *Care Homes for Older People: National Minimum Standards and the Care Homes Regulations 2001*, 3rd edn (London: Stationery Office, 2003).

Donnison, D. V., 'Seebohm: The Report and its Implications', *Social Work* (Britain), 25:4 (1968), pp. 3–8.

Doran, T., F. Drever and M. Whitehead, 'Health of Young and Elderly Informal Carers: Analysis of UK Census Data', *British Medical Journal*, 327:7428 (13 December 2003), p. 1388.

Doyle, B. M., 'Politics, 1835–1945', in C. Rawcliffe and R. Wilson (eds), *Norwich since 1550* (London and New York: Hambledon & London, 2004), pp. 343–60.

Easterbrook, L., *Moving On from Community Care: The Treatment, Care and Support of Older People in England* (London: Age Concern Books, 2003).

Esping-Andersen, G., *The Three Worlds of Welfare Capitalism* (Cambridge: Polity, 1990). Japanese translation available.

—, 'Hybrid or Unique?', *Journal of European Social Policy*, 7:3 (1997), pp. 179–89.

—, *Social Foundations of Postindustrial Economics* (Oxford: Oxford University Press, 1999).

Fisher, M., '"Getting Out of the Asylum": Discharge and Decarceration Issues in Asylum History *c.* 1890–1959' (PhD dissertation, University of East Anglia, 2003).

Fleiss, A., *Home Ownership Alternatives for the Elderly* (London: HMSO, 1985).

Foucault, M., *Madness and Civilization: A History of Insanity in the Age of Reason*, trans. R. Howard, abridged edn (London: Tavistock Publications, 1967).

Fowler, S., *Workhouse: The People, the Places, the Life behind Doors* (Kew: National Archives, 2007).

Fraser, D., *The Evolution of the British Welfare State: A History of Social Policy since the Industrial Revolution* (Basingstoke: Palgrave Macmillan, 2003).

Friedmann, R. R., N. Gilbert and M. Sherer (eds), *Modern Welfare States: A Comparative View of Trends and Prospects* (Brighton: Wheatsheaf, 1987).

Gentleman, A., 'Life in an Old People's Home', *Guardian*, 14 July 2009, *G2*, pp. 5–11.

Gibbs, J., M. Evans and S. Rodway, *Report of the Inquiry into Nye Bevan Lodge* (London: London Borough of Southwark, 1987).

Gilbert, B. B., *British Social Policy 1914–1939* (London: B. T. Batsford, 1970).

Glennerster, H., J. Falkingham and M. Evandrow, 'How Much Do We Care?', *Social Policy and Administration*, 24:2 (1990), pp. 93–103.

Goffman, E., *Asylums: Essays on the Social Situation of Mental Patients and Other Inmates* (New York: Doubleday, 1961). Japanese translation available.

Goodman, R., 'The "Japanese-Style Welfare State" and the Delivery of Personal Social Services', in R. Goodman, G. White and H. Kwon (eds), *The East Asian Welfare Model* (London and New York: Routledge, 1998), pp. 139–58.

Goodman, R., and I. Peng, 'The East Asian Welfare States', in G. Esping-Andersen (ed.), *Welfare States in Transition: National Adaptations in Global Economies* (London: Sage, 1996), pp. 192–224.

Goodman, R., G. White and H. Kwan, 'Editors' Preface', in R. Goodman, G. White and H. Kwan (eds), *The East Asian Welfare Model* (London and New York: Routledge, 1998), pp. xiv–xvii.

Gould, A., *Capitalist Welfare Systems: A Comparison of Japan, Britain and Sweden* (London: Longman, 1993). Japanese translation available.

Gould, F., and B. Roweth, 'Public Spending and Social Policy: The United Kingdom 1950–1977', *Journal of Social Policy*, 9:3 (1980), pp. 337–57.

Great Britain Poor Law Commissioners, *The Poor Law Report of 1834*, ed. and intro. S. G. Checkland and E. O. A. Checkland (Harmondsworth: Penguin, 1974).

Griffith, J. A. G., *Central Departments and Local Authorities* (London: George Allen & Unwin, 1966).

Grundy, E., and T. Arie, 'Falling Rates of Provision of Residential Care for the Elderly', *British Medical Journal*, 284:6318 (1982), pp. 799–802.

Hanson, J., 'Challenge in the Welfare Services', *Municipal Review*, 36:431 (November 1965), p. 666.

Harada, S., 'The Aging Society, the Family, and Social Policy', *University of Tokyo Institute of Social Science Occasional Papers in Law and Society*, 8 (March 1996), pp. 1–70.

Hardy, B., R. Young and G. Wistow, 'Dimensions of Choice in the Assessment and Care Management Process: The Views of Older People, Carers and Care Managers', *Health and Social Care in the Community*, 7:6 (1999), pp. 483–91.

Harris, A. I., *Social Welfare for the Elderly: A Study in Thirteen Local Authority Areas in England, Wales and Scotland*, 2 vols (London: HMSO, 1968).

Harris, B., *The Origins of the British Welfare State: Society, State, and Social Welfare in England and Wales, 1800–1945* (Basingstoke and New York: Palgrave Macmillan, 2004).

Hayashi, M., 'Residential Care for the Elderly in England and Japan in the Twentieth Century: Local Authority Provision in the County of Norfolk and Gifu Prefecture' (PhD dissertation, University of East Anglia, 2010).

—, 'Testing the Limits of Care for Older People', *Society Guardian*, 29 September 2010, p. 3, also available at http://www.guardian.co.uk/society/2010/sep/28/japan-elderly-care-mutual-support [accessed 10 August 2012].

—, 'The Care of Older People in Japan: Myths and Realities of Family "Care"', *History and Policy* (July 2011), at http://www.historyandpolicy.org/papers/policy-paper-121.html [accessed 10 August 2012].

—, *The Care of Older People in Norfolk: Experiences of Social Engagement, Informal Care and Volunteering* (Norwich: University of East Anglia, 2011).

Hennock, E. P., *British Social Reform and German Precedents: The Case of Social Insurance 1880–1914* (Oxford: Clarendon, 1987).

Higgs, P., and C. Victor, 'Institutional Care and the Life Course', in S. Arber and M. Evandrou (eds), *Ageing, Independence and the Life Course* (London: Jessica Kingsley in association with the British Society of Gerontology, 1993), pp. 186–200.

Higginbotham, P., *The Workhouse*, at http://www.workhouses.org.uk [accessed 10 August 2012].

Hill, M., 'Origins of the Local Authority Social Services', in M. Hill (ed.), *Local Authority Social Services: An Introduction* (Oxford: Blackwell, 2000), pp. 22–37.

Hiraoka, K., 'Long-Term Care Insurance in Japan', in H. Yoon and J. Hendricks (eds), *Handbook of Asian Aging* (New York: Baywood Publishing Co., 2006), pp. 123–46.

Holmes, B., *The Realities of Home Life* (Birmingham: National Union of Public Employees, 1986).

Holmes, B., and A. Johnson, *Cold Comfort: The Scandal of Private Rest Homes* (London: Souvenir Press, 1988).

Hoshino, S., 'Paying for the Health and Social Care of the Elderly', *Journal of Aging and Social Policy*, 8:2–3 (1996), pp. 37–55.

Hubback, E. M., *The Population of Britain* (London: Penguin Books, 1947).

Hunt, A., *The Home Help Service in England and Wales* (London: HMSO, 1970).

Ikegami, N., 'Public Long-Term Care Insurance in Japan', *Journal of the American Medical Association*, 278:16 (1997), pp. 1310–14.

Ikegami, N., B. E. Fries, Y. Takagi, S. Ikeda and T. Ibe, 'Applying RUG-III in Japanese Long-Term Care Facilities', *Gerontologist*, 34:5 (1994), pp. 628–39.

Izuhara, M., *Family Change and Housing in Post-War Japanese Society* (Aldershot: Ashgate, 2000).

—, 'Care and Inheritance: Japanese and English Perspectives on the "Generational Contract"', *Ageing and Society*, 22:1 (2002), pp. 61–77.

— (ed.), *Comparing Social Policies: Exploring New Perspectives in Britain and Japan* (Bristol: Policy Press, 2003).

—, 'Ageing and Intergenerational Relations in Japan', in M. Izuhara (ed.), *Comparing Social Policies: Exploring New Perspectives in Britain and Japan* (Bristol: Policy Press, 2003), pp. 73–94.

—, 'Social Inequality under a New Social Contract: Long-Term Care in Japan', *Social Policy and Administration*, 37:4 (2003), pp. 395–410.

Jack, R. (ed.), *Residential Versus Community Care: The Role of Institutions in Welfare Provision* (Basingstoke: Macmillan, 1998). Japanese translation available.

Jerrome, D., 'Introduction', in D. Jerrome (ed.), *Ageing in Modern Society: Contemporary Approaches* (Beckenham: Croom Helm, 1983), pp. 7–10.

Johnson, N., *Voluntary Social Services* (Oxford: Basil Blackwell, 1981). Japanese translation available.

Johnson, P., and P. Thane (eds), *Old Age from Antiquity to Post-Modernity* (London: Routledge, 1998).

Jones, C., 'The Pacific Challenge: Confucian Welfare States', in C. Jones (ed.), *New Perspectives on the Welfare State in Europe* (London: Routledge, 1993), pp. 198–217.

Jones, K., 'The Development of Institutional Care', in E. Butterworth and R. Holman (eds), *Social Welfare in Modern Britain* (London: Fontana, 1975), pp. 286–98.

—, 'Scull's Dilemma', *British Journal of Psychiatry*, 141 (1982), pp. 221–6.

—, 'We Need the Bed', in R. Jack (ed.), *Residential Versus Community Care: The Role of Institutions in Welfare Provision* (Basingstoke: Macmillan, 1998), pp. 140–53.

Kayser-Jones, J., *Old, Alone, and Neglected: Care of the Aged in Scotland and the United States* (Berkeley, CA and London: University of California Press, 1981).

Kelly, E. R. (ed.), *Kelly's Directory of Norfolk* (London: Kelly's Directories, 1883).

— (ed.), *Kelly's Directory of Norfolk*, 20th edn (London: Kelly's Directories, 1933).

Kenny, D., and P. Edwards, *Community Care Trends: The Impact of Funding on Local Authorities* (London: Local Government Management Board, 1996).

Kimura, T., 'From Transfer to Social Service: A New Emphasis on Social Policies for the Aged in Japan', *Journal of Aging and Social Policy*, 8:2–3 (1996), pp. 177–89.

King, S., 'Sickness and Old Age', in S. King, T. Nutt and A. Tomkins, *Narratives of the Poor in Eighteenth-Century Britain*, 5 vols (London: Pickering & Chatto, 2006), vol. 1, pp. 1–125.

Knapp, M., B. Hardy and J. Forder, 'Commissioning for Quality: Ten Years of Social Care Markets in England', *Journal of Social Policy*, 30:2 (2001), pp. 283–306.

Komatsu, R., 'The State and Social Welfare in Japan', in P. Close (ed.), *The State and Caring* (Basingstoke: Macmillan, 1992), pp. 128–47.

Kono, M., 'The Welfare Mix in the Care of Older People in Japan' (PhD dissertation, University of Sheffield, 1997).

Laing, R. D., and A. Esterson, *Sanity, Madness and the Family* (London: Tavistock, 1964).

Laing, W., *Financing Long-Term Care* (London: Age Concern England, 1993).

Laing & Buisson, *Care of Elderly People: UK Market Survey 2003* (London: Laing & Buisson, 2003).

Laing & Buisson, *Care of Elderly People: UK Market Survey 2008* (London: Laing & Buisson, 2008).

Land, H., 'Future Expectations of Care in Old Age', in J. Robinson (ed.), *Towards a New Social Compact for Care in Old Age* (London: King's Fund, 2001), pp. 47–65.

Langley, G. E., 'It May Be "Community" but Is It Comprehensive?', *Psychiatric Bulletin*, 7:4 (1983), pp. 67–9.

Lee, H. K., 'The Japanese Welfare State in Transition', in R. R. Friedmann, N. Gilbert and M. Sherer (eds), *Modern Welfare States* (Brighton: Wheatsheaf, 1987), pp. 243–63.

Lewis, H., G. Wistow, S. Abbott and L. Cotterill, 'Continuing Health Care: The Local Development of Policies and Eligibility Criteria', *Health and Social Care in the Community*, 7:6 (1999), pp. 455–63.

Lewis, J., and H. Glennerster, *Implementing the New Community Care* (Buckingham: Open University Press, 1996).

Long, S. O. (ed.), *Caring for the Elderly in Japan and the US: Practices and Policies* (London: Routledge, 2000).

Longmate, N., *The Workhouse: A Social History* (London: Pimlico, 2003).

Lowe, R., 'The State and the Development of Social Welfare', in M. Pugh (ed.), *A Companion to Modern European History 1871–1945* (Oxford: Blackwell, 1997), pp. 45–69.

Macintyre, S., 'Old Age as a Social Problem', in R. Dingwall, C. Heath, M. Reid and M. Stacey (eds), *Health Care and Health Knowledge* (Beckenham: Croom Helm, 1977), pp. 39–63.

Macnicol, J., *The Politics of Retirement in Britain, 1878–1948* (Cambridge: Cambridge University Press, 1998).

Maeda, D., 'The Socioeconomic Context of Japanese Social Policy for Aging', in S. O. Long (ed.), *Caring for the Elderly in Japan and the US: Practices and Policies* (London: Routledge, 2000), pp. 28–51.

Maher, J., and H. Green, *Carers 2000* (London: Office of National Statistics/Stationery Office, 2002).

Marshall, J. D., *The Old Poor Law, 1795–1834*, 2nd edn (Basingstoke: Macmillan, 1985).

Maruo, N., 'The Development of the Welfare Mix in Japan', in R. Rose and R. Shiratori (eds), *The Welfare State East and West* (Oxford: Oxford University Press, 1986), pp. 64–79.

McCall, C., *Looking Back from the Nineties: An Autobiography* (Norwich: Gliddon Books, 1994).

Meacher, M., *Taken for a Ride: Special Residential Homes for Confused Old People – A Study of Separatism in Social Policy* (London: Longman, 1972).

Means, R., H. Morbey and R. Smith, *From Community Care to Market Care* (Bristol: Policy, 2002).

Means, R., and R. Smith, *From Poor Law to Community Care*, 2nd edn (1985; Bristol: Policy Press, 1998).

Meeres, F., *Norfolk in the Second World War* (Chichester: Phillimore, 2006).

Michael, E. R., *The Relief of Poverty 1834–1914* (London: Macmillan, 1972).

Mitchell, B. R., *International Historical Statistics, Africa, Asia and Oceania 1750–2005*, 5th edn (Basingstoke: Palgrave Macmillan, 2007).

—, *International Historical Statistics, Europe 1750–2005*, 6th edn (Basingstoke: Palgrave Macmillan, 2007).

Money, L. G. C., *Riches and Poverty* (London: Methuen & Co., 1905).

Morrison, K., *The Workhouse: A Study of Poor Law Buildings in England* (Swindon: Royal Commission on the Historical Monuments of England, 1999).

National Association of Health Authorities, *Registration and Inspection of Nursing Homes: A Handbook for Health Authorities* (Birmingham: National Association of Health Authorities, 1985).

Neuman, M., 'Speenhamland in Berkshire', in E. W. Martin (ed.), *Comparative Development in Social Welfare* (London: Allen & Unwin, 1972), pp. 85–127.

NHS Information Centre for Health and Social Care, *Survey of Carers in Households 2009/10* (London: NHS Information Centre for Health and Social Care, 2010), at http://www.ic.nhs.uk/webfiles/publications/009_Social_Care/carersurvey0910/Survey_of_Carers_in_Households_2009_10_England_NS_Status_v1_0a.pdf [accessed 10 August 2012].

Nicholls, G., *A History of the English Poor Law*, 3 vols (London, 1904).

Nishimura, S., 'Financing of Health Care for the Elderly in Japan', *Japan and the World Economy* (1993), pp. 107–20.

Norman, I. J., and S. J. Redfern (eds), *Mental Health Care for Elderly People* (New York and Edinburgh: Churchill Livingstone, 1996).

Nuffield Foundation, *Old People: Report of a Survey Committee on the Problems of Ageing and the Care of Old People* (London: Oxford University Press, 1947).

O'Donnell, R., 'W. J. Donthorn (1799–1859): Architecture with "Great Hardness and Decision in the Edges"', *Architectural History*, 21 (1978), pp. 83–92.

O'Kell, S., 'Short Changed', *Community Care*, 1115 (1996), pp. 26–7.

Ottaway, S. R., 'Providing for the Elderly in Eighteenth-Century England', *Continuity and Change*, 13:3 (1998), pp. 391–418.

Oxley, G. W., *Poor Relief in England and Wales 1601–1834* (Newton Abbot: David & Charles, 1974).

Parker, J., *Local Health and Welfare Services* (London: George Allen & Unwin, 1965).

Parker, R., 'Care and the Private Sector', in I. Sinclair, R. Parker, D. Leat and J. Williams, *The Kaleidoscope of Care: A Review of Research on Welfare Provision for Elderly People* (London: HMSO, 1990), pp. 291–361.

Pelling, M., and R. M. Smith (eds), *Life, Death, and the Elderly* (London: Routledge, 1991).

Peng, I., 'A Fresh Look at the Japanese Welfare State', *Social Policy and Administration*, 34:1 (2000), pp. 87–114.

Perks, R., and A. Thomson, 'Introduction', in R. Perks and A. Thomson (eds), *The Oral History Reader* (London: Routledge, 1998), pp. ix–xiii.

—, 'Part I Critical Developments: Introduction', in R. Perks and A. Thomson (eds), *The Oral History Reader* (London: Routledge, 1998), pp. 1–8.

Phillips, D. R., J. A. Vincent and S. Blacksell, 'Petit Bourgeois Care: Private Residential Care for the Elderly', *Policy and Politics*, 14:2 (1986), pp. 189–208.

Phillips, J., *Private Residential Care: The Admission Process and Reactions of the Public Sector* (Aldershot: Avebury, 1992).

Pinker, R., *Social Theory and Social Policy* (London: Heinemann Educational, 1971).

—, 'Social Welfare in Japan and Britain', in E. Øyen (ed.), *Comparing Welfare States and their Futures* (Aldershot: Gower, 1986), pp. 114–28.

Plath, D. W., 'Japan: The After Years', in D. O. Cowgill and L. D. Holmes (eds), *Aging and Modernization* (New York: Appleton-Century-Crofts, 1972), pp. 133–50.

Player, S., and A. M. Pollock, 'Long-Term Care: From Public Responsibility to Private Good', *Critical Social Policy*, 21:2 (2001), pp. 231–55.

Pope, S., *Gressenhall Farm and Workhouse* (Cromer: Poppyland, 2006).

Poynter, J. R., *Society and Pauperism: English Ideas on Poor Relief, 1795–1834* (London: Routledge & Kegan Paul, 1969).

Qureshi, H., and A. Walker, *The Caring Relationship: Elderly People and their Families* (Basingstoke: Macmillan Education, 1989).

Ribbe, M. W., G. Ljunggren, K. Steel, E. Topinkova, C. Hawes, N. Ikegami, J. Henrard and P. V. Jonnson, 'Nursing Homes in 10 Nations: A Comparison between Countries and Settings', *Age and Aging*, 26:52 (1997), pp. 3–12.

Robb, B., *Sans Everything: A Case to Answer* (London: Nelson, 1967).

Robinson, R., 'Restructuring the Welfare State: An Analysis of Public Expenditure 1979/80–1984/85', *Journal of Social Policy*, 15:1 (1986), pp. 1–21.

Rose, M. E., 'The Allowance System under the New Poor Law', *Economic History Review* (19 December 1966), pp. 607–20.

—, *The English Poor Law 1780–1930* (Newton Abbot: David & Charles, 1971).

—, *The Relief of Poverty: 1834–1914* (London: Macmillan, 1972).

Ross, R. B., 'Regulation of Residential Homes for the Elderly', *Journal of Social Welfare Law* (March 1985), pp. 85–95.

—, 'Keeping the Register Up to Date', *Social Services Insight*, 15:22 (March 1986), pp. 13–15.

—, 'Ways of Keeping Standards High', *Social Services Insight*, 5:12 (April 1986), pp. 14–15.

—, 'Registered Homes and Residents' Well-Being', *Social Work Today*, 19:13 (1987), pp. 12–13.

Rowbotham, S., *Hidden from History: 300 Years of Women's Oppression and the Fight against It* (London: Pluto Press, 1973).

Rowntree, B. S., *Poverty: A Study of Town Life* (London: Macmillan & Co., 1901).

Ruck, S. K., 'A Policy for Old Age', *Political Quarterly*, 31 (1960), pp. 120–31.

Rudd, T. N., 'Basic Problems in Social Welfare of the Elderly', *Almoner*, 10:10 (1958), pp. 348–51.

Samson, E. D., *Old Age in the New World* (London: Pilot Press, 1944).

Samuel, M., 'Poorer People May Not Feel Benefit of Wanless Funding Vision', *Community Care*, 1617 (2006), pp. 16–17.

Savage, W. G., C. Frankau and B. Gibson, *Hospital Survey: The Hospital Services of the Eastern Area* (London: HMSO, 1945).

Serreau, A., *Times and Years: A History of the Blofield Union Workhouse at Lingwood in the County of Norfolk* (Bungay: Morrow & Co., 2000).

Shenfield, B. E., *Social Policies for Old Age: A Review of Social Provision for Old Age in Great Britain* (London: Routledge & Kegan Paul, 1957).

Shiratori, R., 'The Future of the Welfare State', in R. Rose and R. Shiratori (eds), *The Welfare State East and West* (Oxford: Oxford University Press, 1986), pp. 193–206.

Slack, P., *Poverty and Policy in Tudor and Stuart England* (London: Longman, 1988).

—, *The English Poor Law, 1531–1782* (Cambridge: Cambridge University Press, 1995).

Smith, R. M., 'Ageing and Well-Being in Early Modern England', in P. Johnson and P. Thane (eds), *Old Age from Antiquity to Post-Modernity* (London and New York: Routledge, 1998), pp. 64–95.

Sumner, G., and R. Smith, *Planning Local Authority Services for the Elderly* (London: George Allen & Unwin, 1969).

Suzuki, A., 'A Brain Hospital in Tokyo, 1926–45', *History of Psychiatry*, 14 (2003), pp. 337–60.

Tamai, K., 'Development of Social Policy in Japan', in M. Izuhara (ed.), *Comparing Social Policies: Exploring New Perspectives in Britain and Japan* (Bristol: Policy Press, 2003), pp. 35–47.

Tamiya, N., H. Noguchi, A. Nishi, M. R. Reich, N. Ikegami, H. Hashimoto, K. Shibuya, I. Kawachi and J. C. Campbell, 'Population Ageing and Wellbeing: Lessons from Japan's Long-Term Care Insurance Policy', *Lancet*, 378:9797 (24 September 2011), pp. 1183–92.

Taylor, G., *The Problem of Poverty 1660–1834* (Harlow: Longman, 1969).

Taylor, J. S., 'The Unreformed Workhouse 1776–1834', in E. W. Martin (ed.), *Comparative Development in Social Welfare* (London: Allen & Unwin, 1972), pp. 57–84.

Thane, P., 'The Debate on the Declining Birth-Rate in Britain: The "Menace" of an Ageing Population, 1920s–1950s', *Continuity and Change*, 5:2 (1990), pp. 283–305.

—, *Foundations of the Welfare State*, 2nd edn (Harlow: Longman, 1996). Japanese translation available.

—, 'Gender, Welfare and Old Age in Britain 1870s–1940s', in A. Digby and J. Stewart (eds), *Gender, Health and Welfare* (London: Routledge, 1996), pp. 189–207.

—, 'Old People and their Families in the English Past', in M. Daunton (ed.), *Charity, Self-Interest and Welfare in the English Past* (London: UCL Press, 1996), pp. 113–38.

—, *Old Age in English History: Past Experiences, Present Issues* (Oxford and New York: Oxford University Press, 2000).

— (ed.), *The Long History of Old Age* (London: Thames & Hudson, 2005). Japanese translation available.

Thang, L. L., *Generations in Touch: Linking the Old and Young in a Tokyo Neighbourhood* (Ithaca, NY: Cornell University Press, 2001).

Thompson, P., *The Voice of the Past* (Oxford: Oxford University Press, 2000).

Thomson, D., 'Workhouse to Nursing Home: Residential Care of Elderly People in England since 1840', *Ageing and Society*, 3 (1983), pp. 43–69.

—, 'The Decline of Social Security: Falling State Support for the Elderly since Early Victorian Times', *Ageing and Society*, 4 (1984), pp. 451–82.

—, 'Welfare and the Historians', in L. Bonfield, R. M. Smith and K. Wrightson (eds), *The World We Have Gained* (Oxford: Blackwell, 1986), pp. 355–78.

Tinker, A., *The Care of Frail Elderly People in the United Kingdom* (London: HMSO, 1994).

Titmuss, R. M., *Problems of Social Policy* (London: HMSO, 1950).

—, *Essays on 'The Welfare State'*, 2nd edn (London: Unwin University Books, 1963). Japanese translation available.

Townsend, P., *The Last Refuge: A Survey of Residential Institutions and Homes for the Aged in England and Wales*, abridged edn (London: Routledge & Kegan Paul, 1964).

—, 'The Objectives of the New Local Social Service', in P. Townsend, A. Sinfield, B. Kahan, P. Mittler, H. Rose, M. Meacher, J. Agate, T. Lynes and D. Bull, *The Fifth Social Service: A Critical Analysis of the Seebohm Proposals* (London: Fabian Society, 1970), pp. 7–22.

—, 'Social Planning and Treasury', in N. Bosanquet and P. Townsend (eds), *Labour and Equality: A Fabian Study of Labour in Power 1974–79* (London: Heinemann Educational, 1980), pp. 3–23.

—, 'The Structured Dependency of the Elderly: A Creation of Social Policy in the Twentieth Century', *Ageing and Society*, 1 (1981), pp. 5–28.

Townsend, P., and D. Wedderburn, *The Aged in the Welfare State: The Interim Report of a Survey of Persons Aged 65 and Over in Britain, 1962 and 1963* (London: G. Bell & Sons, 1965).

Tsutsui, T., and N. Muramatsu, 'Care-Needs Certification in the Long-Term Care Insurance System of Japan', *International Health Affairs*, 53 (2005), pp. 522–7.

Uehara, Y., *Group Homes in Japan: Approaches to Dementia Care* (Ann Arbor, MI: Proquest, 2006).

United Nations, *World Population Prospects: The 2010 Revision Population Database*, at http://esa.un.org/wpp/unpp/panel_indicators.htm [accessed 10 August 2012].

Uzuhashi, T. K., 'Japan: Bidding Farewell to the Welfare Society', in P. Alcock and G. Craig (eds), *International Social Policy* (Basingstoke: Palgrave Macmillan, 2001), pp. 104–23.

Valios, N., 'Services Cut to Balance Books', *Community Care*, 1117 (1996), p. 3.

Victor, C. R., *Old Age in Modern Society: A Textbook of Social Gerontology*, 2nd edn (London: Chapman & Hall, 1994).

—, *The Social Context of Ageing* (London: Routledge, 2005).

Vincent, J. A., A. D. Tibbenham and D. R. Phillips, 'Choice in Residential Care: Myths and Realities', *Journal of Social Policy*, 16:4 (1987), pp. 435–60.

Wagner, G., *Residential Care: A Positive Choice* (London: HMSO, 1988).

Walker, A., 'The Meaning and Social Division of Community Care', in A. Walker (ed.), *Community Care: The Family, the State and Social Policy* (Oxford: Blackwell, 1982), pp. 13–39.

—, 'Dependent Relativities', *The Times Higher Education Supplement*, 22 April 1988, p. 17.

—, 'Community Care: Past, Present and Future', in S. Lliffe and J. Munro (eds), *Healthy Choices: Future Options for the NHS* (London: Lawrence & Wishart, 1997), pp. 178–200.

Walker, A., and C. Phillipson, 'Introduction', in C. Phillipson and A. Walker (eds), *Ageing and Social Policy: A Critical Assessment* (Aldershot: Gower, 1986), pp. 1–12.

Wanless, D., *Securing Good Care for Older People: Taking a Long-Term View* (London: King's Fund, 2006).

Warburton, R., and J. McCracken, 'An Evidence-Based Perspective from the Department of Health on the Impact of the 1993 Reforms on the Care of Frail, Elderly People', in *Report by the Royal Commission on Long Term Care: With Respect to Old Age*, Cm 4192-I, II/1-3 (London: Stationery Office, 1999), vol. II/3, pp. 25–36.

Weaver, T., D. Willcocks and L. Kellaher, *The Business of Care: A Study of Private Residential Homes for Old People* (London: Polytechnic of North London, 1985).

Webb, A., 'The Personal Social Services', in N. Bosanquet and P. Townsend (eds), *Labour and Equality: A Fabian Study of Labour in Power 1974–79* (London: Heinemann Educational, 1980), pp. 279–95.

Webb, A., and G. Wistow, 'The Personal Social Services: Incrementalism, Expediency or Systematic Social Planning?', in A. Walker (ed.), *Public Expenditure and Social Policy: An Examination of Social Spending and Social Priorities* (London: Heinemann Educational, 1982), pp. 137–64.

—, *Planning, Need and Scarcity: Essays on the Personal Social Services* (London: Allen & Unwin, 1986).

Webb, S., and B. Webb, *English Poor Law History Part 1* (1910; London: Frank Cass & Co., 1963).

Webster, C., *The National Health Service: A Political History* (Oxford: Oxford University Press, 2002).

Wheeler, R., 'Staying Put: A New Development in Policy?', *Ageing and Society*, 2 (1982), pp. 299–329.

White, G., and R. Goodman, 'Welfare Orientalism and the Search for an East Asian Welfare Model', in R. Goodman, G. White and H. Kwan (eds), *The East Asian Welfare Model* (London and New York: Routledge, 1998), pp. 1–24.

White, W., *History, Gazetteer and Directory of Norfolk*, 4th edn (Sheffield: William White, 1883).

Willcocks, A. J. (ed.), *The Care and Housing of the Elderly in the Community: A Report of a Seminar Held at the University of Nottingham on 19–21 September 1979* (Stafford: Hempits, 1981).

Williams, K., *From Pauperism to Poverty* (London: Routledge & Kegan Paul, 1981).

Willmott, P., and M. Young, *Family and Class in a London Suburb* (London: Routledge & Kegan Paul, 1960).

—, *Family and Kinship in East London*, 2nd impression (1957; London: Routledge & Kegan Paul, 1960).

Wright, C. H., and L. Roberts, 'The Place of the Home-Help Service in the Care of the Aged', *Lancet*, 1:7014 (1958), pp. 254–6.

Wright, J., and F. Sheldon, 'Health and Social Services Planning', *Social Policy and Administration*, 19:3 (1985), pp. 258–72.

Wrightson, K., 'The Social Order of Early Modern England', in L. Bonfield, R. M. Smith and K. Wrightson (eds), *The World We Have Gained: Histories of Population and Social Structure* (Oxford: Blackwell, 1986), pp. 177–202.

Wu, Y., *The Care of the Elderly in Japan* (London: RoutledgeCurzon, 2004).

Younghusband, E., *Social Work in Britain 1950–1975: A Follow-up Study*, 2 vols (London: Allen & Unwin, 1978).

In Japanese

Abe, S. and Ioka, T. (eds), *Shakaifukushi no kokusaihikaku* [*International Comparison in Social Welfare*] (Tokyo: Yuhikaku, 2000).

Aida, Y. (ed.), *Dai-ikkai zenkoku yorojigyou chosa sasho* [*The First National Survey of Institutional Care Provision for the Elderly*] (Tokyo: Zenkoku-yoro-jigyo-kyokai, 1933), repr. in Y. Ogasawara (ed.), *Rojinmondai kenkyu kihonbunken shu (Rekishi bunken)* [*Basic Historical Sources for Old Age Research (Historical Sources)*], 29 vols (Tokyo: Ozora-sha, 1990–2), vol. 4.

— (ed.), *Dai-nikai zenkoku yorojigyou chosa sasho* [*The Second National Survey of Institutional Care Provision for the Elderly*] (Tokyo: Zenkoku-yoro-jigyo-kyokai, 1936), repr. in Y. Ogasawara (ed.), *Rekishi bunken* [*Historical Sources*], 29 vols (Tokyo: Ozora-sha, 1990–2), vol. 4.

— (ed.), *Dai-sankai zenkoku yorojigyou chosa sasho* [*The Third National Survey of Institutional Care Provision for the Elderly*] (Tokyo: Zenkoku-yoro-jigyo-kyokai, 1940), repr. in Y. Ogasawara (ed.), *Rekishi bunken* [*Historical Sources*], 29 vols (Tokyo: Ozora-sha, 1990–2), vol. 4.

Ariyoshi, S., *Kokotsu no hito* [*Man in Rapture*] (Tokyo: Shincho-bunko, 1972).

Asai, Y., and S. Miwa, 'Gifu-ken no koreisha ni kansuru kisoteki kenkyu 1: Koreishajinko no suii to sono taisaku o chushin ni' [Research on the Aged in Gifu Prefecture: Ageing Demographical Trends and Reforms], *Gifujoshi-daigaku chiikibunka kenkyujo hokoku* [*Gifu Woman's University Journal*], 11 (1993), pp. 27–43.

Asano, H., 'Koreisha no tameno sogotekihosaku' [Elderly Welfare Services], in Y. Ogasawara, Y. Hashimoto and H. Asano (eds), *Koreisha fukushi* [*Elderly Welfare*], 2nd edn (Tokyo: Yuhikaku, 2003), pp. 95–117.

Central Charity Association, *Zenkoku shakaijigyo meikan soran showa juni-nendo ban* [*National Directory of Social Services 1937/8*], 2 vols (Tokyo: Central Charity Association, 1938), vol. 1, repr. in Shakai-fukushi-chosa-kenkyu-kai (ed.), *Senzen-ki shakaijigyo shiryo syusei* [*Historical Sources for the Pre-War Social Services*], 20 vols, 2nd edn (Tokyo: Nihon-tosho-senta, 1996), vol. 12.

Democratic Party of Japan, *Minshu-to no seiken seisaku manifesto 2009* [*The Democratic Party of Japan, Manifesto 2009*] (Tokyo: Democratic Party of Japan, 2009), at http://www.dpj.or.jp/policies/manifesto2009 [accessed 10 August 2010].

Ebie, N., 'Tokubetsuyogo rojinhomu no genjo to kadai' [Current Situation and Problem of the Nursing Home], in H. Asano and S. Tanaka (eds), *Nihon no shisetsu kea* [*Institutional Care in Japan*] (Tokyo: Chuo-hoki-shuppan, 1993), pp. 28–51.

Ena City Historical Editorial Board (ed.), *Ena-shi shi tsushi-hen* [*History of Ena City*], 5 vols (Ena: Ena City, 1993), vol. 4.

Fujimoto, T., *Igirisu hinkon shi* [*A History of Poverty in Britain*] (Tokyo: Shin-nihon-shuppan-sha, 2000).

Fukazawa, S., *Narayama bushi ko* [*Ballad of Oak Mountain*] (Tokyo: Shincho-sha, 1964).

Fukuchi, Y., and Y. Shimizu (eds), *Koreikataisaku no kokusaihikaku* [*International Comparison in Social Policy for the Elderly*] (Tokyo: Daiichi-hoki-shuppan, 1993).

Fukutake, T., *Nihonshakai no kozo* [*The Structure of Japanese Society*], 2nd edn (Tokyo: Tokyo University Press, 1987).

Gifu City (ed.), *Gifu-shi shi tsushi-hen gendai* [*A History of Gifu City, Contemporary*] (Gifu: Gifu City, 1981).

Gifu City Relief Division, *Showa 7-nen 3-gatsu gifu-shi shakaijigyo yoran* [*Directory of Welfare Work in Gifu City for 1932*] (Gifu: Gifu City, 1932).

Gifu City Welfare Division, *Showa 15-nen 9-gatsu gifu-shi shakaijigyo yoran* [*Directory of Welfare Work in Gifu City for 1940*] (Gifu: Gifu City, 1940).

Gifu Prefecture, *Gifu-ken shi* [*Journal of Gifu Prefecture 1963–91*] (Gifu: Gifu Prefecture, 1963 and various years). Years consulted: 1963; 1966; 1968; 1973; 1976; 1979; 1980; 1981; 1985; 1986; 1987; 1988; 1990; 1991.

—, *Gifu-ken sogo kaihatsu keikaku* [*Gifu Prefecture First Comprehensive Plan 1966–76*] (Gifu: Gifu Prefecture, 1966).

— (ed.), *Gifu-ken shi tsushi-hen kindai* [*History of Gifu Prefecture, Modern*], 3 vols (Gifu: Gifu Prefecture, 1967).

—, *Gifu-ken dai-niji sogo kaihatsu keikaku* [*Gifu Prefecture Second Comprehensive Plan 1972–80*] (Gifu: Gifu Prefecture, 1972).

—, *Gifu-ken dai-sanji sogo kaihatsu keikaku* [*Gifu Prefecture Third Comprehensive Plan 1977–85*] (Gifu: Gifu Prefecture, 1977).

—, *Gifu-ken dai-yoji sogo kaihatsu keikaku* [*Gifu Prefecture Fourth Comprehensive Plan 1984–95*] (Gifu: Gifu Prefecture, 1984).

—, *Rojin no kenko to seikatsu ni kansuru jittaichosa hokokusho* [*Report on the Health and Life of the Prefecture Elderly 1984*] (Gifu: Gifu Prefecture, 1985).

—, *Gifu-ken dai-goji sogo kaihatsu keikaku* [*Gifu Prefecture Fifth Comprehensive Plan 1994–98*] (Gifu: Gifu Prefecture, 1994).

—, *Gifu-ken rojinhokenfukushi keikaku heisei 6-nen* [*Gifu Prefecture Health and Welfare Plan for Older People 1994–2000*] (Gifu: Gifu Prefecture, 1994).

— (ed.), *Gifu-ken shi shiryo-hen gendai* [*Historical Sources for Gifu Prefecture, Post-Contemporary*], 2 vols (Gifu: Gifu Prefecture, 1999).

— (ed.), *Wakariyasui gifu-ken shi* [*Plain History of Gifu Prefecture*] (Gifu: Gifu Prefecture, 2001).

— (ed.), *Gifu-ken shi tsushi-hen zoku-gendai* [*History of Gifu Prefecture, Post-Contemporary*] (Gifu: Gifu Prefecture, 2003).

—, *Gifu-ken rojinhokenfukushi keikaku, kaigohoken jigyoshien keikaku heisei 18-nen* [*Gifu Prefecture Health and Welfare Plan for Older People 2006–15*] (Gifu: Gifu Prefecture, 2006).

Gifu Prefecture Social Welfare Corporation, *Niju-nen no ayumi* [*20-Year History*] (Gifu: Gifu Prefecture Social Welfare Corporation, 1987).

Gifu Prefecture Social Welfare Division, *Gifu-ken ni okeru koreisha no jittai* [*Report on the Conditions of the Prefecture Elderly 1977*] (Gifu: Gifu Prefecture Social Welfare Division, 1978).

— (ed.), *Shakaifukushi shokuin jishukenkyu hokokusho* [*Research Reports by Residential Staff*] (Gifu: Gifu Prefecture Social Welfare Division, 1984).

Gifu Prefecture Statistics Division (ed.), *Gifu ken tokeisho dejitaru a-kaibu* [*Digital Archives Gifu Prefecture Statistics 1874–2011*], at http://www.pref.gifu.lg.jp/kensei-unei/tokei-joho/gifuken-tokeisho/mainendeta [accessed 10 August 2012]. Years consulted: 1925; 1928; 1930; 1935; 1948; 1952; 1953; 1962; 1973; 1974; 1975; 1979; 1980; 1982; 1987; 1992; 2002; 2004.

— (ed.), *Deta ai gifu ga mieru hon, heisei 19-nendo ban* [*Data Gifu Prefecture 2007–8*] (Gifu: Gifu Prefecture, 2008).

Gifu Times (ed.), *Gifu nenkan showa 28-nen ban* [*Gifu Yearbook for 1949–55*] (Gifu: Gifu Times, 1948 and various years). Years consulted: 1949; 1950; 1951; 1955.

Gunji, A. (ed.), *Iryo to fukushi ni okeru shijo no yakuwari to genkai: Igirisu no keiken to nihon no kadai* [*The Role and Limitations of a Medical and Welfare Market: British Experiences and Japanese Problems*] (Ageo City: Seigakuin University Press, 2004).

Hashimoto, H., '"Rojinfukushiho" no hoteki seikaku' [The Margin of Welfare for the Aged in 'The Law for the Welfare of the Aged'], in S. Nasu and Y. Yuzawa (eds), *Rojinkazoku no shakaigaku: Rojinfuyo no kenkyu* [*A Sociological Study on Family Help for the Aged*] (Tokyo: Kakiuchi-shuppan, 1973), pp. 311–52.

Hashimoto, Y., 'Kaigohoken no riyo shisutemu' [Long-Term Care Insurance System], in Y. Ogasawara, Y. Hashimoto and H. Asano (eds), *Koreisha fukushi* [*Elderly Welfare*], 2nd edn (Tokyo: Yuhikaku, 2003), pp. 119–58.

Hidaka, N., *Rojinhomu nikki* [*Old People's Home Diary*] (Tokyo: Asahi-shinbun-sha, 1979).

Hiraoka, K., *Igirisu no syakaifukushi to seisakukenkyu: Igirisumoderu no jizoku to henka* [*Welfare and Social Policy in Britain*] (Kyoto: Minerva, 2003).

Hojo, R., 'Koreisha komyuniti ni okeru kaitekina kenchikukankyo' [Comfortable Living Environments], in K. Hara and M. Oshima (eds), *Koreishashisetsu no mirai o hiraku* [*Explore Future of Facilities for the Elderly*] (Kyoto: Minerva, 2005), pp. 130–60.

Homma, I., *Tokuyohomu de kurasu to iukoto* [*Facts of Life in a Nursing Home*] (Tokyo: Akebi-shobo, 1995).

Ibigawa Town (ed.), *Ibigawa-cho shi tsushi-hen* [*History of Ibigawa Town*] (Ibigawa Town, Gifu: Ibigawa Town, 1971).

Ichibangase, Y. (ed.), *Shakaifukushi chosakushu* [*Historical Sources for Social Welfare*], 5 vols (Tokyo: Rodo-shunpo-sha, 1994).

—, 'Yoikuin hyaku-nen shi to heiwa' [100-Year History of Tokyo Borough Almshouse], in Tokyo Borough Almshouse Committee (ed.), *Nihon no fukushi o kizuite 127-nen: Yoikuin no kaitai wa fukushino kotai* [*127-Year History of Tokyo Borough Almshouse*] (Tokyo: Hobun-sha, 1999), pp. 164–78.

Ikeda, Y., *Nihon shakaifukushi shi* [*History of Japanese Social Welfare*] (Kyoto: Horitsu-bunka-sha, 1986).

—, *Nihon ni okeru shakaifukushi no ayumi* [*History of Welfare in Japan*] (Kyoto: Horitsu-bunka-sha, 1994).

Ikeda, Y., and Y. Doi (eds), *Nihon shakaifukushi sogo nenpyo* [*Comprehensive Chronology of Social Welfare in Japan*] (Kyoto: Horitsu-bunka-sha, 2000).

Ikeda Town (ed.), *Ikeda-cho shi tsushi-hen* [*History of Ikeda Town*] (Ikeda Town, Gifu: Ikeda Town, 1978).

Imura, K., *Nihon no yoroin shi* [*History of Old People's Almshouses in Japan*] (Tokyo: Gakubun-sha, 2005).

Ishida, T., *Kindai nihon no seijibunka to gengoshocho* [*Political Culture and Language Symbolism in Modern Japan*] (Tokyo: Tokyo University Press, 1983).

Ishihara, M., *Ikitete yokatta: Atarashii rojinhomu o motomete* [*Glad to Be Alive*] (Kyoto: Minerva, 1986).

Ito, S., *Shakaihosho shi, onkei kara kenri e: Igirisu to nihon no hikakukenkyu* [*History of Social Security: Comparative Research on Britain and Japan*] (Tokyo: Aoki-shoten, 1994).

Ito, S., 'Kaigohoken'[Long-Term Care Insurance Scheme], in N. Sanada, K. Miyata, S. Kato and K. Kawai (eds), *Zusetsu nihon no shakaifukushi* [*Illustration: Social Welfare in Japan*] (Kyoto: Horitsu-bunka-sha, 2004), pp. 164–77.

Iwata, M., 'Hihogosha cyosa'[Survey of Public Assistance Recipients], in Social Welfare Survey Research Council (ed.), *Senzen nihon no shakaijigyo chosa* [*Pre-War Social Work Survey in Japan*] (Tokyo: Keiso-shobo, 1983), pp. 144–54.

Juroku Bank Research Team, 'Gifu-ken no kaigosabisushijo no doko ni tsuite' [Nursing Care Market Trends in Gifu Prefecture], *Keizaigeppo* [*Monthly Financial Report*], 564 (June 2001), pp. 1–23.

Kagamihara City Educational Board (ed.), *Kagamihara-shi shi shiryo-hen kinsei, gendai* [*Historical Source for Kagamihara City, Contemporary*] (Kagamihara: Kagamihara City, 1986).

— (ed.), *Kagamihara-shi shi tsushi-hen kinsei, kindai, gendai* [*History of Kagamihara City, Contemporary*] (Kagamihara: Kagamihara City, 1987).

Kaigo-rodo-antei-senta, *Heisei 22-nendo kaigorodo jittaichosa kekka ni tsuite* [*Results of the Care Labour Survey 2010–11*] (Tokyo: Kaigorodo-antei-senta, 23 August 2010), at http://www.kaigo-center.or.jp/report/pdf/h22_chousa_kekka.pdf [accessed 10 August 2012].

Kato, E., *Kaigo satsujin: Shihofukushi no shiten kara* [*Care-Giving Murder*] (Tokyo: Kuresu-shuppan, 2005).

Kato, M., 'Rojinhomu ni miru koreijosei no sugata' [Elderly Women in Old People's Homes], in National Council of Social Welfare and National Council of Elderly Homes (eds), *Rojinfukushi nempo 1980-nen* [*Annual Report on Elderly Welfare 1980*] (Tokyo: NCSW, 1982), pp. 105–10.

Kawabata, O., K. Atsumi and S. Shimamura, *Koreisha seikatsu nenpyo 1925–2000* [*Daily Chronology of Older People 1925–2000*] (Tokyo: Nihon Editor School Press, 2001).

Kida, T., 'Sengo ni okeru kotekifujo seido no tenkai sono ichi' [History of Post-War National Assistance System Part 1], in Japan University of Social Work (ed.), *Nihon no kyuhin seido* [*Poor Law System in Japan*] (Tokyo: Keiso-shobo, 1960), pp. 299–342.

Kimura, T., *Nihon kindai shakaijigyo shi* [*A History of Social Services in Modern Japan*] (Kyoto: Minerva, 1964).

Kinoshita, S., 'Rojin no seikatsukukan' [Living Space of the Elderly], in S. Nasu and M. Masuda (eds), *Nihon no rojin* [*Japanese Elderly People*], 3 vols (Tokyo: Kakiuchi-shuppan, 1972), vol. 3, pp. 331–51.

Konuma, A., 'Ryoyo byosho no saihen' [Issue Brief: Restructuring Long-Stay Hospital Beds], *Chosa to joho* [*Research and Information*], 590 (7 June 2007), pp. 1–10, held at Kokuritsu kokkai toshokan [National Diet Library]; also at http://www.ndl.go.jp/jp/data/publication/issue/0590.pdf [accessed 10 August 2012].

Kosei-tokei-kyokai (ed.), *Zusetsu: Tokei de wakaru kaigohoken 2008* [*Illustration: Long-Term Care Insurance Statistics 2008*] (Tokyo: Kosei-tokei-kyokai, 2008).

Kumon, A., 'Nenkin' [Pensions], in N. Sanada, K. Miyata, S. Kato and K. Kawai (eds), *Zusetsu nihon no shakaifukushi* [*Illustration: Social Welfare in Japan*] (Kyoto: Horitsu-bunka-sha, 2004), pp. 178–91.

Kure, S., *Wagakuni ni okeru seishinbyo ni kansuru saikin no shisetsu* [*Contemporary Institutions for the Insane in Japan*] (publisher unknown, 1920), Kokuristu kokkai toshokan dejitaru a-kaibu potaru [National Diet Library Digital Archive Portal], at http://kindai.ndl.go.jp [accessed 10 August 2012].

Mahoroba (ed.), *Zenkoku rojinfukushi shisetsu meibo heisei 12-nendo ban* [*Directory of Elderly Welfare Facilities in Japan 2000/1*] (Tokyo: Daiichi-hoki-shuppan, 2001).

Masuda, K. (ed.), *Shin waei dai-jiten* [*Kenkyusha's New Japanese–English Dictionary*], 4th edn (Tokyo: Kenkyusha, 1987).

Mitaka Town Historical Editorial Board (ed.), *Mitaka-cho shi tsushi-hen* [*History of Mitaka Town*], 2 vols (Mitaka Town, Gifu: Mitaka Town, 1992).

Mitoki, K., *Igirisu no komyuniti-kea to kaigosha: Kaigosha shien no kokusai teki tenkai* [*Community Care and Carers in the UK: International Development of Support for Carers*] (Kyoto: Minerva, 2008).

Miyazaki, E., 'Roreisha chosa: Yohogorojin to yorojigyo no doko' [Survey of the Elderly], in Social Welfare Survey Research Council (ed.), *Senzen nihon no shakaijigyo chosa* [*Pre-War Social Work Survey in Japan*] (Tokyo: Keiso-shobo, 1983), pp. 336–52.

Miyazaki, M., 'Koreishafukushi' [Welfare for the Elderly], in N. Sanada, K. Miyata, S. Kato and K. Kawai (eds), *Zusetsu nihon no shakaifukushi* [*Illustration: Social Welfare in Japan*] (Kyoto: Horitsu-bunka-sha, 2004), pp. 92–109.

Ministry of Health and Welfare, *Rojinfukushi 10-nen no ayumi* [*Ten-Year History of Elderly Welfare*] (Tokyo: Ministry of Health, Labour and Welfare, 1974).

—, *Showa 50-nendo shakaifukushi shisetsu chosahokoku* [*Summary of the Year 1975/6 Social Welfare Facilities Survey*], 2 vols (Tokyo: Ministry of Health, Labour and Welfare Statistics Bureau, 1975 and successive years).

— (ed.), *Wagakuni no shakaifukushi shisetsu* [*Welfare Institutions in Japan*] (Tokyo: Shakai-fukushi-chosa-kai, 1981).

—, *Zenkoku rojinfukushi shisetsu heisei 2-nendo ban* [*National Directory of Elderly Welfare Facilities 1990*] (Tokyo: Daiichi-hoki-shuppan, 1990).

Ministry of Health, Labour and Welfare, *Kaigohoken seido kaikaku no gaiyo* [*Summary of the Long-Term Care Insurance Act Reform*] (Tokyo: Ministry of Health, Labour and Welfare, March 2006), at http://www.mhlw.go.jp/topics/kaigo/topics/0603/dl/data.pdf [accessed 10 August 2012].

—, *Heisei 12-nen kaigo sabisu shisetsu jigyosho chosa* [*The 2000 Survey of Long-Term Care Insurance Residential Facility Providing Agencies*] (Tokyo: Kosei-tokei-kyokai, 2002).

—, *Heisei 14-nen kanja chosa* [*Patient Survey 2002*], 2 vols (Tokyo: Ministry of Health, Labour and Welfare, 2004).

—, *Heisei 16-nen kaigo sabisu shisetsu jigyosho chosa* [*The 2004 Survey of Long-Term Care Insurance Residential Facility Providing Agencies*] (Tokyo: Kosei-tokei-kyokai, 2004).

—, 'Tokubetsu yogorojin homu no nyusho moshikomisha no jokyo' [Current State of Nursing Home Waiting Lists] (Tokyo: Ministry of Health, Labour and Welfare, 22 December 2009), at http://www.mhlw.go.jp/stf/houdou/2r98520000003byd.html [accessed 10 August 2012].

—, *Heisei 22-nendo kaigokyufuhi jittai chosa no gaikyo* [*Summary of the Year 2010/11 Long-Term Care Insurance Expenditure Survey*] (Tokyo: MoHLW, 23 August 2011), at http://www.mhlw.go.jp/toukei/saikin/hw/kaigo/kyufu/10/ [accessed 10 August 2012].

—, *Heisei 22-nen shakaifukushi shisetsutou chosa kekkano gaikyo* [*Summary of the Year 2010 Social Welfare Facilities Survey*] (Tokyo: Ministry of Health, Labour and Welfare, 30 November 2011), at http://www.mhlw.go.jp/toukei/saikin/hw/fukushi/10/index.html [accessed 10 August 2012].

—, *Heisei 22-nendo kaigohoken jigyo jokyo hokoku* [*Annual Report on the Year 2010/11 Long-Term Care Insurance Scheme*], at http://www.mhlw.go.jp/topics/kaigo/osirase/jigyo/10/dl/h22_gaiyou.pdf [accessed 10 August 2012].

—, *Kaigohoken sei kaisei no gaiyo oyobi chiikihokatsu kea no rinen* [*Summary of the Long-Term Care Insurance Reform and Philosophy of Comprehensive Community Care*] (Tokyo: Ministry of Health, Labour and Welfare, 2012), at http://www.mhlw.go.jp/stf/shingi/2r98520000026b0a-att/2r98520000026b4b.pdf [accessed 10 August 2012].

Ministry of Health and Welfare Fifty-Year Historical Editorial Board (ed.), *Koseisho goju-nen shi, kijutsu hen* [*Fifty-Year History of Ministry of Health and Welfare, Description*] (Tokyo: Chuo-hoki-shuppan, 1988).

Momose, T., *Nihon fukushiseido shi* [*History of the Welfare System in Japan*] (Kyoto: Minerva, 1997).

—, *Nihon rojinfukushi shi* [*History of Elderly Welfare in Japan*] (Tokyo: Chuo-hoki-shuppan, 1997).

—, *Shakaifukushi no seiritsu* [*The Establishment of 'Social Welfare'*] (Kyoto: Minerva, 2002).

Mori, M., *Nihon no rojin sekaino rojin* [*Old People in Japan and the World*] (Tokyo: Shakai-hoken-shuppan-sha, 1974).

—, *Rojin homu ron* [*Theory of the Old People's Home*] (Osaka: Rojin-seikatsu-kenkyu-jo, 1978).

—, *'Roikiron' no shintenkai: Gendai ronengaku hihan* [*A New Evolution of the 'Aged Theory': Criticism of Current Gerontology*] (Higashimurayama: Kirisutokyo-tosho-shuppan, 1995).

Mori, U., *Gendainihon no kaigohoken kaikaku* [*Long-Term Care Insurance Reform in Contemporary Japan*] (Kyoto: Horitsu-bunka-sha, 2008).

Motosu Town (ed.), *Motosu-cho shi tsushi-hen* [*History of Motosu Town*] (Motosu Town, Gifu: Motosu City, 1975).

Murota, H., 'Shisetsu kea' [Residential Care], in T. Ota (ed.), *Koreishafukushi ron* [*Introduction to Welfare for the Elderly*], 3rd edn (Tokyo: Koseikan, 2005), pp. 117–36.

Nakamura, R., 'Yokaigo koreisha no zoka to kaigomondai' [Nursing Problems], in Y. Ogasawara, Y. Hashimoto and H. Asano (eds), *Koreisha fukushi* [*Elderly Welfare*], 2nd edn (Tokyo: Yuhikaku, 2003), pp. 41–57.

National Council of Elderly Homes (ed.), *Dai-nikai zenkoku rojinhomu kisochosa hokokusyo* [*The Second National Survey on Elderly Homes*] (Tokyo: National Council of Elderly Homes, 1982).

— (ed.), *Dai-sankai zenkoku rojinhomu kisochosa hokokusyo* [*The Third National Survey of Elderly Homes*] (Tokyo: National Council of Social Welfare and National Council of Elderly Homes, 1988).

— (ed.), *Dai-yonkai zenkoku rojinhomu kisochosa hokokusyo* [*The Fourth National Survey of Elderly Homes*] (Tokyo: National Council of Elderly Homes, 1993).

National Council of Social Welfare, *Akarui yorojigyo* [*Cheerful Elderly Welfare*] (Tokyo: National Council of Social Welfare, 1953), repr. in Y. Ogasawara (ed.), *Rekishi bunken* [*Historical Sources*], 29 vols (Tokyo: Ozora-sha, 1990–2), vol. 29.

National Council of Social Welfare and National Council of Elderly Homes (eds), *Rojinfukushi nenpo 1980-nen* [*Annual Report on Elderly Welfare 1980*] (Tokyo: National Council of Social Welfare, 1980).

Noguchi, N., 'Wagakuni no koreishafukushi ni okeru shisetsu kea no kiseki to kadai: Yoroin, yoroshisetsu soshite "rojinhomu" e' [Residential Care for the Elderly in Japan: History and Issues] (PhD dissertation, Nihon Fukushi University, 2003).

Ogaki City, *Ogaki-shi sogo keikaku* [*Ogaki City First Comprehensive Plan 1970–85*] (Ogaki: Ogaki City, 1970).

—, *Ogaki-shi dai-niji sogo keikaku* [*Ogaki City Second Comprehensive Plan 1986–95*] (Ogaki: Ogaki City, 1981).

— (ed.), *Shinshu ogaki-shi shi tsushi-hen* [*History of Ogaki City*], 3 vols (1968; Kyoto: Rinkawa-shoten, 1987).

—, *Ogaki-shi roujinhokenfukushi keikaku heisei 6-nen* [*Ogaki City Health and Welfare Plan 1994–2000*] (Ogaki: Ogaki City, 1994).

Ogaki City Council Secretariats, *Shisei no aramashi* [*Ogaki City Government History*] (Ogaki: Ogaki City, 2001).

Ogasawara, Y., 'Rojinhomu no rekishi to sono isan' [History and Remnants of Old People's Homes], in National Council of Social Welfare and National Council of Elderly Home (eds), *Rojinfukushi nenpo 1982-nen* [*Annual Report on Elderly Welfare 1982*] (Tokyo: National Council of Social Welfare, 1982), pp. 140–55.

—, 'Shakaijigyo shisetsu chosa' [Research on Pre-War Social Welfare Institutions], in Social Welfare Survey Research Council (ed.), *Senzen nihon no shakaijigyo chosa* [*Pre-War Social Work Survey in Japan*] (Tokyo: Keiso-shobo, 1983), pp. 354–68.

—, 'Rojinhomu hyaku-nen no ayumi' [100-Year History of Homes for the Elderly], in National Council of Social Welfare and National Council of Elderly Homes (eds), *Rojinfukushi shisetsu kyogikai goju-nen shi* [*Fifty-Year History of National Council of Elderly Homes*] (Tokyo: National Council of Social Welfare, 1984), pp. 3–154.

—, 'Rojinhomu kono ju-nen' [Homes for the Elderly in the Past Decade], in National Council of Social Welfare and National Council of Elderly Home (eds), *Zenkoku rojinfukushi shisetsu kyogikai rokuju-nen shi, gekido no ju-nen* [*Sixty-Year History of National Council of Elderly Homes*] (Tokyo: National Council of Social Welfare and National Council of Elderly Homes, 1995), pp. 25–74.

—, *Kaigo no kihon to kangaekata: Rojin homu no shikumi to seikatsushien* [*Basics and Theory of Nursing Care: Function and Living Assistance of Old People's Homes*] (Tokyo: Chuo-hoki-shuppan, 1995).

—, *'Seikatsu no ba' to shiteno rojin homu: sono kako, genzai, ashita* [*Old People's Home as a 'Place for Living'*] (Tokyo: Chuo-hoki-shuppan, 1999).

Ogasawara, Y., N. Hirue, H. Yabe, K. Moritsugi, M. Tsuda, O. Nishioka and F. Yasuoka, *Rojinhomu wa darenomono: Seikatsuno ba toshiteno rojinhomu o kangaeru* [*For Whom Are Old People's Homes?*] (Tokyo: Akebi-shobo, 1985).

Ogawa, M., 'Taisho demokurashi-ki no kyuhintaisei' [Poor Relief System, 1912–26], in Japan University of Social Work (ed.), *Nihon no kyuhin seido* [*Poor Law System in Japan*] (Tokyo: Keiso-shobo, 1960), pp. 153–222.

—, 'Senso no nakano shakaijigyo' [Social Work in Wartime], in Tokyo Borough Almshouse Committee (ed.), *Nihon no fukushi o kizuite 127-nen: Yoikuin no kaitai wa fukushino kotai* [*127-Year History of Tokyo Borough Almshouse*] (Tokyo: Hobun-sha, 1999), pp. 179–201.

Okada, Y., *Shisetsu: Matsuzawa byoin shi, 1879–1980* [*Matsuzawa Hospital: A Private History, 1879–1980*] (Tokyo: Iwasaki-gakujutsu-shuppan-sha, 1981).

Okamoto, T., 'Senchuki no yorojigyo ni kansuru ichikosatsu (1931–1945)' [Wartime History of Institutional Care for the Elderly], *Shakaironengaku* [*Social Gerontology*], 21 (1984), pp. 84–95.

—, *Rojinfukushiho no seitei* [*Establishment of the Elderly Welfare Act*] (Tokyo: Seishin-shobo, 1993).

Okamoto, Y., *Koreishairyo to fukushi* [*Medical Care and Welfare for the Elderly*] (Tokyo: Iwanami-shinsho, 1996).

—, *Kaigohoken no ayumi: Jiritsu wo mezasu kaigo eno chosen* [*History of the Long-Term Care Insurance System*] (Kyoto: Minerva, 2009).

Okitoh, N., *Kaigohoken wa oi wo mamoruka* [*Can Long-Term Care Insurance Guarantee Old Age?*] (Tokyo: Iwanami-shoten, 2010).

Okuma, K., *Rupo: Seishin byoto* [*Non-fiction Report: Psychiatric Hospitals*] (Tokyo: Asahi-shinbun-sha, 1973).

—, *Rupo: Rojin byoto* [*Non-fiction Report: Geriatric Hospitals*] (Tokyo: Asahi-shinbun-sha, 1988).

—, *Rupo: Yuryo rojin homu* [*Non-fiction Report: Private Nursing Homes*] (Tokyo: Asahi-shinbun-sha, 1995).

Omata, W., *Seishin igaku no rekishi* [*History of Psychiatry*] (Tokyo: Daisan-bunmei-sha, 2005).

Onizaki, N., M. Masuda and H. Inagawa (eds), *Sekai no kaigojijo* [*Long-Term Care in the World*] (Tokyo: Chuo-hoki-shuppan, 2002).

Otsuka, N., 'Rojin senmonbyoin no genjo to kaikaku: Shakaiteki nyuin no shomondai' [Current Situation and Reforms of Old People's Hospitals: Problems of Social Hospitalization], in H. Asano and S. Tanaka (eds), *Nihon no shisetsu kea* [*Institutional Care in Japan*] (Tokyo: Chuo-hoki-shuppan, 1993), pp. 200–22.

Sakahogi Town Educational Board (ed.), *Sakahogi-cho shi tsushi-hen* [*History of Sakahogi Town*] (Sakahogi Town, Gifu: Sakahogi Town, 2005).

Sakai, J., 'Shisetsu kea no shomondai: Hiyo futan to shakaika o medutte' [Problems of Institutional Care], in National Council of Social Welfare and National Council of Elderly Homes (eds), *Rojinfukushi nenpo 1980-nen* [*Annual Report on Elderly Welfare 1980*] (Tokyo: National Council of Social Welfare, 1980), pp. 67–71.

Seikatsu-kagaku-chosa-kai (ed.), *Rogomondai no kenkyu* [*Research on the Old Age Problem*] (Tokyo: Ishiyaku-shuppan, 1961).

Seki, T., 'Shisetsu shi' [History of Institutions], in K. Imura and M. Fujiwara (eds), *Nihon shakaifukushi shi* [*Modern History of Japanese Social Welfare*] (Tokyo: Keiso-shobo, 2007), pp. 113–22.

Seki City Educational Board (ed.), *Shinshu seki-shi shi tsushi-hen Kinsei, kinndai, gendai* [*Revised Version: History of Seki City, Post-modern*] (Seki: Seki City, 1999).

Shakai-fukushi-jigyo-shinko-kai (ed.), *Atarashii rojinhomu* [*The New Old People's Home*] (Tokyo: Shakai-fukushi-shinko-kenkyu-kai, 1964), repr. in Y. Ogasawara (ed.), *Rekishi bunken* [*Historical Sources*], 29 vols (Tokyo: Ozora-sha, 1990–2), vol. 9.

Statistics Bureau, *Jinkosuikei shiryo no. 76: Wagakuni no suikeijinko, taisyo 9-nen kara heisei 12-nen* [*Population Estimates of Japan 1920–2000*] (Tokyo: Japan Statistical Association, 2003).

Sugimoto, K., *Nihon jin to koreika* [*The Japanese and Ageing*] (Tokyo: Nihon-shakai-bunka-kenkyu-kai, 2001).

Tabata, T., *Igirisu chiikifukushi no keisei to tenkai* [*The Making and Development of Community-Based Social Services in Britain*] (Tokyo: Yuhikaku, 2003).

Tajimi City (ed.), *Tajima-shi shi* [*History of Tajimi City*], 2 vols (Tajimi: Tajimi City, 1987).

Takagi, T., and Y. Takama, 'Koreishafukushi to fukushishisetsu nyushosha no seikatsu ni tuiteno genjo to kadai' [Living Situation in Homes for the Elderly in Gifu Prefecture, Compared to National Trends], *Tokaijoshi-tankidaigaku kiyo* [*Journal of Tokai Woman's Junior College*], 27 (2001), pp. 25–36.

Takahashi, B., 'Yoikusha' [Youikusha Old People's Almshouse], in Central Charity Association (ed.), *Yoronenkinsei oyobi ippan yoroshisestu shiryo* [*Historical Sources for the Old-Age Pension System and Almshouse*] (Tokyo: Central Charity Association, 1937), repr. in Y. Ogasawara (ed.), *Rekishi bunken* [*Historical Sources*], 29 vols (Tokyo: Ozora-sha, 1990–2), vol. 3, pp. 1–8.

Takashima, S., *Igirisu fukushi hattatsushi ron* [*History of British Welfare Development*] (Kyoto: Minerva, 1979).

Takayama City (ed.), *Takayama-shi shi fukkoku ban* [*Reprinted: History of Takayama City*], 2 vols (1952–3; Takayama: Takayama-insatsu Co., 1981).

— (ed.), *Takayama–shi shi* [*History of Takayama City*], 3 vols (Takayama: Takayama-insatsu Co., 1983).

Takegawa, S., *Fukushikokka to shiminshakai* [*Welfare State and Civil Society*] (Kyoto: Horitsu-bunka-sha, 1992).

Tanaka, S., 'Nihon ni okeru shisetsu kea seido: rekishiteki kosatsu' [The Institutional Care System in Japan], in H. Asano and S. Tanaka (eds), *Nihon no shisetsu kea* [*Institutional Care in Japan*] (Tokyo: Chuo-hoki-shuppan, 1993), pp. 245–85.

Tanikawa, S., 'Gendai "Narayama bushi" ko: Rojinhomu wa dokoe ikuka' [A Modern Reading of 'Ballad of Oak Mountain'], in National Council of Social Welfare and National Council of Elderly Homes (eds), *Rojinfukushi nenpo 1976-nen* [*Annual Report on Elderly Welfare 1976*] (Tokyo: National Council of Social Welfare, 1976), pp. 50–6.

Tarui Town History Editorial Board (ed.), *Tarui-cho shi tsushi-hen* [*History of Tarui Town*] (Tarui Town, Gifu: Tarui Town Mayor Mr Yagino, 1969).

Terawaki, T., 'Hikyugosha, yohogosha chosa' [Survey of Poor Relief Recipients and Eligible People], in Social Welfare Survey Research Council (ed.), *Senzen nihon no shakaijigyo chosa* [*Pre-War Social Work Survey in Japan*] (Tokyo: Keiso-shobo, 1983), pp. 94–143.

Toyama, T., 'Seikatsukukan to shiteno koshitsu no hitsuyosei' [The Necessity of Single Rooms as Living Space], in W. Omori (ed.), *Shingata tokubetsuyogo rojinhomu: Koshitsuka, yunitto kea eno tenkan* [*New-Style Nursing Homes*] (Tokyo: Chuo-hoki-shuppan, 2002), pp. 44–73.

Tsuruta, H., *Hogoshisetsu jittai chosa kaisekisho* [*Analysis of Old People's Institution Survey*] (Tokyo: Shakai-fukushi-shisetsu-kenkyu-kai, 1956), repr. in Y. Ogasawara (ed.), *Rekishi bunken* [*Historical Sources*], 29 vols (Tokyo: Ozora-sha, 1990–2), vol. 9.

Umemura, S., 'Yamamoto-kyugosho no rekishi' [History of Yamamoto Relief Institution], *Kyodokenkyu gifu* [*Gifu Local History Journal*], 14 (1976), pp. 13–17.

—, 'Gifu-ken shakaijigyo shoshi sono ichi [A Short History of Gifu Prefecture Social Work], *Chubujoshi-tankidaigaku kiyo* [*Journal of Chubu Woman's Junior College*], 13 (1983), pp. 53–69.

Uzuhashi, T., (ed.), *Hikaku no nakano fukushikokka* [*The Welfare State in Comparative Perspective*] (Kyoto: Minerva, 2003).

Washiya, Y., 'Showa kyoko-ki ni okeru kyuhin seido' [The Wartime Poor Relief System], in Japan University of Social Work (ed.), *Nihon no kyuhin seido* [*Poor Law System in Japan*] (Tokyo: Keiso-shobo, 1960), pp. 223–68.

Wedge, 'Iede oite iede shinu niwa' [How to Age and Die at Home?], *Wedge*, 22:11 (November 2010), pp. 20–8.

Yabe, H., 'Tokyo-to yoikuin no rekishi to seikatsu no dampen 1872–1975' [History and Life of Tokyo Borough Almshouse 1872–1975], in Tokyo Borough Almshouse Committee (ed.), *Nihon no fukushi o kizuite 127-nen: Yoikuin no kaitai wa fukushino kotai* [*127-Year History of Tokyo Borough Almshouse*] (Tokyo: Hobun-sha, 1999), pp. 217–58.

Yamagiwa, T., 'Showa 53-nendo kenkyukaihatsu kekka no gaiyo: Koreikashakai deno rojin-fukushi to ikigai' [The 1978 Survey of Elderly Welfare], *Shinku tanku: Gifu o kangaeru* [*Think-Tank Gifu Journal*], 23 (November 1979), pp. 3–13.

Yamato Town (ed.), *Yamato-cho shi tsushi-hen* [*History of Yamato Town*], 2 vols (Yamato Town, Gifu: Yamato Town, 1988).

Yorojigyo [*Journal of Social Work for the Elderly*], 18 (1937), repr. in Y. Ogasawara (ed.), *Rekishi bunken* [*Historical Sources*], 29 vols (Tokyo: Ozora-sha, 1990–2), vol. 11, pp. 36–42.

Yorojigyo [*Journal of Social Work for the Elderly*], 24 (1943), repr. in Y. Ogasawara (ed.), *Rekishi bunken* [*Historical Sources*], 29 vols (Tokyo: Ozora-sha, 1990–2), vol. 12, p. 32.

Yoshida, K., 'Meijiishin ni okeru kyuhin seido' [The Poor Relief System, 1868–1911], in Japan University of Social Work (ed.), *Nihon no kyuhin seido* [*Poor Law System in Japan*] (Tokyo: Keiso-shobo, 1960), pp. 49–100.

—, 'Nihon hinkon shi' [A History of Poverty in Japan], in Social Welfare Survey Research Council (ed.), *Senzen nihon no shakaijigyo chosa* [*Pre-War Social Work Survey in Japan*] (Tokyo: Keiso-shobo, 1983), pp. 3–26.

—, *Shin nihon shakaijigyo no rekishi* [*New Edition: History of Japanese Social Services*] (Tokyo: Keiso-shobo, 2004).

Yoshida, T., *Rojinhomu wa ima: Genba karano houkoku* [*Old People's Homes Now*] (Kyoto: Minerva, 1980).

Yuki, Y., *Kaigo: Genbakara no kensho* [*Long-Term Care: Analysis from Grassroots Evidence*] (Tokyo: Iwanami-shinsho, 2008).

Zenkoku-yoro-jigyo-kyokai, *Zenkoku yoroshisetsu ichiran showa 27-nen 8-gatsu* [*National Directory of Old People's Institutions 1952*] (Tokyo: Zenkoku-yoro-jigyo-kyokai, 1952), repr. in Y. Ogasawara (ed.), *Rekishi bunken* [*Historical Sources*], 29 vols (Tokyo: Ozora-sha, 1990–2), vol. 29.

—, *Zenkoku yoroshisetsu chosa showa 24-nen 12-gatsu matsu* [*National Survey of Elderly Institutions 1949*] (Tokyo: Zenkoku-yoro-jigyo-kyokai, 1950), repr. in Y. Ogasawara (ed.), *Rekishi bunken* [*Historical Sources*], 29 vols (Tokyo: Ozora-sha, 1990-2), vol. 29.

Japanese Translations

Campbell, J. C., *How Policies Change: The Japanese Government and the Aging Society* (Princeton, NJ and Oxford: Princeton University Press, 1992), trans. F. Miura and S. Sakata, *Nihonseifu to koreishashakai: Seisaku tenkan no riron to kensho* (Tokyo: Chuo-hoki-shuppan, 1995).

Centre for Policy on Ageing, *A Better Home Life* (London: Centre for Policy on Ageing, 1996), trans. N. Hisada, K. Oda, N. Onizaki and T. Sugimoto, *Koreishashisetsu kea no jissen koryo: Igirisu no koreisha kyoju shisetsu to nashingu homu no uneikijun* (Tokyo: Gakuensha, 1999).

Esping-Andersen, G., *The Three Worlds of Welfare Capitalism* (Cambridge: Polity, 1990), trans. T. Miyamoto and N. Okazawa, *Fukushi shihonshugi no mittsu no sekai: Hikakufukushi kokka no riron to dotai* (Kyoto: Minerva, 2001).

Goffman, E., *Asylums: Essays on the Social Situation of Mental Patients and Other Inmates* (New York: Doubleday, 1961), trans. T. Ishiguro, *Goffuman no syakaigaku: Shisetsu hishuyosha no nichijo seikai* (Tokyo: Seishin-shobo, 1984).

Gould, A., *Capitalist Welfare Systems: A Comparison of Japan, Britain and Sweden* (London: Longman, 1993), trans. M. Nimonji, S. Takashima and Y. Yamane, *Fukushikokka wa doko e ikunoka: Nihon, igirisu, sueden* (Kyoto: Minerva, 1997).

Jack, R. (ed.), *Residential versus Community Care: The Role of Institutions in Welfare Provision* (Basingstoke: Macmillan, 1998), trans. N. Hisada, K. Oda, C. Saito and T. Sugimoto, *Shisetsu kea tai komyuniti kea: Fukushi shin-jidai ni okeru shisetsu kea no yakuwari to kino*, 2nd edition (Tokyo: Keiso-shobo, 2001).

Johnson, N., *Voluntary Social Services* (Oxford: Basil Blackwell, 1981), trans. T. Tabata, *Igirisu no minkan shakaifukushi katudo: Sono rekishi to genjo* (Tokyo: National Council of Social Welfare, 1989).

Thane, P., *Foundations of the Welfare State*, 2nd edn (Harlow: Longman, 1996), trans. K. Fukasawa and A. Fukasawa, *Igirisu fukushikokka no shakai shi: Keizai, shakai, seiji, bunkateki haikei* (Kyoto: Minerva, 2000).

Thane, P. (ed.), *The Long History of Old Age* (London: Thames & Hudson, 2005), trans. Y. Kinoshita, *Rojin no rekishi* (Tokyo: Toyoshorin, 2009).

Titmuss, R. M., *Essays on 'The Welfare State'*, 2nd edn (London: Unwin University Books, 1963), trans. M. Tani, *Fukushikokka no riso to genjitsu* (Tokyo: Tokyo University Press, 1967).

INDEX

Page numbers in bold type refer to figures and tables.